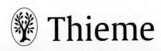

Duus'
Topical Diagnosis
in Neurology

Anatomy · Physiology · Signs · Symptoms
4th completely revised edition

Mathias Baehr, M.D.
Professor of Neurology and Chairman
Department of Neurology
University of Goettingen
Goettingen, Germany

Michael Frotscher, M.D.
Professor of Anatomy and Chairman
Department of Anatomy and Cell Biology
University of Freiburg
Freiburg, Germany

With contributions by
Wilhelm Kueker

Founding author Peter Duus

Translated by Ethan Taub, M.D.

400 illustrations, most in color,
by Professor Gerhard Spitzer and Barbara Gay

Thieme
Stuttgart · New York

Library of Congress Cataloging-in-Publication Data

Baehr, Mathias.
[Duus' neurologisch-topische Diagnostik. English]
Duus' topical diagnosis in neurology : anatomy,
physiology, signs, symptoms/Mathias Baehr,
Michael Frotscher ; with contributions by
Wilhelm Kueker ; translated by Ethan Taub ;
illustrated by Gerhard Spitzer. - 4th, rev. ed.
  p. ; cm.
Rev. translation of the 8th German ed. c2003.
Includes index.
ISBN 3-13-612804-4 (GTV : alk. paper) -
ISBN 1-58890-215-3 (TNY : alk. paper)
1. Nervous system-Diseases-Diagnosis.
2. Neuroanatomy. 3. Anatomy, Pathological.
4. Nervous system-Pathophysiology. I. Frotscher,
M. (Michael), 1947- . II. Duus, Peter, 1908-. Topical
diagnosis in neurology. III. Title. IV. Title: Topical
diagnosis in neurology. [DNLM: 1. Nervous System
Diseases-diagnosis. 2. Nervous System-anatomy &
histology.
3. Nervous System-physiopathology.
WL 141 B139d 2005a]
RC347.D8813 2005
616.8'04754-dc22   2005013120

1st Brazilian (Portuguese) edition 1985	1st Greek edition 1992
2nd Brazilian (Portuguese) edition 1990	1st Indonesian edition 1996
1st Chinese edition 1996	1st Italian edition 1987
1st English edition 1983	1st Japanese edition 1982
2nd English edition 1989	2nd Japanese edition 1984
3rd English edition 1998	3rd Japanese edition 1988
	4th Japanese edition 1999
1st French edition 1998	1st Korean edition 1990
1st German edition 1976	
2nd German edition 1980	1st Polish edition 1990
3rd German edition 1983	1st Russian edition 1996
4th German edition 1987	
5th German edition 1990	1st Spanish edition 1985
6th German edition 1995	1st Turkish edition 2001
7th German edition 2001	
8th German edition 2003	

© 2005 Georg Thieme Verlag,
Rüdigerstrasse 14, 70469 Stuttgart,
Germany
http://www.thieme.de

Thieme New York, 333 Seventh Avenue,
New York, NY 10001 USA
http://www.thieme.com

Cover design: Cyclus, Stuttgart
Typesetting by primustype Hurler, Notzingen
Printed in Germany by Appl, Wemding

ISBN 3-13-612804-4 (GTV)
ISBN 1-58890-215-3 (TNY)   1 2 3 4 5

Important note: Medicine is an ever-changing science undergoing continual development. Research and clinical experience are continually expanding our knowledge, in particular our knowledge of proper treatment and drug therapy. Insofar as this book mentions any dosage or application, readers may rest assured that the authors, editors, and publishers have made every effort to ensure that such references are in accordance with **the state of knowledge at the time of production of the book.**

Nevertheless, this does not involve, imply, or express any guarantee or responsibility on the part of the publishers in respect to any dosage instructions and forms of applications stated in the book. **Every user is requested to examine carefully** the manufacturers' leaflets accompanying each drug and to check, if necessary in consultation with a physician or specialist, whether the dosage schedules mentioned therein or the contraindications stated by the manufacturers differ from the statements made in the present book. Such examination is particularly important with drugs that are either rarely used or have been newly released on the market. Every dosage schedule or every form of application used is entirely at the user's own risk and responsibility. The authors and publishers request every user to report to the publishers any discrepancies or inaccuracies noticed.

This book is an authorized and revised translation of the 8th German edition published and copyrighted 2003 by Georg Thieme Verlag, Stuttgart, Germany. Title of the German edition: Duus' Neurologisch-topische Diagnostik

Contributor: Wilhem Küker, M.D., Radiological Clinic, Department of Neuroradiology, University Hospital Tübingen, Germany

Translator: Ethan Taub, M.D., Klinik im Park, Zurich, Switzerland

Illustrators: Gerhard Spitzer, Frankfurt/M; Barbara Gay, Stuttgart

Preface

This is the first complete revision of Duus' textbook of topical diagnosis in neurology since the death of its original author, Professor Peter Duus, in 1994. As is well known, the intervening time has witnessed major developments, both in the clinical neurosciences and in basic research. In particular, modern imaging techniques such as magnetic resonance imaging and positron emission tomography on the one hand, and the new molecular biological understanding of the development, plasticity, and pathology of the nervous system on the other, have brought about substantial progress in our knowledge in the field of neuroscience. Yet, despite all of the advances in ancillary diagnostic techniques, topical neurological diagnosis—the correct attribution of symptoms or syndromes to lesions at specific sites in the nervous system—remains today the primary task of the clinical neurologist.

In this entirely new, thoroughly revised edition of "Duus," we have tried to preserve the remarkably effective didactic conception of the book while bringing it up to date. We have replaced older case studies based mainly on history by new ones more closely reflecting current practice, provided multicolored illustrations to ease and enhance comprehension, and added state-of-the-art neuroradiological images to demonstrate the correlation of structure and function in nervous system lesions. We have also newly color-coded the section headings to enable readers to distinguish at a glance between neuroanatomical (blue) and clinical (green) material, without having to disrupt the thematic continuity of the text.

Welcome changes in the undergraduate medical curriculum over the past two decades have vastly increased the exposure of medical students in the so-called "preclinical" years to clinical case material. To make the book more accessible to these students, we have written a new first chapter entitled "Elements of the Nervous System," and we have also added a brief summary of basic concepts at the beginning of each of the other chapters.

The authors thank Georg Thieme Verlag and Dr. Kundmueller for their diligence and for many constructive discussions, as well as Mrs. Gay for her outstanding work on the illustrations.

We hope that this "new Duus," like the earlier editions, will merit the appreciation of its audience, and we look forward to receiving readers' comments in any form that they choose.

Professor M. Baehr   Professor M. Frotscher   Associate Professor W. Küker

Contents

Abbreviations

5-HT$_3$	serotonin
ACTH	adrenocorticotropic hormone (corticotropin)
AIDS	acquired immunodeficiency syndrome
AMPA	α-amino-3-hydroxy-5-methyl-4-isoxazolepropionate acid
ARAS	ascending reticular activating system
BAEP	brainstem auditory evoked potentials
BPPV	benign paroxysmal positioning vertigo
CNS	central nervous system
CRF	corticotropin-releasing factor
CSF	cerebrospinal fluid
CT	computed tomography
DREZ	dorsal root entry zone (also called the Redlich-Obersteiner zone)
ECG	electrocardiography/electrocardiogram
EEG	electroencephalography/electroencephalogram
EMG	electromyography/electromyogram
EPSP	excitatory postsynaptic potential
FLAIR	fluid-attenuated inversion recovery
fMRI	functional magnetic resonance imaging
FSH	follicle-stimulating hormone
GABA	γ-aminobutyric acid
GH (STH)	growth hormone (somatotropic hormone)
GHRH	growth-hormone-releasing hormone
GnRH	gonadotropin-releasing hormone
HIV	human immunodeficiency virus
HMSN	hereditary motor and sensory polyneuropathy
INO	internuclear ophthalmoplegia
IP	interphalangeal
IPSP	inhibitory postsynaptic potential
LH	luteninizing hormone
LPH	lipotropin
LTM	long-term memory
MEG	magnetoencephalography
MIF	melanocyte-stimulating hormone-inhibiting factor
MLF	medial longitudinal fasciculus
MP	metacarpophalangeal
MRF	melanocyte-stimulating hormone-releasing factor
MRI	magnetic resonance imging

MSH	melanocyte-stimulating hormone
NMDA	*N*-methyl-D-aspartate
PET	positron emission tomography
PICA	posterior inferior cerebellar artery
PIF	prolactin-inhibiting factor (= dopamine)
PPRF	paramedian pontine reticular formation
PRF	prolactin-releasing factor
PRL	prolactin
rCBF	regional cerebral blood flow
SCD	subacute combined degeneration
SRIF	somatotropin inhibiting factor
STM	short-term memory
T_3	triiodothyronine
T_4	tetraiodothyronine (thyroxine)
TRH	thyrotropin-releasing hormone
TSH	thyroid-stimulating hormone
VEP	visual evoked potentials
VOR	vestibulo-ocular reflex
VPL	ventral posterolateral nucleus of the thalamus
VPM	ventral posteromedial nucleus of the thalamus

1   Elements of the Nervous System

1   Elements of the Nervous System

The nervous system is composed of cells, called **neurons**, that are specialized for information processing and transmission. Neurons make contact with each other at junctions called **synapses**, at which information is transferred from one neuron to the next by means of chemical messenger substances called **neurotransmitters**. In general, neurons can be divided into two classes: **excitatory** and **inhibitory**. The organization of the nervous system is easier to understand after a brief consideration of its (ontogenetic) development.

Information Flow in the Nervous System

Information flow in the nervous system can be broken down schematically into three steps (Fig. 1.1): an external or internal stimulus impinging on the sense organs induces the generation of nerve impulses that travel toward the central nervous system (CNS) (**afferent impulses**); complex processing occurs within the CNS (**information processing**); and, as the product of this processing, the CNS generates impulses that travel toward the periphery (**efferent impulses**) and effect the (motor) response of the organism to the stimulus. Thus, when a pedestrian sees a green traffic light, afferent impulses are generated in the optic nerves and visual system that convey information about the specific color present. Then, at higher levels in the CNS, the stimulus is interpreted and assigned a meaning (green light = go). Efferent impulses to the legs then effect the motor response (crossing the street).

In the simplest case, information can be transferred directly from the afferent to the efferent arm, without any intervening complex processing in the CNS; this is what happens, for example, in an intrinsic muscle reflex such as the knee-jerk (patellar) reflex.

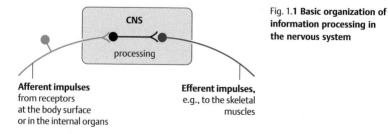

Afferent impulses
from receptors
at the body surface
or in the internal organs

Efferent impulses,
e.g., to the skeletal
muscles

Fig. 1.1 **Basic organization of information processing in the nervous system**

Neurons and Synapses

Neurons

The **neurons** and their processes (see below) and the **synapses** (see p. 7) are responsible for the flow of information in the nervous system. At the synapses, information is transferred from one neuron to the next by means of chemical substances called neurotransmitters.

Dendrites and axons. Neurons transfer information in one direction only because they are **bipolar**: they receive information from other neurons at one end, and transmit information to other neurons at the other end.

The **receptive structures** of a nerve cell, called **dendrites**, are branched processes attached to the cell body. Neurons vary considerably with regard to the number and branching pattern of their dendrites. The **forward conducting structure** is the **axon**, which in humans can be up to a meter in length. In contrast to the variable number of dendrites, each neuron possesses only a *single* axon. "Axis cylinder" is an older and now little-used term for "axon" that refers to its long, cylindrical shape. At its distal end, the axon splits into a number of terminal branches, each of which ends in a so-called terminal bouton that makes contact with the next neuron (Fig. 1.**2**).

The long peripheral processes of the pseudounipolar neurons of the spinal ganglia are an important special case. These are the fibers that relay information regarding touch, pain, and temperature from the body surface to the CNS. Although they are receptive structures, they nonetheless possess the structural characteristics of axons and are designated as such.

The trophic (nutritive) center of the neuron is its cell body (**soma** or **perikaryon**), which contains the cell nucleus and various different types of subcellular organelles.

Axonal transport. The neurotransmitters, or the enzymes catalyzing their biosynthesis, are synthesized in the perikaryon and then carried down axonal microtubules to the end of the axon in a process known as axoplasmic transport. The neurotransmitter molecules are stored in synaptic vesicles inside the terminal boutons (each bouton contains many synaptic vesicles). Axoplasmic transport, generally speaking, can be in either direction—from the cell body toward the end of the axon (**anterograde transport**), or in the reverse direction (**retrograde transport**). Rapid axoplasmic transport proceeds at a speed of 200-400 mm/day. This is distinct from axoplasmic flow, whose speed is 1-5 mm/day. Axoplasmic transport is exploited in the research laboratory by anterograde and retrograde tracer techniques for the anatomical demonstration of neural projections (Fig. 1.**3**).

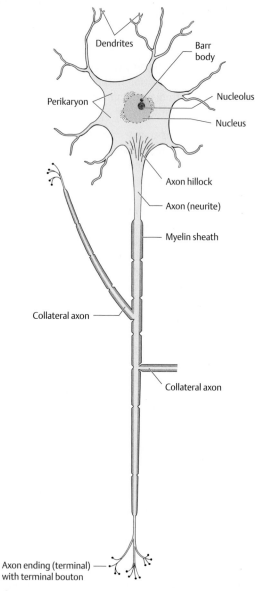

Fig. 1.**2 Structure of a neuron** (schematic drawing). From: Kahle W and Frotscher M: Taschenatlas der Anatomie, vol. 3, 8th ed., Thieme, Stuttgart, 2002.

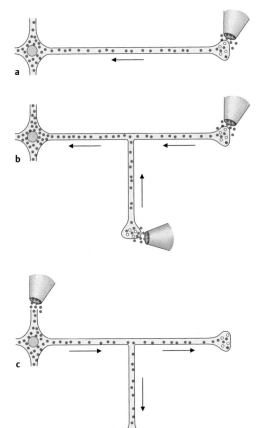

Fig. 1.**3 Tracing of neuronal projections with retrograde and anterograde tracer substances.** Tracer substances, such as fluorescent dyes, are injected either at the site of origin or at the destination of the neuronal pathway in question. The tracer substances are then transported along the neurons, either from the cell bodies to the axon terminals (anterograde transport) or in the reverse direction (retrograde transport). It is thus possible to trace the entire projection from one end to the other.

a Retrograde transport.
b Retrograde transport from multiple projection areas of a single neuron.
c Anterograde transport from a single cell body into multiple projection areas.

From: Kahle W and Frotscher M: Taschenatlas der Anatomie, vol. 3, 8th ed., Thieme, Stuttgart, 2002.

Axon myelination. Axons are surrounded by a sheath of myelin (Fig. 1.**4**). The myelin sheath, which is formed by **oligodendrocytes** (a special class of glial cells) in the central nervous system and by **Schwann cells** in the peripheral nervous system, is a sheetlike continuation of the oligodendrocyte or Schwann cell membrane that wraps itself around the axon multiple times, providing electrical insulation. Many oligodendrocytes or Schwann cells form the myelin surrounding a single axon. The segments of myelin sheath formed by two adjacent cells are separated by an area of uncovered axonal membrane called a *node of Ranvier*. Because of the insulating property of myelin, an action potential causes *depolarization* only at the nodes of Ranvier; thus, neural excitation

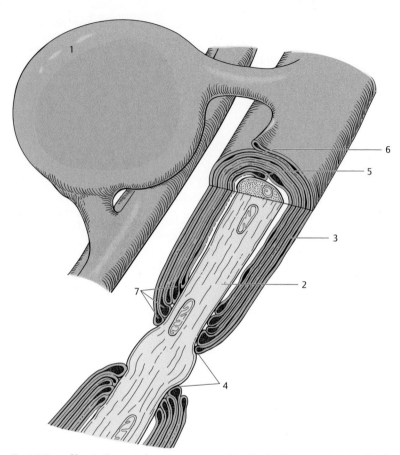

Fig. 1.4 Nerve fiber in the central nervous system, with oligodendrocyte and myelin sheath (schematic drawing). **1**, Oligodendrocyte. **2**, Axon. **3**, Myelin sheath. **4**, Node of Ranvier. **5**, Inner mesaxon. **6**, Outer mesaxon. **7**, Pockets of cytoplasm. From: Kahle W and Frotscher M: Taschenatlas der Anatomie, vol. 3, 8th ed., Thieme, Stuttgart, 2002.

jumps from one node of Ranvier to the next, a process known as **saltatory conduction.** It follows that neural conduction is fastest in neurons that have thick insulating myelin with nodes of Ranvier spaced widely apart. On the other hand, in axons that lack a myelin covering, excitation must travel relatively slowly down the entire axonal membrane. Between these two extremes there are axons with myelin of intermediate thickness. Thus, axons are divided into **thickly myelinated**, **thinly myelinated**, and **unmyelinated axons** (nerve fibers);

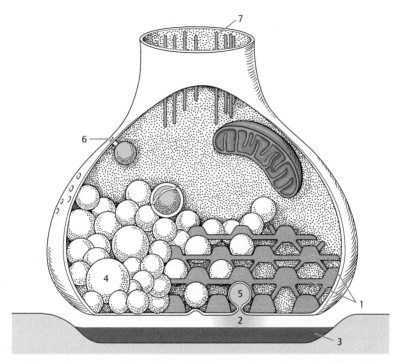

Fig. 1.**5 Synaptic structure** (schematic drawing). **1**, Presynaptic membrane with gridlike thickening, leaving hexagonal spaces in between. **2**, Synaptic cleft. **3**, Postsynaptic membrane. **4**, Synaptic vesicle. **5**, Fusion of a synaptic vesicle with the presynaptic membrane (so-called Ω [omega] figure), with release of the neurotransmitter (green) into the synaptic cleft. **6**, Vesicle with neurotransmitter molecules taken back up into the terminal bouton. **7**, Axon filaments. From: Kahle W and Frotscher M: Taschenatlas der Anatomie, vol. 3, 8th ed., Thieme, Stuttgart, 2002.

these classes are also designated by the letters A, B, and C. The thickly myelinated A fibers are of 3-20 µm diameter and conduct at speeds up to 120 m/s. The thinly myelinated B fibers are up to 3 µm thick and conduct at speeds up to 15 m/s. The unmyelinated C fibers conduct no faster than 2 m/s.

Synapses

General structure. As late as the 1950s, it was still unclear whether neurons were connected to each other in a continuous network (syncytium), which would theoretically allow rapid electrical communication between neurons, or whether each neuron was entirely enclosed in its own membrane. Subsequent visualization of synapses under the electron microscope settled the question: there is no direct spatial continuity between neurons. The axon ends on one side of the synapse, and neural impulses are conveyed across it by special transmitter substances (Fig. 1.**5**). The axon terminal (bouton) is the **presynaptic** part of the synapse, and the membrane of the cell receiving the transmitted information is the **postsynaptic** part. The presynaptic and postsynaptic membranes are separated by the synaptic cleft. The bouton contains vesicles filled with the neurotransmitter substance.

Examination of synapses under the electron microscope reveals specialized, osmiophilic thickenings of the presynaptic and postsynaptic membranes, which are more pronounced on the postsynaptic side in so-called **asymmetrical synapses**, and are approximately equally thick on both sides in so-called **symmetrical synapses**. These two types of synapse are also known, after their original describer, as *Gray type I* and *Gray type II synapses*, respectively. Asymmetrical synapses were found to be excitatory and symmetrical synapses to be inhibitory (see below for the concepts of excitation and inhibition). This hypothesis was later confirmed by immunocytochemical studies using antibodies directed against neurotransmitter substances and the enzymes involved in their biosynthesis.

Synaptic transmission (Fig. 1.**6**) is essentially a sequence of three different processes:

- The excitatory impulse (*action potential*) arriving at the axon terminal depolarizes the presynaptic membrane, causing voltage-dependent calcium channels to open. As a result, calcium ions flow into the terminal bouton and then interact with various proteins to cause fusion of synaptic vesicles with the presynaptic membrane. The neurotransmitter molecules within the vesicles are thereby released into the synaptic cleft.
- The neurotransmitter molecules diffuse across the synaptic cleft and bind to specific *receptors* on the postsynaptic membrane.
- The binding of neurotransmitter molecules to receptors causes ion channels to open, inducing ionic currents that cause either a depolarization or a hyperpolarization of the postsynaptic membrane—i.e., either an *excitatory postsynaptic potential* (*EPSP*) or an *inhibitory postsynaptic potential* (*IPSP*). Thus, synaptic transmission results in either an excitation or an inhibition of the postsynaptic neuron.

In addition to these fast-acting transmitter-gated or *ligand-gated ion channels*, there are also *G-protein-coupled receptors* that generate a much slower response by means of an intracellular signal cascade.

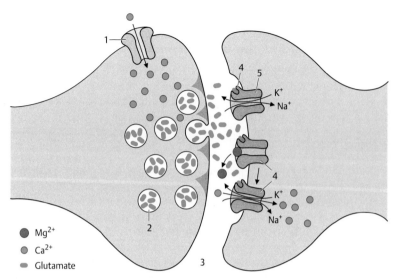

Fig. 1.6 Synaptic transmission at a glutamatergic (excitatory) synapse (schematic drawing). The arriving action potential induces an influx of Ca^{2+} (**1**), which, in turn, causes the synaptic vesicles (**2**) to fuse with the presynaptic membrane, resulting in the release of neurotransmitter (in this case, glutamate) into the synaptic cleft (**3**). The neurotransmitter molecules then diffuse across the cleft to the specific receptors in the postsynaptic membrane (**4**) and bind to them, causing ion channels (**5**) to open, in this case Na^+ channels. The resulting Na^+ influx, accompanied by a Ca^{2+} influx, causes an excitatory depolarization of the postsynaptic neuron (excitatory postsynaptic potential, EPSP). This depolarization also removes a blockade of the so-called NMDA receptor by Mg^{2+} ions. From: Kahle W and Frotscher M: Taschenatlas der Anatomie, vol. 3, 8th ed., Thieme, Stuttgart, 2002.

Chemical and electrical synapses. The type of synaptic transmission described above, involving the release and receptor binding of a neurotransmitter, is the type most commonly found. There are also so-called electrical synapses in which the excitation is transmitted directly to the next neuron across a *gap junction.*

Types of synapses. Synapses mediate the transfer of information from one neuron to the next; the synapses that bring information to a particular cell are known as its **input synapses.** Most input synapses are to be found on a cell's dendrites (**axodendritic synapses**). The dendrites of many neurons (e. g., cortical pyramidal cells) possess thornlike processes, the *dendritic spines*, that enable the compartmentalization of synaptic input. Many spines contain a *spine apparatus* for the internal storage of calcium ions. The synapses on dendritic spines are mainly asymmetrical, excitatory synapses.

Input synapses are found not only on the dendrites but also on the cell body itself (perikaryon; **axosomatic synapses**) and even on the axon and its initial segment, the axon hillock (**axo-axonal synapses**).

Convergence and divergence of synaptic connections. In general, each individual neuron receives information through synapses from many different neurons and neuron types (**convergence** of information transfer). The neuron can, in turn, make synaptic contact with a large number of other neurons through numerous collateral axonal branches (**divergence** of information transfer).

Excitation and inhibition. The nervous system is constructed in such a way that each neuron can be in one of two basic states at any moment: either the neuron is electrically discharging and transmitting information via synapses to other neurons, or else it is silent. Excitatory input to the neuron causes it to discharge, while inhibitory input causes it to be silent.

It follows that neurons can be classified as excitatory and inhibitory in terms of their effect on the neurons to which they provide input. **Excitatory neurons** are usually principal neurons (e. g., the pyramidal cells of the cerebral cortex), which often project over long distances and thus have long axons. **Inhibitory neurons,** on the other hand, are often interneurons and have short axons.

Principles of neuronal inhibition (Fig. 1.7). Collaterals of excitatory cells can activate inhibitory interneurons, which then inhibit the principal neuron itself (**recurrent inhibition**, a form of negative feedback). In **forward inhibition**, collaterals of principal neurons activate inhibitory interneurons that then inhibit other principal neurons. When an inhibitory neuron inhibits another inhibitory neuron, the resulting decrease in inhibition of the postsynaptic principal cell causes a net increase in its activity (**disinhibition**).

Neurotransmitters and Receptors

Excitatory and inhibitory neurotransmitters. In classic neuroanatomical studies, neurons were divided into two major types on the basis of their shape and the length of their projections: principal neurons with distant projections were called Golgi type I neurons, while interneurons with short axons were called Golgi type II neurons. Currently, neurons are usually classified according to their *neurotransmitter phenotype*, which generally determines whether they

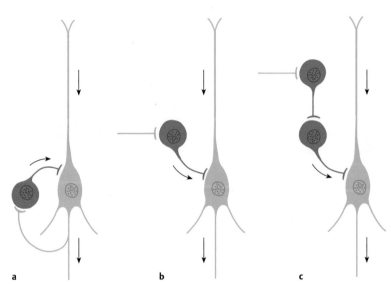

a   b   c

Fig. 1.7 Three types of neuronal inhibition. a, Recurrent inhibition. **b,** Forward inhibition. **c,** Disinhibition. From: Kahle W and Frotscher M: Taschenatlas der Anatomie, vol. 3, 8th ed., Thieme, Stuttgart, 2002.

are excitatory or inhibitory. The commonest excitatory neurotransmitter in the CNS is **glutamate**, while the commonest inhibitory neurotransmitter is γ-**aminobutyric acid** (GABA). The inhibitory neurotransmitter in the spinal cord is **glycine**. **Acetylcholine** and **norepinephrine** are the most important neurotransmitters in the autonomic nervous system but are also found in the CNS. Other important neurotransmitters include **dopamine, serotonin,** and various **neuropeptides,** many of which have been (and continue to be) identified; these are found mainly in interneurons.

Ligand-gated receptors. Ligand-gated ion channels are constructed of multiple subunits that span the cell membrane. The binding of neurotransmitter to the receptor opens the ion channel (i.e., makes it permeable) for one or more particular species of ion.

Excitatory amino acid receptors. Glutamate receptors are subdivided into three types called *AMPA, NMDA,* and *kainate receptors.* Glutamate binding to an AMPA receptor results in an influx of Na^+ ions, which depolarizes the cell. The activation of an NMDA receptor also causes an Na^+ influx, accompanied by a Ca^{2+} influx. The NMDA receptor, however, can be activated only after the blockade of its ion channel by a magnesium ion is removed; this, in turn, is accomplished through an AMPA-receptor-induced membrane depolarization (Fig. 1.**6**). The excitatory neurotransmitter glutamate thus has a graded effect: it activates AMPA receptors first and NMDA receptors later, after the membrane has been depolarized.

Inhibitory GABA and glycine receptors. The activation of either of these two types of receptor causes an influx of negatively charged chloride ions, and thus a hyperpolarization of the postsynaptic cell. Other types of ligand-gated ion channel include the *nicotinic acetylcholine receptor* and the serotonin (5-HT$_3$) receptor.

G-protein-coupled receptors. The response to a stimulus acting through a G-protein-coupled receptor lasts considerably longer, as it results from the activation of an intracellular signal cascade. The response may consist of changes in ion channels or in gene expression. Examples of G-protein-coupled receptors include muscarinic acetylcholine receptors and metabotropic glutamate receptors.

Functional Groups of Neurons

As discussed on p. 10, neurons are currently classified according to the neurotransmitters that they release. Thus, one speaks of the *glutamatergic, GABA-ergic, cholinergic,* and *dopaminergic systems,* among others. These systems have distinct properties. Glutamatergic neurons make point-to-point connections with their target cells, while the dopaminergic system, for example, has rather more diffuse connections: a single dopaminergic neuron generally projects to a large number of target neurons. The connections of the GABAergic system are particularly highly specialized. Some GABAergic neurons (basket cells) make numerous synaptic connections onto the cell body of the postsynaptic neuron, forming a basketlike structure around it; others form mainly axodendritic or axo-axonal synapses. The latter are found at the axon hillock.

Neurotransmitter analogues or receptor blockers can be applied pharmacologically for the specific enhancement or weakening of the effects of a particular neurotransmitter on neurons.

Glial Cells

The numerically most common cells in the nervous system are, in fact, not the neurons, but the glial cells (also called glia or neuroglia). These cells do not participate directly in information processing and transmission; rather, they play an indispensable supportive role for the function of neurons. The three types of glial cells in the CNS are the astroglial cells (astrocytes), oligodendroglia (oligodendrocytes), and microglial cells.

Astrocytes are divided into two types: protoplasmic and fibrillary. In the intact nervous system, astrocytes are responsible for the maintenance of the internal environment (homeostasis), particularly with respect to ion concentrations. Fine astrocyte processes surround each synapse, sealing it off from its surroundings so that the neurotransmitter cannot escape from the synaptic cleft. When the central nervous system is injured, astrocytes are responsible for the formation of scar tissue (gliosis).

The **oligodendrocytes** form the myelin sheaths of the CNS (see above). The **microglial cells** are phagocytes that are activated in inflammatory and degenerative processes affecting the nervous system.

Development of the Nervous System

A detailed discussion of the development of the nervous system would be beyond the scope of this book and not directly relevant to its purpose. The physician should understand some of the basic principles of neural development, however, as developmental disturbances account for a large number of diseases affecting the nervous system.

The nervous system develops from the (initially) longitudinally oriented *neural tube*, which consists of a solid wall and a central fluid-filled cavity. The cranial portion of the neural tube grows more extensively than the rest to form **three distinct brain vesicles**, the *rhombencephalon* (hindbrain), the *mesencephalon* (midbrain), and the *prosencephalon* (forebrain). The prosencephalon, in turn, becomes further differentiated into a caudal part, the *diencephalon*, and the most cranial portion of the entire neural tube, the paired *telencephalon* (endbrain). The central cavity of the two telencephalic ventricles communicates with that of the diencephalon through the interventricular foramen (destined to become the foramen of Monro). The central cavity undergoes its greatest enlargement in the areas where the neural tube has its most pronounced growth; thus, the lateral ventricles form in the two halves of the telencephalon, the third ventricle within the diencephalon, and the fourth ventricle in the brainstem. In those segments of the neural tube that grow to a relatively lesser extent, such as the mesencephalon, no ventricle is formed (in the fully developed organism, the cerebral aqueduct runs through the mesencephalon).

Over the course of vertebrate phylogeny, progressive enlargement of the telencephalon has caused it to overlie the brainstem and to rotate back on itself in semicircular fashion. This rotation is reflected in the structure of various components of the telencephalic gray matter, including the caudate nucleus and hippocampus; in the course of certain white matter tracts, such as the fornix; and in the shape of the lateral ventricles, each of which is composed of a frontal horn, a central portion (atrium), and a temporal horn, as shown in Fig. 10.**3**, p. 407.

Cellular proliferation. Immature neurons (neuroblasts) proliferate in the ventricular zone of the neural tube, i.e., the zone neighboring its central cavity. It is a major aim of current research in neuroembryology to unveil the molecular mechanisms controlling neuronal proliferation.

Neuronal migration. Newly formed nerve cells leave the ventricular zone in which they arise, migrating along radially oriented glial fibers toward their definitive location in the cortical plate. Migratory processes are described in greater detail on pp. 350 ff.

Growth of cellular processes. Once they have arrived at their destinations, the postmigratory neuroblasts begin to form dendrites and axons. One of the major questions in neurobiology today is how the newly sprouted axons find their way to their correct targets over what are, in some cases, very long distances. Important roles are played in this process by membrane-bound and soluble factors that are present in a concentration gradient, as well as by extracellular matrix proteins. There are ligand-receptor systems that exert both attractive and repulsive influences to steer the axon into the appropriate target area. These systems cannot be described in greater detail here.

Synaptogenesis. The axon terminals, having found their way to their targets, proceed to form synaptic contacts. Recent studies have shown that the formation of synapses, and of dendritic spines, is activity-dependent. Much evidence suggests that new synapses can be laid down throughout the lifespan of the individual, providing the basis of adaptive processes such as learning and memory.

Physiological neuronal death (programmed cell death, apoptosis). Many neurons die as the CNS develops, presumably as part of the mechanism enabling the precise and specific formation of interneuronal connections. The regulation of neuronal survival and neuronal death is a major topic of current research.

2 Somatosensory System

2 Somatosensory System

After a preliminary chapter on the structural elements of the nervous system, the discussion of its major functional components and mechanisms now begins with the **perceptual processes** mediated by **receptor organs**: as depicted earlier in Figure 1.**1**, these organs are the site of origin of information flow in the nervous system, in accordance with the basic organizing principle, perception → processing → response. Somatosensory impulses from the periphery are conducted along an **afferent nerve fiber** to its neuronal cell body, which lies in a **dorsal root ganglion (spinal ganglion)**. The impulses are then conducted onward into the **central nervous system**, without any intervening synapses, along the central process (axon) of the same neuron. This axon makes synaptic contact with a **second neuron** in the spinal cord or brainstem, whose axon, in turn, proceeds further centrally, and **crosses the midline** to the opposite side at some level along its path. The **third neuron** lies in the **thalamus**, the so-called "gateway to consciousness"; it projects to various cortical areas, most importantly the primary somatosensory cortex, which is located in the **postcentral gyrus** of the parietal lobe.

Peripheral Components of the Somatosensory System and Peripheral Regulatory Circuits

Receptor Organs

Receptors are specialized sensory organs that register physical and chemical changes in the external and internal environment of the organism and convert (transduce) them into the electrical impulses that are processed by the nervous system. They are found at the peripheral end of afferent nerve fibers. Some receptors inform the body about changes in the nearby external environment (**exteroceptors**) or in the distant external environment (**teleceptors**, such as the eye and ear). **Proprioceptors**, such as the labyrinth of the inner ear, convey information about the position and movement of the head in space, tension in muscles and tendons, the position of the joints, the force needed to carry out a particular movement, and so on. Finally, processes within the body are reported on by **enteroceptors**, also called **visceroceptors** (including **osmoceptors**, **chemoceptors**, and **baroceptors**, among others). Each type of receptor responds to a stimulus of the appropriate, specific kind, provided that the intensity of the stimulus is above threshold.

Sensory receptor organs are abundantly present in the skin but are also found in deeper regions of the body and in the viscera.

Receptors in the Skin

Most receptors in the skin are exteroceptors. These are divided into two classes: (1) free nerve endings and (2) encapsulated end organs.

The encapsulated, differentiated end organs are probably mainly responsible for the mediation of epicritic sensory modalities such as fine touch, discrimination, vibration, pressure, and so forth, while the free nerve endings mediate protopathic modalities such as pain and temperature. The evidence for this functional distinction is incomplete, however (see below).

Various receptor organs of the skin and its appendages are depicted in Figure 2.**1**, including **mechanoreceptors** (for touch and pressure), **thermoreceptors** (for warm and cold), and **nociceptors** (for pain). These receptors are located mainly in the zone between the epidermis and the connective tissue. The skin can thus be regarded as a sensory organ that covers the entire body.

Special receptor organs. The **peritrichial nerve endings** around the hair follicles are found in all areas of hair-bearing skin and are activated by the movement of hairs. In contrast, the **tactile corpuscles of Meissner** are found only on glabrous skin, particularly on the palms and soles but also on the lips, the tip of the tongue, and the genitals, and respond best to touch and light pressure. The **laminated Vater-Pacini corpuscles** (pacinian corpuscles) are found in deeper layers of the skin, especially in the area between the cutis and the subcutis, and mediate pressure sensations. The **end bulbs of Krause** were once thought to be cold receptors, while the **corpuscles of Ruffini** were thought to be warm receptors, but there is some doubt about this at present. Free nerve endings have been found to be able to transmit information about warmth and cold as well as about position. In the cornea, for example, only free nerve endings are present to transmit information about all of these sensory modalities. Aside from the receptor types specifically mentioned here, there are also many others in the skin and elsewhere whose function mostly remains unclear.

Free nerve endings (Fig. 2.1) are found in the clefts between epidermal cells, and sometimes also on more specialized cells of neural origin, such as the tactile disks of Merkel. Free nerve endings are present, however, not just in the skin but in practically all organs of the body, from which they convey nociceptive and thermal information relating to cellular injury. Merkel's disks are mainly located in the pads of the fingers and respond to touch and light pressure.

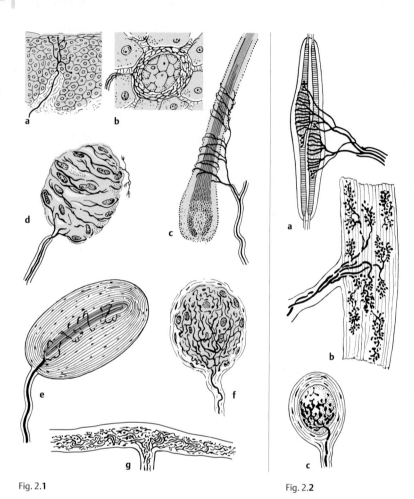

Fig. 2.**1**

Fig. 2.**2**

Fig. 2.**1 Somatosensory receptors in the skin. a** Free nerve ending (pain, temperature). **b** Tactile disk of Merkel. **c** Peritrichial nerve endings around a hair follicle (touch). **d** Tactile corpuscle of Meissner. **e** Vater–Pacini corpuscle (pressure, vibration). **f** End bulb of Krause (cold?). **g** Ruffini corpuscle (warmth?).

Fig. 2.**2 Receptors in muscle, tendons, and fascia. a** Annulospiral ending of a muscle spindle (stretch). **b** Golgi tendon organ (tension). **c** Golgi–Mazzoni corpuscle (pressure).

Receptors in Deeper Regions of the Body

A second group of receptor organs lies deep to the skin, in the muscles, tendons, fasciae, and joints (Fig. 2.**2**). In the muscles, for example, one finds muscle spindles, which respond to stretching of the musculature. Other types of receptors are found at the transition between muscles and tendons, in the fasciae, or in joint capsules.

Muscle spindles are very thin, spindle-shaped bodies that are enclosed in a connective-tissue capsule and lie between the striated fibers of the skeletal musculature. Each muscle spindle itself usually contains 3-10 fine striated muscle fibers, which are called **intrafusal muscle fibers** in contrast to the extrafusal fibers of the muscular tissue proper. The two ends of each spindle, composed of connective tissue, are fixed within the connective tissue between muscle fascicles, so that they move in conjunction with the muscle. An afferent nerve fiber called an annulospiral ending or primary ending winds around the middle of the muscle spindle. This afferent fiber has a very thick myelin sheath and belongs to the most rapidly conducting group of nerve fibers in the body, the so-called Ia fibers. For further details, see p. 30 (monosynaptic intrinsic muscle reflex; polysynaptic reflexes).

Golgi tendon organs contain fine nerve endings, derived from branches of thickly myelinated nerve fibers, that surround a group of collagenous tendon fibers. They are enclosed in a connective-tissue capsule, are located at the junction between tendon and muscle, and are connected in series to the adjacent muscle fibers. Like muscle spindles, they respond to stretch (i.e., tension), but at a higher threshold (see Fig. 2.**12**, p. 34).

Other receptor types. In addition to the muscle spindles and Golgi tendon organs, receptor types in the deep tissues include the laminated Vater-Pacini corpuscles and the Golgi-Mazzoni corpuscles as well as other terminal nerve endings that mediate pressure, pain, etc.

Peripheral Nerve, Dorsal Root Ganglion, Posterior Root

The further "way stations" through which an afferent impulse must travel as it makes its way to the CNS are the peripheral nerve, the dorsal root ganglion, and the posterior nerve root, through which it enters the spinal cord.

Peripheral nerve. Action potentials arising in a receptor organ of one of the types described above are conducted centrally along an afferent fiber, which is the peripheral process of the first somatosensory neuron, whose cell body is located in a dorsal root ganglion (see below). The afferent fibers from a circum-

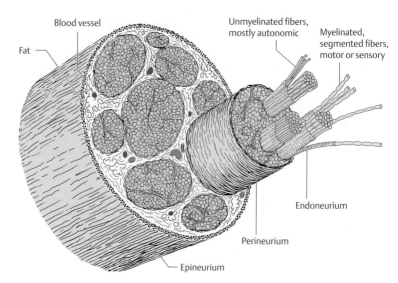

Fig. 2.**3 Cross section of a mixed peripheral nerve**

scribed area of the body run together in a peripheral nerve; such nerves contain not only fibers for superficial and deep sensation (*somatic afferent fibers*) but also efferent fibers to striated muscle (*somatic efferent fibers*) and fibers innervating the internal organs, the sweat glands, and vascular smooth muscle (*visceral afferent* and *visceral efferent fibers*). Fibers (axons) of all of these types are bundled together inside a series of connective-tissue coverings (endoneurium, perineurium, and epineurium) to form a "nerve cable" (Fig. 2.**3**). The perineurium also contains the blood vessels that supply the nerve (*vasa nervorum*).

Nerve plexus and posterior root. Once the peripheral nerve enters the spinal canal through the intervertebral foramen, the afferent and efferent fibers go their separate ways: the peripheral nerve divides into its two "sources," the anterior and posterior spinal roots (Fig. 2.**4**). The anterior root contains the efferent nerve fibers exiting the spinal cord, while the posterior root contains the afferent fibers entering it. A direct transition from the peripheral nerve to

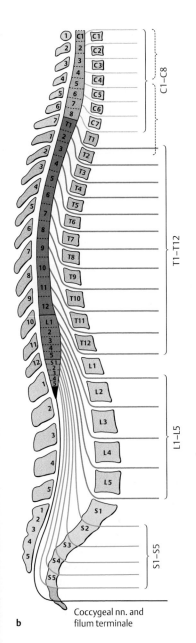

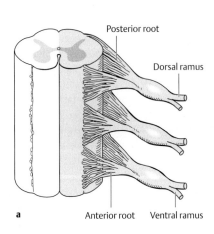

Fig. 2.**4 Nerve root segments and their relationship to the vertebral bodies. a** Anatomy of the anterior and posterior spinal roots. **b** Enumeration of the nerve root segments and the levels of exit of the spinal nerves from the spinal canal. The spinal cord grows to a shorter final length than the vertebral column, so that the nerve roots (proceeding caudally) must travel increasingly long distances to reach their exit foramina. See also p. 70, Chapter 3 (Motor System).

the spinal nerve roots is found, however, only in the thoracic region. At cervical and lumbosacral levels, nerve plexuses are interposed between the peripheral nerves and the spinal nerve roots (the cervical, brachial, lumbar, and sacral plexuses). In these plexuses, which are located outside the spinal canal, the afferent fibers of the peripheral nerves are redistributed so that fibers from each individual nerve ultimately join spinal nerves at multiple segmental levels (Fig. 2.**5**). (In analogous fashion, the motor fibers of a single segmental nerve root travel to multiple peripheral nerves; cf. Fig. 2.**5** and p. 100 ff. in Chapter 3.) The redistributed afferent fibers then enter the spinal cord at multiple levels and ascend a variable distance in the spinal cord before making synaptic contact with the second sensory neuron, which may be at or near the level of the entering afferent fibers or, in some cases, as high as the brainstem. Thus, in general, a peripheral nerve is composed of fibers from multiple radicular segments; this is true of both afferent and efferent fibers.

Digression: Anatomy of the spinal roots and nerves. In total, there are 31 pairs of spinal nerves; each spinal nerve is formed by the junction of an anterior and a posterior nerve root within the spinal canal. The numbering of the spinal nerves is based on that of the vertebral bodies (Fig. 2.**4**). Even though there are only *seven* cervical vertebrae, there are *eight* pairs of cervical nerves, because the highest spinal nerve exits (or enters) the spinal canal just above the first cervical vertebra. Thus, this nerve, the first cervical nerve (C1), exits the spinal canal between the occipital bone and the first cervical vertebra (atlas); the remaining cervical nerves, down to C7, exit *above* the correspondingly numbered vertebra; and C8 exits between the seventh (lowest) cervical vertebra and the first thoracic vertebra. At thoracic, lumbar, and sacral levels, each spinal nerve exits (or enters) the spinal canal *below* the correspondingly numbered vertebra. There are, therefore, just as many pairs of nerves in each of these regions as there are vertebrae (12 thoracic, 5 lumbar, and 5 sacral) (Fig. 2.**4**). Lastly, there is a single pair of coccygeal nerves (or, occasionally, more than one pair).

Spatial organization of somatosensory fibers in the posterior root. Nerve impulses relating to different somatosensory modalities originate in different types of peripheral receptor and are conducted centrally in separate groups of afferent fibers, which are spatially arranged in the posterior root in a characteristic pattern. As shown in Figure 2.**15** (p. 40), the most thickly myelinated nerve fibers, which originate in muscle spindles, run in the medial portion of the root; these fibers are responsible for proprioception. Fibers originating in receptor organs, which mediate the senses of touch, vibration, pressure, and discrimination, run in the central portion of the root, and the small and thinly myelinated fibers mediating pain and temperature sensation run in its lateral portion.

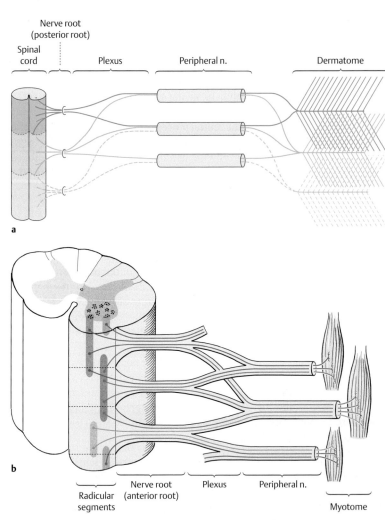

Fig. 2.**5 Redistribution of afferent and efferent nerve fibers in a nerve plexus.** The sensory fibers contained in a single peripheral nerve are distributed to multiple dorsal spinal nerve roots, and, analogously, the motor fibers of a single nerve root are distributed to multiple peripheral nerves. **a** In the periphery, the sensory fibers of a single radicular segment are grouped together once again to supply a characteristic segmental region of the skin (dermatome). **b** Radicular and peripheral nerve innervation of muscle: each muscle is supplied by a single peripheral nerve, which, however, generally contains fibers from multiple nerve roots (so-called polyradicular or plurisegmental innervation).

Dorsal root ganglion. The dorsal root ganglion is macroscopically visible as a swelling of the dorsal root, immediately proximal to its junction with the ventral root (Fig. 2.**4**). The neurons of the dorsal root ganglion are pseudounipolar, i.e., they possess a single process that divides into two processes a short distance from the cell, in a T-shaped configuration. One of these two processes travels to the receptor organs of the periphery, giving off numerous collateral branches along the way, so that a single ganglion cell receives input from multiple receptor organs. The other process (the central process) travels by way of the posterior root into the spinal cord, where it either makes synaptic contact with the second sensory neuron immediately, or else ascends toward the brainstem (see Fig. 2.**17**, p. 43). There are no synapses within the dorsal root ganglion itself.

Somatosensory Innervation by Nerve Roots and Peripheral Nerves

The fibers of individual nerve roots are redistributed into multiple peripheral nerves by way of the plexuses (cf. p. 24), and each nerve contains fibers from multiple adjacent radicular segments (see also Figs. 3.**31**, 3.**32**, and 3.**33**, p. 100-102). The fibers of each radicular segment regroup in the periphery, however (Fig. 2.**5**), to innervate a particular segmental area of the skin (**dermatome**). Each dermatome corresponds to a single radicular segment, which, in turn, corresponds to a single "spinal cord segment." The latter term is used even though the mature spinal cord no longer displays its original metameric segmentation.

The dermatomes on the anterior and posterior body surfaces are shown in Figure 2.**6**. The metameric organization of the dermatomes is easiest to see in the thoracic region.

As shown in Figure 2.**5**, the dermatomes of neighboring roots overlap considerably, so that a lesion confined to a single root often causes a barely discernible sensory deficit, or none at all.

Sensory deficits due to radicular lesions. A demonstrable sensory deficit in a segmental distribution is usually found only when multiple adjacent nerve roots are involved by a lesion. As each dermatome corresponds to a particular spinal cord or radicular level, the dermatome(s) in which a sensory deficit is located is a highly valuable indicator of the level of a lesion involving the spinal cord or one or more nerve roots. The schematic representation of Figure 2.**7** is intended for didactic purposes, to help the student remember where the boundaries between the cervical, thoracic, lumbar, and sacral dermatomal areas are located.

The dermatomes for the sense of touch overlap to a greater extent than those for pain and temperature. It follows that, in a lesion of one or two adja-

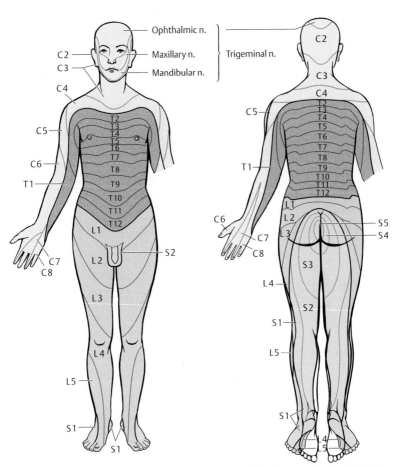

Fig. 2.**6 Segmental innervation of the skin** (after Hansen–Schliack). **a** Anterior view. **b** Posterior view.

cent roots, a dermatomal deficit of touch is generally hard to demonstrate, while one of pain and temperature sensation is more readily apparent. Thus, nerve root lesions can be more sensitively detected by testing for hypalgesia or analgesia, rather than hypesthesia or anesthesia.

Sensory deficits due to peripheral nerve lesions. It is easy to see why a lesion affecting a nerve plexus or a peripheral nerve produces a sensory deficit of an entirely different type than a radicular lesion. As plexus lesions usually cause a

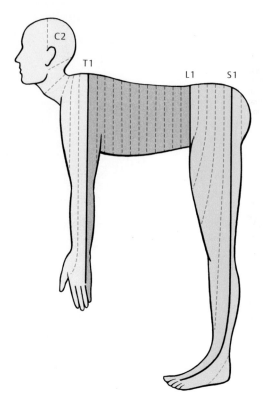

Fig. 2.**7 Segmental innervation of the skin: simplified diagram of dermatomal topography**

prominent motor deficit in addition, we will defer further discussion of plexus lesions to the next chapter on the motor system (p. 100).

When a peripheral nerve is injured, the fibers within it, derived from multiple nerve roots, can no longer rejoin in the periphery with fibers derived from the same nerve roots but belonging to other peripheral nerves—in other words, the fibers in the injured nerve can no longer reach their assigned dermatomes. The sensory deficit thus has a different distribution from that of the dermatomal deficit seen after a radicular injury (Fig. 2.**8**). Furthermore, the cutaneous areas innervated by individual peripheral nerves overlap much less that those innervated by adjacent nerve roots. Sensory deficits due to peripheral nerve lesions are, therefore, more readily apparent than those due to radicular lesions.

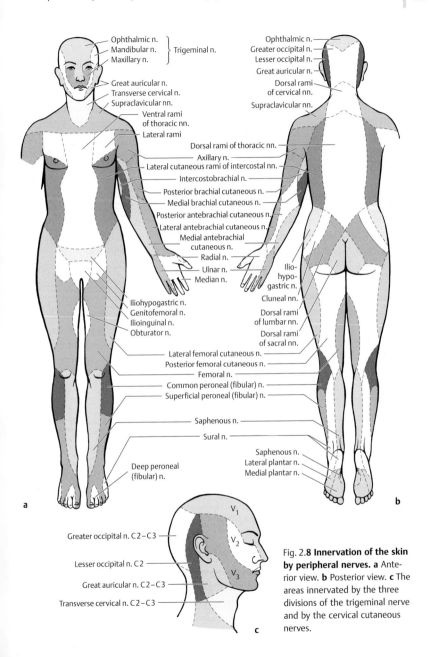

Ophthalmic n.
Mandibular n. } Trigeminal n.
Maxillary n.

Great auricular n.
Transverse cervical n.
Supraclavicular nn.
Ventral rami of thoracic nn.
Lateral rami

Dorsal rami of thoracic nn.
Axillary n.
Lateral cutaneous rami of intercostal nn.
Intercostobrachial n.
Posterior brachial cutaneous n.
Medial brachial cutaneous n.
Posterior antebrachial cutaneous n.
Lateral antebrachial cutaneous n.
Medial antebrachial cutaneous n.
Radial n.
Ulnar n.
Median n.

Iliohypogastric n.
Genitofemoral n.
Ilioinguinal n.
Obturator n.

Lateral femoral cutaneous n.
Posterior femoral cutaneous n.
Femoral n.
Common peroneal (fibular) n.
Superficial peroneal (fibular) n.

Saphenous n.
Sural n.

Deep peroneal (fibular) n.

a

Ophthalmic n.
Greater occipital n.
Lesser occipital n.
Great auricular n.
Dorsal rami of cervical nn.
Supraclavicular nn.

Ilio-hypo-gastric n.
Cluneal nn.
Dorsal rami of lumbar nn.
Dorsal rami of sacral nn.

Saphenous n.
Lateral plantar n.
Medial plantar n.

b

Greater occipital n. C2–C3
Lesser occipital n. C2
Great auricular n. C2–C3
Transverse cervical n. C2–C3

V₁
V₂
V₃

c

Fig. 2.8 Innervation of the skin by peripheral nerves. a Anterior view. **b** Posterior view. **c** The areas innervated by the three divisions of the trigeminal nerve and by the cervical cutaneous nerves.

Peripheral Regulatory Circuits

In the next section after this one, we will trace the ascending fiber pathways responsible for pain and temperature sensation, and for sensory modalities such as touch and pressure, as they travel up the spinal cord and into the brain. Before doing so, however, we will explain the function of a number of important peripheral regulatory circuits. Even though the current chapter is devoted to the sensory system, it will be useful, in this limited context, to describe not only the afferent (sensory) arm of these regulatory circuits, but their efferent (motor) arm as well.

Monosynaptic and Polysynaptic Reflexes

Monosynaptic intrinsic reflex. As illustrated in Figure 2.**11** (p. 34), the large-diameter **afferent fiber** arising in a muscle spindle gives off many terminal branches shortly after entering the spinal cord; some of these branches make direct synaptic contact onto neurons in the gray matter of the anterior horn. These neurons, in turn, are the origin of efferent motor fibers, and are therefore called **motor anterior horn cells**. The **efferent neurites** exit the spinal cord by way of the anterior root and then travel, along peripheral nerves, to the skeletal muscles.

A neural loop is thus created from a skeletal muscle to the spinal cord and back again, composed of two neurons—an afferent sensory neuron and an efferent motor neuron. This loop constitutes a simple, monosynaptic reflex arc. Because the arc begins and ends in the *same* muscle, the associated reflex is called an **intrinsic** (or **proprioceptive**) **muscle reflex**.

Such monosynaptic reflex arcs provide the neuroanatomical basis for the regulation of muscle length (see below).

Reflex relaxation of antagonist muscles. In a strict sense, the monosynaptic reflex is not truly monosynaptic, because it also has a polysynaptic component. The reflex is manifested not only in contraction of the muscle in question, but also in relaxation of its antagonist muscle(s). The inhibition of muscle cells that leads these muscles to relax is a polysynaptic process occurring by way of interneurons in the spinal gray matter. Were this not the case, tension in the antagonist muscles would counteract agonist contraction (see Fig. 2.**14**, p. 37).

Polysynaptic flexor reflex. Another important reflex arc is that of the polysynaptic flexor reflex, a **protective and flight reflex** that is mediated by many interneurons and is thus **polysynaptic**.

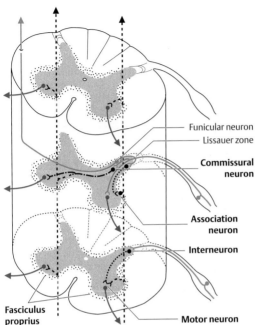

Fig. 2.**9 Intrinsic neurons and polysynaptic connections in the spinal cord.** Note: interneurons are also called "intercalated" or "internuncial" neurons (from Latin *nuntius*, messenger).

Funicular neuron
Lissauer zone
Commissural neuron
Association neuron
Interneuron
Fasciculus proprius
Motor neuron

When a finger touches a hot stove, the hand is pulled back with lightning speed, before any pain is felt. The action potentials that arise in the cutaneous receptor (nociceptor) for this reflex travel by way of afferent fibers to the substantia gelatinosa of the spinal cord, where they are then relayed, across synapses, into cells of various types belonging to the cord's intrinsic neuronal apparatus (interneurons, association neurons, and commissural neurons). Some of these cells—particularly the association neurons—project their processes multiple spinal levels upward and downward, in the so-called fasciculus proprius (Fig. 2.**9**). After crossing multiple synapses, excitatory impulses finally reach the motor neurons and travel along their efferent axons into the spinal nerve roots, peripheral nerves, and muscle, producing the muscular contraction that pulls the hand back from the stove.

A reflex of this type requires the coordinated contraction of multiple muscles, which must contract in the right sequence and with the right intensity, while others (the antagonist muscles) must relax at the appropriate times. The intrinsic neuronal apparatus of the spinal cord is the computerlike, interconnected network of cells that makes this process possible.

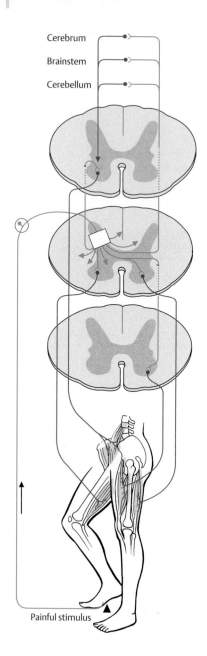

Cerebrum

Brainstem

Cerebellum

Painful stimulus

Fig. 2.**10 Flexor reflex with polysynaptic connections**

In another paradigmatic situation, stepping on a sharp rock generates noci-ceptive impulses that initiate a complex but unvarying sequence of events (Fig. 2.**10**): the painful foot is raised by flexion of the hip, knee, and ankle, while the opposite leg is extended so that the individual can stand on it alone (**crossed extensor reflex**). The sudden redistribution of weight does not cause the individual to fall over, because it is immediately compensated for by reflex contraction of muscles of the trunk, shoulders, arms, and neck, maintaining the body's upright posture. This process requires synaptic communication among many different neurons in the spinal cord, with simultaneous participation of the brainstem and cerebellum. All of this happens in a fraction of a second; only afterward does the individual feel pain, look to see what caused it, and check whether the foot has been injured.

These monosynaptic and polysynaptic reflexes are unconscious processes occurring mainly in the spinal cord, yet the last example shows that higher components of the CNS must often be activated at the same time, e. g., to pre-serve balance (as in the example).

Regulation of Muscle Length and Tension

As discussed above, monosynaptic and polysynaptic reflex arcs serve different purposes: polysynaptic reflex arcs mediate protective and flight responses, while monosynaptic reflex arcs are incorporated in functional circuits that regulate the length and tension of skeletal muscle. Each muscle, in fact, con-tains two servo-control (feedback) systems:

- A **control system for length**, in which the nuclear bag fibers of the muscle spindles serve as length receptors
- A **control system for tension**, in which the Golgi tendon organs and the nu-clear chain fibers of the muscle spindles serve as tension receptors

Stretch and tension receptors. **Muscle spindles** are receptors for both stretch (length) and tension. These two distinct modalities are subserved by two different kinds of intrafusal fibers, the so called nuclear bag and nuclear chain fibers (Figs. 2.**11** and 2.**12**). Fibers of both of these types are typically shorter and thinner than extrafusal muscle fibers. The two types of intrafusal fiber are depicted separately for didactic reasons in Figures 2.**11** and 2.**12**, but, in reality, the shorter and thinner nuclear chain fibers are directly attached to the some-what longer nuclear bag fibers. Muscle spindles generally consist of two nu-clear bag fibers and four or five nuclear chain fibers. In the middle of a nuclear bag fiber, the intrafusal muscle fibers widen to a form a bag containing about 50 nuclei, which is covered by a network of sensory nerve fibers known as a primary or annulospiral ending (from Latin *annulus*, ring). This spiral ending

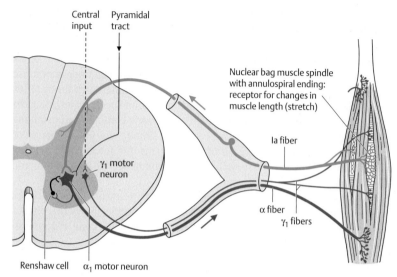

Fig. 2.**11 Regulatory circuit for muscle length**

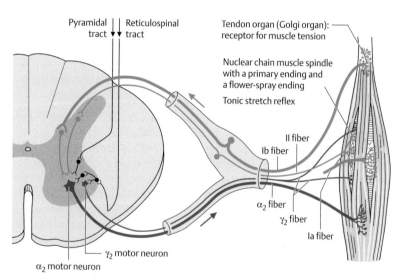

Fig. 2.**12 Regulatory circuit for muscle tension**

reacts very sensitively to muscle stretch, mainly registering *changes* in muscle length; the nuclear bag fibers are thus stretch receptors. The nuclear chain fibers, on the other hand, mainly register a persistently stretched *state* of the muscle, and are thus tension receptors.

Maintenance of constant muscle length. The extrafusal muscle fibers have a certain length at rest, which the organism always tries to maintain constant. Whenever the muscle is stretched beyond this length, the muscle spindle is stretched along with it. This generates action potentials in the annulospiral ending, which travel very rapidly in Ia afferent fibers and are then relayed across a synapse to motor neurons in the anterior horn of the spinal cord (Fig. 2.**11**). The excited motor neurons fire impulses that travel in equally rapidly conducting, large-diameter α_1 efferent fibers back to the working extrafusal muscle fibers, causing them to contract to their former length. Any stretch of the muscle induces this response.

The physician tests the intactness of this regulatory circuit with a quick tap on a muscle tendon, e. g., the patellar tendon for elicitation of the quadriceps (knee-jerk) reflex. The resulting muscular stretch activates the monosynaptic reflex arc. Intrinsic muscle reflexes are of major value for localization in clinical neurology because the reflex arc for a particular muscle occupies only one or two radicular or spinal cord segments; thus, a finding of an abnormal reflex enables the physician to infer the level of the underlying radicular or spinal lesion. The more important intrinsic muscle reflexes in clinical practice, the manner in which they are elicited, and the segments that participate in their reflex arcs are shown in Figure 2.**13**. It should be realized that the clinical elicitation of intrinsic muscle reflexes is an artificial event: a brief muscular stretch such as that produced with a reflex hammer is a rarity in everyday life.

Reflex relaxation of antagonist muscles. The reflex contraction of a stretched muscle to maintain constant length is accompanied by reflex relaxation of its antagonist muscle(s). The regulatory circuit for this likewise begins in the muscle spindles. The nuclear chain fibers of many muscle spindles contain secondary endings called *flower-spray endings* in addition to the primary (annulospiral) endings discussed above. These secondary endings react to stretch as the primary endings do, but the afferent impulses generated in them travel centrally in II fibers, which are thinner than the Ia fibers associated with the primary endings. The impulses are relayed via spinal interneurons to produce a net inhibition—and thus relaxation—of the antagonist muscle(s) (reciprocal antagonist inhibition, Fig. 2.**14**).

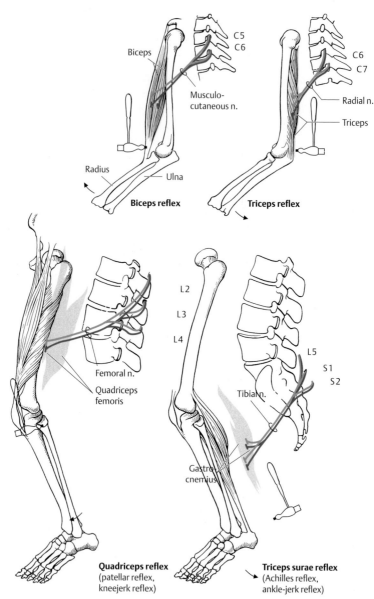

Biceps

C5
C6

Musculo-
cutaneous n.

Radius

Ulna

Biceps reflex

C6
C7

Radial n.

Triceps

Triceps reflex

L2
L3
L4

Femoral n.

Quadriceps
femoris

L5
S1
S2

Tibial n.

Gastro-
cnemius

Quadriceps reflex
(patellar reflex,
kneejerk reflex)

Triceps surae reflex
(Achilles reflex,
ankle-jerk reflex)

Fig. 2.**13 The most important intrinsic muscle reflexes**

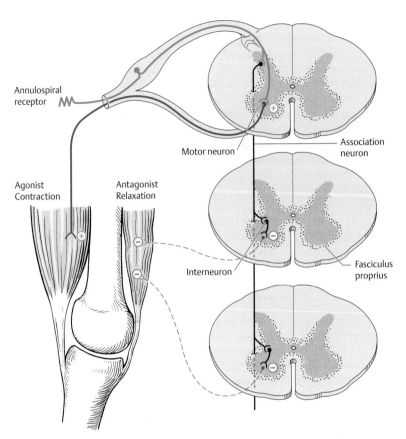

Fig. 2.14 Monosynaptic reflex with polysynaptic inhibition of antagonist muscles

Setting of target values for muscle length. There is a special motor system whose function is to set adjustable target values in the regulatory circuit for muscle length.

As shown in Figure 2.**11**, the anterior horn of the spinal cord contains not only the large α motor neurons but also the smaller γ motor neurons. These cells project their axons (γ fibers) to the small, striated intrafusal fibers of the muscle spindles. Excitation by γ fibers induces contraction of the intrafusal muscle fibers at either end of a muscle spindle. This stretches the midportion of the spindle, leading the annulospiral ending to fire action potentials, which, in turn, elevate tension in the working muscle.

The γ motor neurons are under the influence of several descending motor pathways, including the pyramidal, reticulospinal, and vestibulospinal tracts. They thus serve as intermediaries for the control of muscle tone by higher motor centers, which is clearly an important aspect of voluntary movement. The γ efferents enable precise control of voluntary movements and also regulate the sensitivity of the stretch receptors. When the intrafusal muscle fibers contract and stretch the midportion of a muscle spindle, the threshold of the stretch receptors is lowered, i.e., they require much less muscular stretch to be activated. In the normal situation, the target muscle length that is to be maintained is automatically set by the fusimotor (γ) innervation of the muscle.

If both the primary receptors (nuclear bag fibers with annulospiral endings) and the secondary receptors (nuclear chain fibers with flower-spray endings) are slowly stretched, the response of the spindle receptors is static, i.e., unchanging in time. On the other hand, if the primary receptors are very rapidly stretched, a dynamic (rapidly changing) response ensues. Both the static and the dynamic responses are controlled by efferent γ neurons.

Static and dynamic γ motor neurons. There are presumed to be two types of γ motor neurons, dynamic and static. The former innervate mainly the intrafusal nuclear bag fibers, the latter mainly the intrafusal nuclear chain fibers. Excitation of nuclear bag fibers by dynamic γ neurons induces a strong, dynamic response mediated by the annulospiral ending, while excitation of nuclear chain fibers by static γ neurons induces a static, tonic response.

Muscle tone. Every muscle possesses a certain degree of tone, even in its maximally relaxed (resting) state. In the clinical neurological examination, the physician assesses muscle tone by noting the resistance to passive movement of the limbs (e. g., flexion and extension).

Total loss of muscle tone can be produced experimentally either by transection of all of the anterior roots or, perhaps more surprisingly, by transection of all of the posterior roots. Resting tone, therefore, is not a property of the muscle itself, but rather is maintained by the reflex arcs described in this section.

Adaptation of muscle tone to gravity and movement. The human body is continually subject to the earth's gravitational field. When an individual stands or walks, anti-gravity muscles must be activated (among them the quadriceps femoris, the long extensors of the trunk, and the cervical muscles) to keep the body erect.

When a heavy object is lifted, the tone normally present in the quadriceps muscle no longer suffices to keep the body erect. Buckling at the knees can be prevented only by an immediate increase in quadriceps tone, which occurs as a result of tonic intrinsic reflexes induced by the stretching of the muscle and of the muscle spindles within it. This feedback mechanism or servomechanism enables automatic adaptation of the tension in a muscle to the load that is placed upon it. Thus, whenever an individual stands, walks, or lifts, action potentials are constantly being relayed back and forth to ensure the maintenance of the correct amount of muscle tension.

Central Components of the Somatosensory System

Having traced the path of afferent impulses from the periphery to the spinal cord in the preceding sections, we will now proceed to discuss their further course within the central nervous system.

Root entry zone and posterior horn. Individual somatosensory fibers enter the spinal cord at the dorsal root entry zone (DREZ; also called the Redlich-Obersteiner zone) and then give off numerous collaterals that make synaptic contact with other neurons within the cord. Fibers subserving different sensory modalities occupy different positions in the spinal cord (Fig. 2.**15**). It is important to note that the myelin sheaths of all afferent fibers become considerably thinner as the fibers traverse the root entry zone and enter the posterior horn. The type of myelin changes from peripheral to central, and the myelinating cells are no longer Schwann cells, but rather oligodendrocytes.

The afferent fiber pathways of the spinal cord subserving individual somatosensory modalities (Fig. 2.**16**) will now be described individually.

Posterior and Anterior Spinocerebellar Tracts

Some of the afferent impulses arising in organs of the musculoskeletal system (the muscles, tendons, and joints) travel by way of the spinocerebellar tracts to the organ of balance and coordination, the cerebellum. There are two such tracts on each side, one anterior and one posterior (Fig. 2.**16a**).

Posterior spinocerebellar tract. Rapidly conducting Ia fibers from the muscle spindles and tendon organs divide into numerous collaterals after entering the spinal cord. Some of these collateral fibers make synaptic contact directly onto the large α motor neurons of the anterior horn (monosynaptic reflex arc,

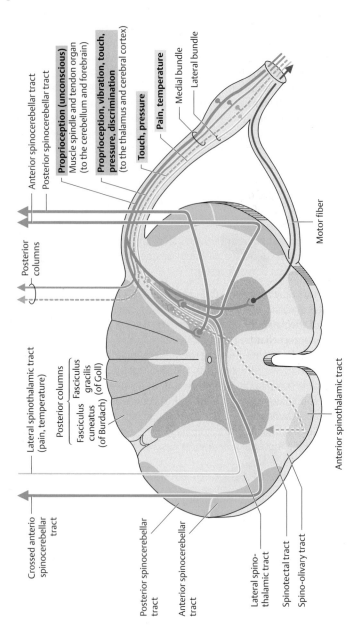

Anterior spinocerebellar tract
Posterior spinocerebellar tract

Proprioception (unconscious)
Muscle spindle and tendon organ
(to the cerebellum and forebrain)

**Proprioception, vibration, touch,
pressure, discrimination**
(to the thalamus and cerebral cortex)

Touch, pressure

Pain, temperature

Medial bundle

Lateral bundle

Motor fiber

Posterior columns

Lateral spinothalamic tract
(pain, temperature)

Posterior columns

Fasciculus   Fasciculus
cuneatus   gracilis
(of Burdach) (of Goll)

Crossed anterior
spinocerebellar
tract

Posterior spinocerebellar
tract

Anterior spinocerebellar
tract

Lateral spino-
thalamic tract

Spinotectal tract

Spino-olivary tract

Anterior spinothalamic tract

Fig. 2.15 **Position of fibers of different somatosensory modalities in the posterior root and root entry zone, and their further course in the spinal cord**

Figs. 2.**15** and 2.**11**). Other collateral fibers arising at thoracic, lumbar, and sacral levels terminate in a column-shaped nucleus occupying the base of the posterior horn at levels C8-L2, which is variously named the intermediolateral cell column, thoracic nucleus, Clarke's column, and Stilling's nucleus. The post-synaptic second neurons with cell bodies lying in this nucleus are the origin of the posterior spinocerebellar tract, whose fibers are among the most rapidly conducting of any in the body. The posterior spinocerebellar tract ascends the spinal cord *ipsilaterally* in the posterior portion of the lateral funiculus and then travels by way of the inferior cerebellar peduncle to the *cerebellar vermis* (p. 253; Figs. 2.**16a** and 2.**17**). Afferent fibers arising at cervical levels (i.e., above the level of the intermediolateral cell column) travel in the fasciculus cuneatus to make a synapse onto their corresponding second neurons in the accessory cuneate nucleus of the medulla (Fig. 2.**17**), whose output fibers ascend to the cerebellum.

Anterior spinocerebellar tract. Other afferent Ia fibers entering the spinal cord form synapses with funicular neurons in the posterior horns and in the central portion of the spinal gray matter (Figs. 2.**15**, 2.**16a**, and 2.**17**). These second neurons, which are found as low as the lower lumbar segments, are the cells of origin of the anterior spinocerebellar tract, which ascends the spinal cord *both ipsilaterally and contralaterally* to terminate in the cerebellum. In contrast to the posterior spinocerebellar tract, the anterior spinocerebellar tract traverses the floor of the fourth ventricle to the midbrain and then turns in a posterior direction to reach the *cerebellar vermis* by way of the superior cerebellar peduncle and the superior medullary velum. The cerebellum receives afferent proprioceptive input from all regions of the body; its polysynaptic efferent output, in turn, influences muscle tone and the coordinated action of the agonist and antagonist muscles (synergistic muscles) that participate in standing, walking, and all other movements. Thus, in addition to the lower regulatory circuits in the spinal cord itself, which were described in earlier sections, this higher functional circuit for the regulation of movement involves other, nonpyramidal pathways and both α and γ motor neurons. All of these processes occur unconsciously.

Posterior Columns

We can feel the position of our limbs and sense the degree of muscle tension in them. We can feel the weight of the body resting on our soles (i.e., we "feel the ground under our feet"). We can also perceive motion in the joints. Thus, at least some proprioceptive impulses must reach consciousness. Such impulses are derived from receptors in muscles, tendons, fasciae, joint capsules, and

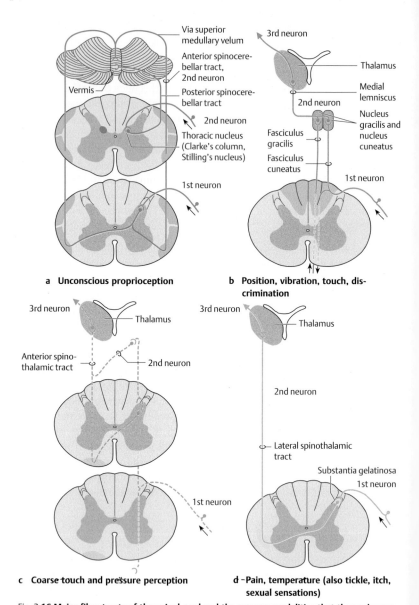

a   **Unconscious proprioception**

b   **Position, vibration, touch, discrimination**

c   **Coarse touch and pressure perception**

d – **Pain, temperature (also tickle, itch, sexual sensations)**

Fig. 2.**16 Major fiber tracts of the spinal cord and the sensory modalities that they subserve.**
a The anterior and posterior spinocerebellar tracts. **b** The posterior funiculus (posterior columns).
c The anterior spinothalamic tract. **d** The lateral spinothalamic tract.

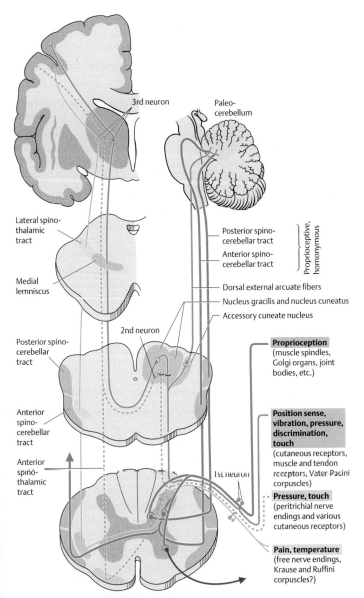

Fig. 2.**17 Spinal cord with major ascending pathways and their further course to target structures in the cerebrum and cerebellum** (schematic drawing)

connective tissue (Vater-Pacini and Golgi-Mazzoni corpuscles), as well as cutaneous receptors. The afferent fibers conveying them are the distal processes of pseudounipolar neurons in the spinal ganglia. The central processes of these cells, in turn, ascend the spinal cord and terminate in the posterior column nuclei of the lower medulla (Figs. 2.**16b** and 2.**17**).

Central continuation of posterior column pathways. In the posterior funiculus of the spinal cord, the afferent fibers derived from the lower limbs occupy the most medial position. The afferent fibers from the upper limbs join the cord at cervical levels and lie more laterally, so that the posterior funiculus here consists of two columns (on either side): the medial *fasciculus gracilis* (column of Goll), and the lateral *fasciculus cuneatus* (column of Burdach). The fibers in these columns terminate in the correspondingly named nuclei in the lower medulla, i.e., the nucleus gracilis and the nucleus cuneatus, respectively. These posterior column nuclei contain the second neurons, which project their axons to the *thalamus* (bulbothalamic tract). All of the bulbothalamic fibers cross the midline to the other side as they ascend, forming the so-called *medial lemniscus* (Figs. 2.**16b** and 2.**17**). These fibers traverse the medulla, pons, and midbrain and terminate in the *ventral posterolateral nucleus* of the thalamus (VPL, Fig. 6.**4**, p. 266). Here they make synaptic contact with the third neurons, which, in turn, give off the *thalamocortical tract*; this tract ascends by way of the *internal capsule* (posterior to the pyramidal tract) and through the *corona radiata* to the primary somatosensory cortex in the *postcentral gyrus*. The somatotopic organization of the posterior column pathway is preserved all the way up from the spinal cord to the cerebral cortex (Fig. 2.**19a**). The somatotopic projection on the postcentral gyrus resembles a person standing on his head—an inverted "homunculus" (Fig. 9.**19**, p. 374).

Posterior column lesions. The posterior columns mainly transmit impulses arising in the proprioceptors and cutaneous receptors. If they are dysfunctional, the individual can no longer feel the position of his or her limbs; nor can he or she recognize an object laid in the hand by the sense of touch alone or identify a number or letter drawn by the examiner's finger in the palm of the hand. Spatial discrimination between two stimuli delivered simultaneously at different sites on the body is no longer possible. As the sense of pressure is also disturbed, the floor is no longer securely felt under the feet; as a result, both stance and gait are impaired (gait ataxia), particularly in the dark or with the eyes closed. These signs of posterior column disease are most pronounced when the posterior columns themselves are affected, but they can also be seen in lesions of the posterior column nuclei, the medial lemniscus, the thalamus, and the postcentral gyrus.

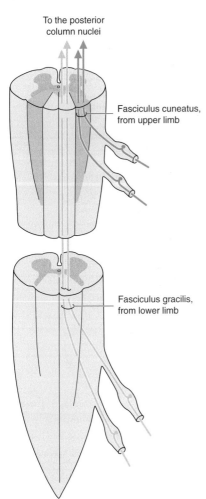

To the posterior
column nuclei

Fasciculus cuneatus,
from upper limb

Fasciculus gracilis,
from lower limb

Fig. 2.**18 Posterior funiculus,** containing the posterior columns: fasciculus gracilis (medial, afferent fibers from lower limb) and fasciculus cuneatus (lateral, afferent fibers from upper limb)

The clinical signs of a posterior column lesion are, therefore, the following:

- *Loss of the sense of position and movement* (kinesthetic sense): the patient cannot state the position of his or her limbs without looking.
- *Astereognosis:* the patient cannot recognize and name objects by their shape and weight using the sense of touch alone.

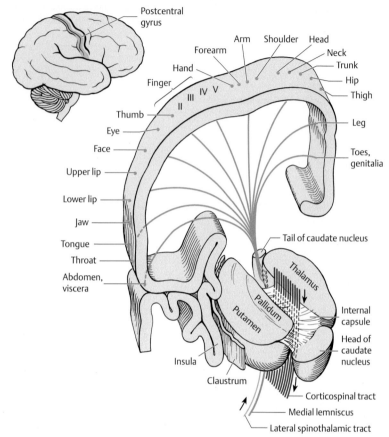

Fig. 2.**19 Course of the sensory pathways by way of the thalamus and internal capsule to the cerebral cortex**

- *Agraphesthesia:* the patient cannot recognize by touch a number or letter drawn in the palm of the hand by the examiner's finger.
- *Loss of two-point discrimination.*
- *Loss of vibration sense:* the patient cannot perceive the vibration of a tuning fork placed on a bone.
- *Positive Romberg sign:* The patient cannot stand for any length of time with feet together and eyes closed without wobbling and perhaps falling over.

The loss of proprioceptive sense can be compensated for, to a considerable extent, by opening the eyes (which is not the case, for example, in a patient with a cerebellar lesion).

The fibers in the posterior columns originate in the pseudounipolar neurons of the spinal ganglia, but the fibers in the anterior and posterior spinothalamic tracts do not; they are derived from the *second* neurons of their respective pathways, which are located within the spinal cord (Fig. 2.**16c,d**, p. 42).

Anterior Spinothalamic Tract

The impulses arise in cutaneous receptors (peritrichial nerve endings, tactile corpuscles) and are conducted along a moderately thickly myelinated peripheral fiber to the pseudounipolar dorsal root ganglion cells, and thence by way of the posterior root into the spinal cord. Inside the cord, the central processes of the dorsal root ganglion cells travel in the posterior columns some 2-15 segments upward, while collaterals travel 1 or 2 segments downward, making synaptic contact onto cells at various segmental levels in the *gray matter of the posterior horn* (Fig. 2.**16c**, p. 42). These cells (the second neurons) then give rise to the anterior spinothalamic tract, whose fibers *cross* in the anterior spinal commissure, ascend in the contralateral anterolateral funiculus, and terminate in the *ventral posterolateral nucleus* of the *thalamus*, together with the fibers of the lateral spinothalamic tract and the medial lemniscus (Fig. 2.**17**, p. 43). The third neurons in this thalamic nucleus then project their axons to the *postcentral gyrus* in the *thalamocortical tract*.

Lesions of the anterior spinothalamic tract. As explained above, the central fibers of the first neurons of this tract ascend a variable distance in the *ipsilateral* posterior columns, giving off collaterals along the way to the second neurons, whose fibers then cross the midline and ascend further in the *contralateral* anterior spinothalamic tract. It follows that a lesion of this tract at a lumbar or thoracic level generally causes minimal or no impairment of touch, because many ascending impulses can circumvent the lesion by way of the ipsilateral portion of the pathway. A lesion of the anterior spinothalamic tract at a *cervical* level, however, will produce mild hypesthesia of the contralateral lower limb.

Lateral Spinothalamic Tract

The free nerve endings of the skin are the peripheral receptors for noxious and thermal stimuli. These endings constitute the end organs of thin group A fibers and of nearly unmyelinated group C fibers that are, in turn, the peripheral processes of pseudounipolar neurons in the spinal ganglia. The central processes pass in the lateral portion of the posterior roots into the spinal cord and then divide longitudinally into short collaterals that terminate within one or two segments in the substantia gelatinosa, making synaptic contact with *funicular neurons* (second neurons) whose processes form the lateral spinothalamic tract (Fig. 2.**16d**, p. 42). These processes *cross* the midline in the anterior spinal commissure before ascending in the contralateral lateral funiculus to the thalamus. Like the posterior columns, the lateral spinothalamic tract is somatotopically organized; here, however, the fibers from the lower limb lie laterally, while those from the trunk and upper limb lie more medially (Fig. 2.**20**).

The fibers mediating pain and temperature sensation lie so close to each other that they cannot be anatomically separated. Lesions of the lateral spinothalamic tract thus impair both sensory modalities, though not always to the same degree.

Central continuation of the lateral spinothalamic tract. The fibers of the lateral spinothalamic tract travel up through the brainstem together with those of the medial lemniscus in the *spinal lemniscus*, which terminates in the *ventral posterolateral nucleus* of the thalamus (*VPL*, p. 265; see Fig. 6.**4**, p. 266, and Fig. 2.**19**). The third neurons in the VPL project via the *thalamocortical tract* to the *postcentral gyrus* in the parietal lobe (Fig. 2.**19**). Pain and temperature are perceived in a rough manner in the thalamus, but finer distinctions are not made until the impulses reach the cerebral cortex.

Lesions of the lateral spinothalamic tract. The lateral spinothalamic tract is the main pathway for pain and temperature sensation. It can be neurosurgically transected to relieve pain (**cordotomy**); this operation is much less commonly performed today than in the past, because it has been supplanted by less invasive methods and also because the relief it provides is often only temporary. The latter phenomenon, long recognized in clinical experience, suggests that pain-related impulses might also ascend the spinal cord along other routes, e. g., in spinospinal neurons belonging to the fasciculus proprius.

If the lateral spinothalamic tract is transected in the ventral portion of the spinal cord, pain and temperature sensation are deficient on the opposite side one or two segments below the level of the lesion, while the sense of touch is preserved (*dissociated sensory deficit*).

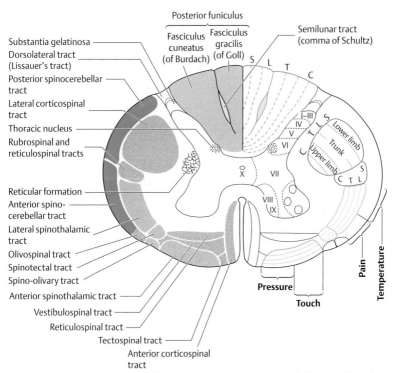

Fig. 2.**20 Somatotopic organization of spinal cord tracts in cross section.** The laminae of Rexed are also designated with Roman numerals (cytoarchitectural organization of the spinal gray matter).

Other Afferent Tracts of the Spinal Cord

In addition to the spinocerebellar and spinothalamic tracts discussed above, the spinal cord contains yet other fiber pathways ascending to various target structures in the brainstem and deep subcortical nuclei. These pathways, which originate in the dorsal horn of the spinal cord (second afferent neuron) and ascend in its anterolateral funiculus, include the **spinoreticular**, **spinotectal**, **spino-olivary**, **and spinovestibular tracts**. The spinovestibular tract is found in the cervical spinal cord, from C4 upward, in the area of the (descending) vestibulospinal tract and is probably a collateral pathway of the posterior spinocerebellar tract.

Figure 2.**20** is a schematic drawing of the various sensory (ascending) tracts, as seen in a cross section of the spinal cord. The motor (descending) tracts are also indicated, so that the spatial relationships between the various tracts can be appreciated. Finally, in addition to the ascending and descending tracts, the spinal cord also contains a so-called intrinsic apparatus, consisting of neurons that project upward and downward over several spinal segments in the fasciculus proprius (Fig. 2.**9**, p. 31).

Central Processing of Somatosensory Information

Figure 2.**17** traces all of the sensory pathways discussed above, in schematically simplified form and in spatial relation to one another, as they ascend from the posterior roots to their ultimate targets in the brain. The sensory third neurons in the thalamus send their axons through the posterior limb of the internal capsule (posterior to the pyramidal tract) to the primary somatosensory cortex, which is located in the postcentral gyrus (Brodmann cytoarchitectural areas 3a, 3b, 2, and 1). The third neurons that terminate here mediate superficial sensation, touch, pressure, pain, temperature, and (partly) proprioception (Fig. 2.**19**, p. 46).

Sensorimotor integration. In fact, not all of the sensory afferent fibers from the thalamus terminate in the somatosensory cortex; some terminate in the primary motor cortex of the precentral gyrus. Thus, the sensory and motor cortical fields overlap to some extent, so that the precentral and postcentral gyri are sometimes together designated the **sensorimotor area**. The integration of function occurring here enables incoming sensory information to be immediately converted to outgoing motor impulses in sensorimotor regulatory circuits, about which we will have more to say later. The descending pyramidal fibers emerging from these circuits generally terminate directly—without any intervening interneurons—on motor neurons in the anterior horn. Finally, even though their functions overlap, it should be remembered that the precentral gyrus remains almost entirely a motor area, and the postcentral gyrus remains almost entirely a (somato)sensory area.

Differentiation of somatosensory stimuli by their origin and quality. It has already been mentioned that somatosensory representation in the cerebral cortex is spatially segregated in somatotopic fashion: the inverted sensory homunculus has been encountered in Figure 2.**19** and will be seen again in Figure 9.**19**, p. 374. But somatosensory representation in the cerebral cortex is also spatially segregated by *modality*: pain, temperature, and the other modalities are represented by distinct areas of the cortex.

Although the different sensory modalities are already spatially segregated in the thalamus, conscious differentiation among them requires the participation of the cerebral cortex. Higher functions, such as discrimination or the exact determination of the site of a stimulus, are cortex-dependent.

A unilateral *lesion of the somatosensory cortex* produces a subtotal impairment of the perception of noxious, thermal, and tactile stimuli on the opposite side of the body; contralateral discrimination and position sense, however, are totally lost, as they depend on an intact cortex.

Stereognosis. The recognition by touch of an object laid in the hand (stereognosis) is mediated not just by the primary sensory cortex, but also by association areas in the parietal lobe, in which the individual sensory features of the object, such as its size, shape, consistency, temperature, sharpness/dullness, softness/hardness, etc., can be integrated and compared with memories of earlier tactile experiences.

Astereognosis. Injury to an area in the inferior portion of the parietal lobe impairs the ability to recognize objects by touch with the contralateral hand. This is called astereognosis.

Somatosensory Deficits due to Lesions at Specific Sites along the Somatosensory Pathways

Figure 2.**21** shows some typical sites of lesions along the somatosensory pathways; the corresponding sensory deficits are discussed below.

- A **cortical or subcortical lesion** in the sensorimotor area corresponding to the arm or leg (**a** and **b**, respectively, in Fig. 2.**21**) causes paresthesia (tingling, etc.) and numbness in the contralateral limb, which are more pronounced distally than proximally. An irritative lesion at this site can produce a sensory focal seizure; because the motor cortex lies directly adjacent, there are often motor discharges as well (jacksonian seizure).
- A **lesion of all sensory pathways below the thalamus** (**c**) eliminates all qualities of sensation on the opposite side of the body.
- If all somatosensory pathways are affected except the pathway for pain and temperature (**d**), there is hypesthesia on the opposite side of the body and face, but pain and temperature sensation are unimpaired.
- Conversely, a **lesion of the trigeminal lemniscus** and of the lateral spinothalamic tract (**e**) in the brainstem impairs pain and temperature sen-

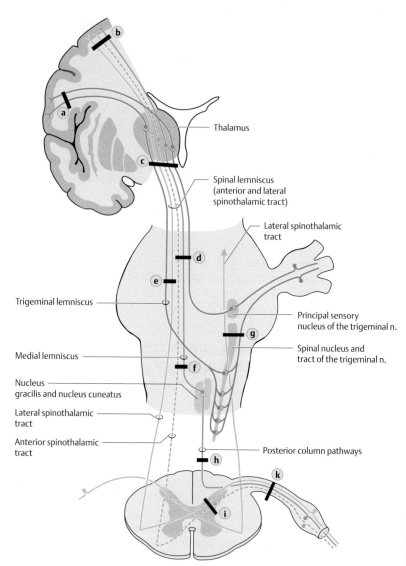

Thalamus

Spinal lemniscus
(anterior and lateral
spinothalamic tract)

Lateral spinothalamic
tract

Trigeminal lemniscus

Principal sensory
nucleus of the trigeminal n.

Medial lemniscus

Spinal nucleus and
tract of the trigeminal n.

Nucleus
gracilis and nucleus cuneatus

Lateral spinothalamic
tract

Anterior spinothalamic
tract

Posterior column pathways

Fig. 2.21 Potential sites of lesions along the somatosensory pathways. For the corresponding clinical syndromes, see text.

sation on the opposite side of the body and face, but does not impair other somatosensory modalities.

- If the **medial lemniscus and anterior spinothalamic tract** (**f**) are affected, all somatosensory modalities of the contralateral half of the body are impaired, except pain and temperature.
- **Lesions of the spinal nucleus and tract of the trigeminal nerve** and of the **lateral spinothalamic tract** (**g**) impair pain and temperature sensation on the ipsilateral half of the face and the contralateral half of the body.
- **Posterior column lesions** (**h**) cause loss of position and vibration sense, discrimination, etc., combined with ipsilateral ataxia.
- If the **posterior horn of the spinal cord** is affected by a lesion (**i**), ipsilateral pain and temperature sensation are lost, but other modalities remain intact (dissociated sensory deficit).
- A lesion affecting **multiple adjacent posterior roots** (**j**) causes radicular pain and paresthesiae, as well as impairment or loss of all sensory modalities in the affected area of the body, in addition to hypotonia or atonia, areflexia, and ataxia if the roots supply the upper or lower limb.

3 Motor System

3 Motor System

The motor impulses for voluntary movement are mainly generated in the **precentral gyrus** of the frontal lobe (primary motor cortex, Brodmann area 4) and in the adjacent cortical areas (**first motor neuron**). They travel in the long fiber pathways (mainly the **corticonuclear and corticospinal tracts**/pyramidal pathway), passing through the **brainstem** and down the **spinal cord** to the **anterior horn**, where they make synaptic contact with the **second motor neuron**—usually by way of one or more intervening interneurons.

The nerve fibers emerging from area 4 and the adjacent cortical areas together make up the **pyramidal tract**, which is the quickest and most direct connection between the primary motor area and the motor neurons of the anterior horn. In addition, other cortical areas (especially the premotor cortex, area 6) and subcortical nuclei (especially the basal ganglia, cf. p. 330) participate in the neural control of movement. These areas form complex feedback loops with one another and with the primary motor cortex and cerebellum; they exert an influence on the anterior horn cells by way of several distinct fiber pathways in the spinal cord. Their function is mainly to modulate movement and to regulate muscle tone.

Impulses generated in the second motor neurons of the motor cranial nerve nuclei and the anterior horn of the spinal cord pass through the **anterior roots**, the **nerve plexuses** (in the cervical and lumbosacral regions), and the **peripheral nerves** on their way to the skeletal muscles. The impulses are conveyed to the muscle cells through the **motor end plates** of the neuromuscular junction.

Lesions of the first motor neuron in the brain or spinal cord usually produce **spastic paresis**, while lesions of the second motor neuron in the anterior horn, anterior root, peripheral nerve, or motor end plate usually produce **flaccid paresis**. Motor deficits rarely appear in isolation as the result of a lesion of the nervous system; they are usually accompanied by sensory, autonomic, cognitive, and/or neuropsychological deficits of various kinds, depending on the site and nature of the causative lesion.

Central Components of the Motor System and Clinical Syndromes of Lesions Affecting Them

The central portion of the motor system for voluntary movement consists of the *primary motor cortex (area 4)* and the *adjacent cortical areas* (particularly the premotor cortex, area 6), and the *corticobulbar* and *corticospinal tracts* to which these cortical areas give rise (Figs. 3.**1** and 3.**2**).

Motor Cortical Areas

The *primary motor cortex* (precentral gyrus, Fig. 3.**1**) is a band of cortical tissue that lies on the opposite side of the central sulcus from the primary somatosensory cortex (in the postcentral gyrus) and, like it, extends upward and past the superomedial edge of the hemisphere onto its medial surface. The area representing the throat and larynx lies at the inferior end of the primary motor cortex; above it, in sequence, are the areas representing the face, upper limbs, trunk, and lower limbs (Fig. 3.**2**). This is the inverted "*motor homunculus*," corresponding to the "somatosensory homunculus" of the postcentral gyrus that was discussed in Chapter 2 (see Fig. 9.**19**, p. 374).

Motor neurons are found not only in area 4 but also in the adjacent cortical areas. The fibers mediating fine voluntary movements, however, originate mainly in the precentral gyrus. This is the site of the characteristic, large *pyramidal neurons (Betz cells)*, which lie in the fifth cellular layer of the cortex and send their rapidly conducting, thickly myelinated axons (Fig. 3.**3**) into the pyramidal tract. The pyramidal tract was once thought to be entirely composed of Betz cell axons, but it is now known that these account for only 3.4-4% of its fibers. The largest fiber contingent in fact originates from the smaller pyramidal and fusiform cells of Brodmann areas 4 and 6. Axons derived from area 4 make up about 40% of all pyramidal tract fibers; the remainder come from other frontal areas, from areas 3, 2, and 1 of the parietal somatosensory cortex (sensorimotor area), and from other areas in the parietal lobe (Fig. 3.**1**). The motor neurons of area 4 subserve fine, voluntary movement of the contralateral half of the body; the pyramidal tract is, accordingly, crossed (see Fig. 3.**4**). Direct electrical stimulation of area 4, as during a neurosurgical procedure, generally induces contraction of an individual muscle, while stimulation of area 6 induces more complex and extensive movements, e. g., of an entire upper or lower limb.

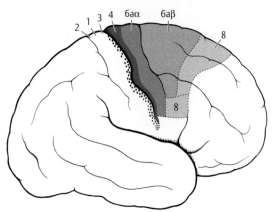

Fig. 3.**1 Primary motor area/precentral gyrus** (area 4), **premotor cortex** (area 6), and **prefrontal eye field** (area 8). For the functions of these areas, see text.

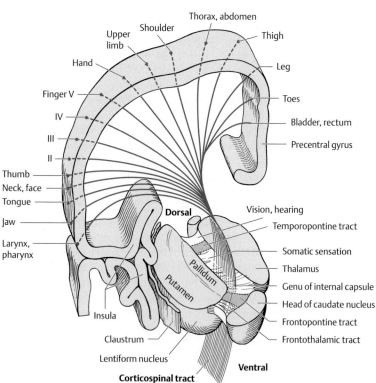

Fig. 3.**2 Course of the pyramidal tract**, upper portion: the corona radiata and internal capsule

Corticospinal Tract (Pyramidal Tract)

This tract originates in the *motor cortex* and travels through the *cerebral white matter* (corona radiata), the posterior limb of the *internal capsule* (where the fibers lie very close together), the central portion of the *cerebral peduncle* (crus cerebri), the *pons*, and the base (i.e., the anterior portion) of the *medulla*, where the tract is externally evident as a slight protrusion called the pyramid. The medullary pyramids (there is one on either side) give the tract its name. At the lower end of the medulla, 80–85% of the pyramidal fibers cross to the other side in the so-called *decussation of the pyramids*. The fibers that do not cross here descend the spinal cord in the ipsilateral anterior funiculus as the *anterior corticospinal tract*; they cross farther down (usually at the level of the segment that they supply) through the anterior commissure of the spinal cord (cf. Fig. 3.**6**). At cervical and thoracic levels, there are probably also a few fibers that remain uncrossed and innervate ipsilateral motor neurons in the anterior horn, so that the nuchal and truncal musculature receives a bilateral cortical innervation.

The majority of pyramidal tract fibers cross in the decussation of the pyramids, then descend the spinal cord in the contralateral lateral funiculus as the *lateral corticospinal tract*. This tract shrinks in cross-sectional area as it travels down the cord, because some of its fibers terminate in each segment along the way. About 90% of all pyramidal tract fibers end in synapses onto interneurons, which then transmit the motor impulses onward to the large α motor neurons of the anterior horn, as well as to the smaller γ motor neurons (Fig. 3.**4**).

Corticonuclear (Corticobulbar) Tract

Some of the fibers of the pyramidal tract branch off from the main mass of the tract as it passes through the midbrain and then take a more dorsal course toward the motor cranial nerve nuclei (Figs. 3.**4** and 4.**54**, p. 212). The fibers supplying these brainstem nuclei are partly crossed and partly uncrossed (for further details, cf. Chapter 4, section 4.4 "Cranial Nerves"). The nuclei receiving pyramidal tract input are the ones that mediate voluntary movements of the cranial musculature through cranial nerves V (the trigeminal nerve), VII (the facial nerve), IX, X, and XI (the glossopharyngeal, vagus, and accessory nerves), and XII (the hypoglossal nerve).

Corticomesencephalic tract. There is also a contingent of fibers traveling together with the corticonuclear tract that arises, not in areas 4 and 6, but rather in area 8, the frontal eye field (Figs. 3.**1** and 3.**4**). The impulses in these fibers mediate conjugate eye movements (p. 46), which are a complex motor process.

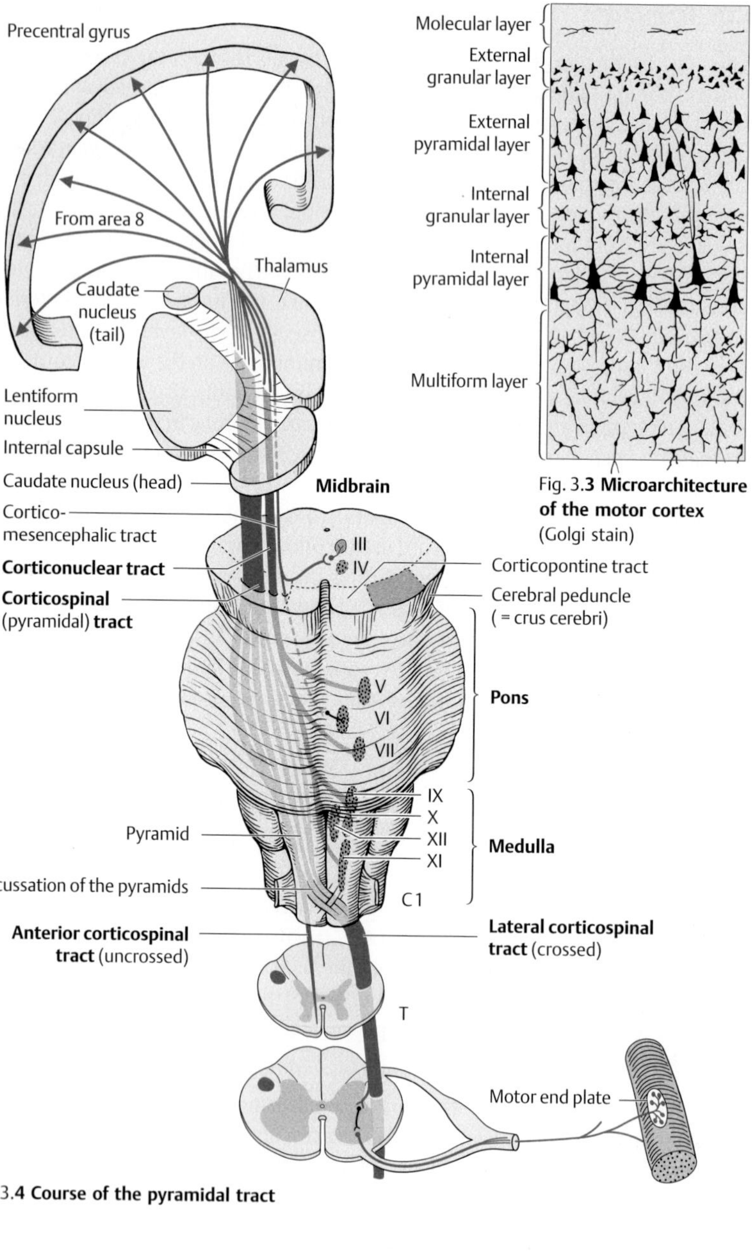
Molecular layer
External granular layer
External pyramidal layer
Internal granular layer
Internal pyramidal layer
Multiform layer
Precentral gyrus
From area 8
Thalamus
Caudate nucleus (tail)
Lentiform nucleus
Internal capsule
Caudate nucleus (head)
Midbrain
Cortico-mesencephalic tract
Corticonuclear tract
Corticospinal (pyramidal) tract
III
IV
Corticopontine tract
Cerebral peduncle (= crus cerebri)
V
VI
VII
Pons
IX
X
XII
XI
Medulla
Pyramid
Decussation of the pyramids
C1
Anterior corticospinal tract (uncrossed)
Lateral corticospinal tract (crossed)
T
Motor end plate

Fig. 3.**3 Microarchitecture of the motor cortex** (Golgi stain)

Fig. 3.**4 Course of the pyramidal tract**

Because of its special origin and function, the pathway originating in the frontal eye fields has a separate name (the corticomesencephalic tract), though most authors consider it a part of the corticonuclear tract.

The corticomesencephalic tract runs in tandem with the pyramidal tract (just rostral to it, in the posterior limb of the internal capsule) and then heads dorsally toward the nuclei of the cranial nerves that mediate eye movements, i.e., cranial nerves III, IV, and VI (the oculomotor, trochlear, and abducens nerves). Area 8 innervates the eye muscles exclusively in synergistic fashion, rather than individually. Stimulation of area 8 induces conjugate gaze deviation to the opposite side. The fibers of the corticomesencephalic tract do not terminate directly onto the motor neurons of cranial nerve nuclei III, IV, and VI; the anatomical situation here is complicated and incompletely understood, and is discussed further in Chapter 4 (p. 46 ff).

Other Central Components of the Motor System

A number of central pathways beside the pyramidal tract play major roles in the control of motor function (Fig. 3.**5**). One important group of fibers (the **corticopontocerebellar tract**) conveys information from the cerebral cortex to the cerebellum, whose output in turn modulates planned movements (cf. Chapter 5 "Cerebellum"). Other fibers travel from the cortex to the **basal ganglia** (mainly the corpus striatum = caudate nucleus and putamen), the **substantia nigra**, the brainstem **reticular formation**, and other nuclei (e. g., in the midbrain tectum). In each of these structures, the impulses are processed and conveyed onward, via interneurons, to efferent tracts that project to the motor neurons of the anterior horn—the tectospinal, rubrospinal, reticulospinal, vestibulospinal, and other tracts (Fig. 3.**6**). These tracts enable the cerebellum, basal ganglia, and brainstem motor nuclei to influence motor function in the spinal cord. (For further details, see Chapter 4 "Brainstem," and Chapter 8 "Basal Ganglia.")

Lateral and medial motor tracts in the spinal cord. The motor tracts in the spinal cord are anatomically and functionally segregated into two groups: a *lateral group*, comprising the corticospinal and rubrospinal tracts, and a *medial group*, comprising the reticulospinal, vestibulospinal, and tectospinal tracts (Kuypers, 1985). The lateral tracts mainly project to the distal musculature (especially in the upper limbs) and also make short propriospinal connections. They are primarily responsible for voluntary movements of the forearms and hands, i.e., for precise, highly differentiated, fine motor control. The medial tracts, in contrast, innervate motor neurons lying more medially in the anterior horn and make relatively long propriospinal connections. They are primarily responsible for movements of the trunk and lower limbs (*stance and gait*).

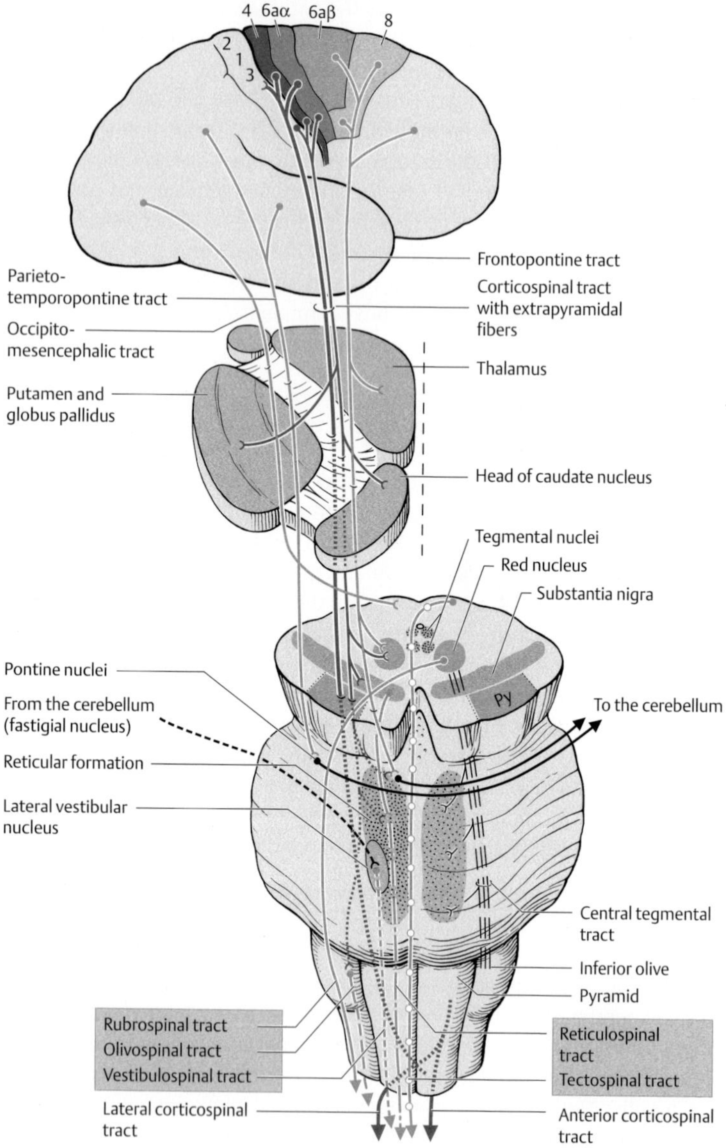

Fig. 3.**5 Brain structures involved in motor function and the descending tracts that originate in them**

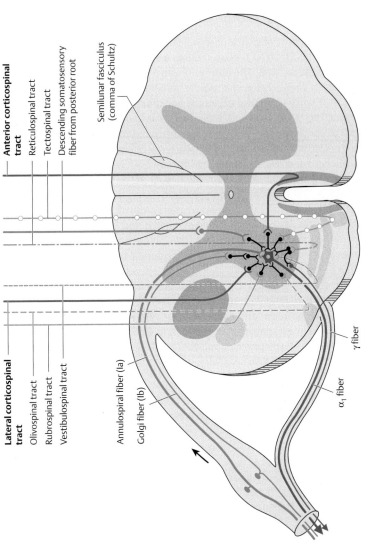

Lateral corticospinal tract

Olivospinal tract

Rubrospinal tract

Vestibulospinal tract

Annulospiral fiber (Ia)

Golgi fiber (Ib)

Anterior corticospinal tract

Reticulospinal tract

Tectospinal tract

Descending somatosensory fiber from posterior root

Semilunar fasciculus (comma of Schultz)

γ fiber

$α_1$ fiber

Fig. 3.6 Synapses of the descending motor tracts onto anterior horn neurons

Lesions of Central Motor Pathways

Pathogenesis of central spastic paresis. In the acute phase of a lesion of the corticospinal tract, the deep tendon reflexes are hypoactive and there is flaccid weakness of the muscles. The reflexes return a few days or weeks later and become hyperactive, because the muscle spindles respond more sensitively to stretch than normal, particularly in the upper limb flexors and the lower limb extensors. This hypersensitivity is due to a loss of descending central inhibitory control of the fusimotor cells (γ motor neurons) that innervate the muscle spindles. The intrafusal muscle fibers are, therefore, permanently activated (prestretched) and respond more readily than normal to further stretching of the muscle. A disturbance of the *regulatory circuit for muscle length* probably occurs (cf. p. 33 ff.), in which the upper limb flexors and lower limb extensors are set to an abnormally short target length. The result is *spastic increased tone* and *hyperreflexia*, as well as so-called *pyramidal tract signs* and *clonus*. Among the pyramidal tract signs are certain well-known findings in the fingers and toes, such as the *Babinski sign* (tonic extension of the big toe in response to stroking of the sole of the foot).

Spastic paresis is always due to a lesion of the central nervous system (brain and/or spinal cord) and is more pronounced when both the lateral and the medial descending tracts are damaged (e. g., in a spinal cord lesion). The pathophysiology of spasticity is still poorly understood, but the *accessory motor pathways* clearly play an important role, because an isolated, purely cortical lesion does not cause spasticity.

Syndrome of central spastic paresis. This syndrome consists of:
- Diminished muscular strength and impaired fine motor control
- Spastic increased tone
- Abnormally brisk stretch reflexes, possibly with clonus
- Hypoactivity or absence of exteroceptive reflexes (abdominal, plantar, and cremasteric reflexes)
- Pathological reflexes (Babinski, Oppenheim, Gordon, and Mendel-Bekhterev reflexes, as well as disinhibition of the flight response), and
- (initially) Preserved muscle bulk

Localization of Lesions in the Central Motor System

A lesion involving the cerebral cortex (**a** in Fig. 3.**7**), such as a tumor, an infarct, or a traumatic injury, causes weakness of part of the body on the opposite side. Hemiparesis is seen in the face and hand (*brachiofacial weakness*) more frequently than elsewhere, because these parts of the body have a large cortical

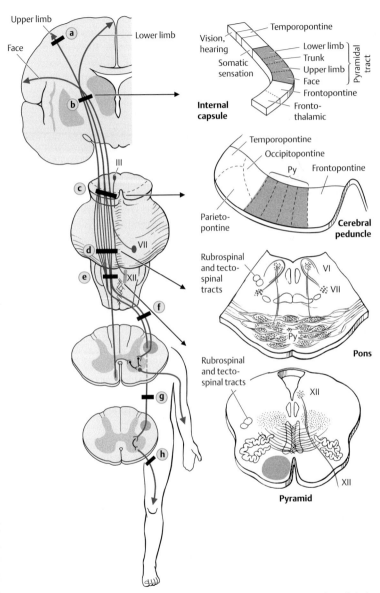

Fig. 3.**7 Sites of potential lesions of the pyramidal tract.** For the corresponding clinical syndromes, see text.

representation. The typical clinical finding associated with a lesion in site (**a**) is a predominantly distal paresis of the upper limb, most serious functional consequence of which is an impairment of fine motor control. The weakness is incomplete (paresis rather than plegia), and it is flaccid, rather than spastic, because the accessory (nonpyramidal) motor pathways are largely spared. An irritative lesion at site (**a**) can cause focal (jacksonian) seizures (which are described further in neurology textbooks).

If the internal capsule (**b** in Fig. 3.7) is involved (e. g., by hemorrhage or ischemia), there will be a *contralateral spastic hemiplegia*—lesions at this level affect both pyramidal and nonpyramidal fibers, because fibers of the two types are in close proximity here. The corticonuclear tract is involved as well, so that a contralateral *facial palsy* results, perhaps accompanied by a central *hypoglossal nerve palsy*. No other cranial nerve deficits are seen, however, because the remaining motor cranial nerve nuclei are bilaterally innervated. The contralateral paresis is flaccid at first (in the "shock phase") but becomes spastic within hours or days because of concomitant damage to nonpyramidal fibers.

Lesions at the level of the cerebral peduncle (**c** in Fig. 3.7), such as a vascular process, a hemorrhage, or a tumor, produce contralateral *spastic hemiparesis,* possibly accompanied by an ipsilateral oculomotor nerve palsy (cf. Weber syndrome, p. 235).

Pontine lesions involving the pyramidal tract (**d** in Fig. 3.7; e. g., a tumor, brainstem ischemia, a hemorrhage) cause *contralateral* or possibly *bilateral hemiparesis.* Typically, not all of the fibers of the pyramidal tract are involved, because its fibers are spread over a wider cross-sectional area at the pontine level than elsewhere (e. g., at the level of the internal capsule). Fibers innervating the facial and hypoglossal nuclei have already moved to a more dorsal position before reaching this level; thus, an accompanying central facial or hypoglossal palsy is rare, though there may be an accompanying ipsilateral trigeminal nerve deficit or abducens palsy (see Figs. 4.**66** and 4.**67**, p. 233 f.).

A lesion of the medullary pyramid (**e** in Fig. 3.7; usually a tumor) can damage the pyramidal tract fibers in isolation, as the nonpyramidal fibers are further dorsal at this level. *Flaccid contralateral hemiparesis* is a possible result. The weakness is less than total (i.e., paresis rather than plegia), because the remaining descending pathways are preserved.

Lesions of the pyramidal tract in the spinal cord. A lesion affecting the pyramidal tract at a **cervical** level (**f** Fig. 3.7; e. g., a tumor, myelitis, trauma) causes *ipsilateral spastic hemiplegia*: ipsilateral because the tract has already crossed at a higher level, and spastic because it contains nonpyramidal as well as pyramidal fibers at this level. A bilateral lesion in the upper cervical spinal cord can cause quadriparesis or quadriplegia.

A lesion affecting the pyramidal tract in the **thoracic** spinal cord (**g** in Fig. 3.7; e.g., trauma, myelitis) causes spastic ipsilateral monoplegia of the lower limb. Bilateral involvement causes paraplegia.

Peripheral Components of the Motor System and Clinical Syndromes of Lesions Affecting Them

The peripheral portion of the motor system comprises the motor cranial nerve nuclei of the brainstem, the motor anterior horn cells of the spinal cord, the anterior roots, the cervical and lumbosacral nerve plexuses, the peripheral nerves, and the motor end plates in skeletal muscle.

Anterior horn cells (α *and* γ *motor neurons*). The fibers not only of the pyramidal tract but also of the nonpyramidal descending pathways (the reticulospinal, tectospinal, vestibulospinal, and rubrospinal tracts, among others), as well as afferent fibers from the posterior roots, terminate on the cell bodies or dendrites of the larger and smaller α motor neurons. Fibers of all of these types also make synaptic contact with the small γ motor neurons, partly directly, and partly through intervening interneurons and the association and commissural neurons of the intrinsic neuronal apparatus of the spinal cord (Fig. 3.**6**). Some of these synapses are excitatory, others inhibitory. The thin, unmyelinated neurites of the γ motor neurons innervate the intrafusal muscle fibers. In contrast to the pseudounipolar neurons of the spinal ganglia, the anterior horn cells are multipolar. Their dendrites receive synaptic contact from a wide variety of afferent and efferent systems (Fig. 3.**6**).

The functional groups and nuclear columns of neurons in the anterior horn are not separated from one another by anatomically discernible borders (cf. Fig. 2.**5b**, p. 25). In the cervical spinal cord, the motor neurons for the upper limbs lie in the lateral portion of the gray matter of the anterior horn; those for the truncal muscles lie in its medial portion. The same somatotopic principle applies in the lumbar spinal cord, where the lower limbs are represented laterally, the trunk medially.

Inhibition of anterior horn cells by Renshaw cells. Among the various types of interneurons of the anterior horn, the Renshaw cells deserve special mention (Fig. 2.**11**, p. 34). These small cells receive synaptic contact from collateral axons of the large α motor neurons. Their axons then project back onto the anterior horn cells and inhibit their activity. Renshaw inhibition is an example of a spinal negative feedback loop that stabilizes the activity of motor neurons.

Anterior roots. The neurites of the motor neurons exit the anterior aspect of the spinal cord as rootlets (fila radicularia) and join together, forming the anterior roots. Each anterior root joins the corresponding posterior root just distal to the dorsal root ganglion to form a spinal nerve, which then exits the spinal canal through the intervertebral foramen.

Peripheral nerve and motor end plate. There is one pair of spinal nerves for each segment of the body. The spinal nerves contain afferent somatosensory fibers, efferent somatic motor fibers, efferent autonomic fibers from the lateral horns of the spinal gray matter, and afferent autonomic fibers (cf. p. 22). At cervical and lumbosacral levels, the spinal nerves join to form the nerve plexuses, which, in turn, give rise to the peripheral nerves that innervate the musculature of the neck and limbs (Figs. 3.**31**, 3.**32**, and 3.**34**).

The thick, myelinated, rapidly conducting neurites of the large α motor neurons are called α_1 fibers (Fig. 2.**11**, p. 34). These fibers travel to the working musculature, where they divide into a highly variable number of branches that terminate on muscle fibers. Synaptic impulse transmission occurs at the neuromuscular junctions (motor end plates).

Motor unit. An anterior horn cell, its neurites, and the muscle fibers it innervates are collectively termed a motor unit (Sherrington). Each motor unit constitutes the final common pathway for movement-related impulses arriving at the anterior horn cell from higher levels: its activity is influenced by impulses in a wide variety of motor tracts that originate in different areas of the brain, as well as by impulses derived from intrasegmental and intersegmental reflex neurons of the spinal cord. All of these movement-related impulses are integrated in the motor unit, and the result of this integration is transmitted to the muscle fibers.

Muscles participating in finely differentiated movements are supplied by a large number of anterior horn cells, each of which innervates only a few (5-20) muscle fibers; such muscles are thus composed of *small motor units*. In contrast, large muscles that contract in relatively undifferentiated fashion, such as the gluteal muscles, are supplied by relatively few anterior horn cells, each of which innervates 100-500 muscle fibers (*large motor units*).

Clinical Syndromes of Motor Unit Lesions

Flaccid paralysis is caused by interruption of motor units at any site, be it in the anterior horn, one or more anterior roots, a nerve plexus, or a peripheral nerve. Motor unit damage cuts off the muscle fibers in the motor unit from both voluntary and reflex innervation. The affected muscles are extremely weak (*plegic*), and there is a marked diminution of muscle tone (*hypotonia*), as well as a loss of reflexes (*areflexia*) because the monosynaptic stretch reflex loop has been interrupted. Muscle atrophy sets in within a few weeks, as the muscle is gradually replaced by connective tissue; after months or years of progressive atrophy, this replacement may be complete. Thus, the anterior horn cells exert a trophic influence on muscle fibers, which is necessary for the maintenance of their normal structure and function.

The syndrome of flaccid paralysis consists of the following:
- Diminution of raw strength
- Hypotonia or atonia of the musculature
- Hyporeflexia or areflexia
- Muscle atrophy

The lesion can usually be localized more specifically to the anterior horn, the anterior root(s), the nerve plexus, or the peripheral nerve with the aid of electromyography and electroneurography (nerve conduction studies). If paralysis in a limb or limbs is accompanied by somatosensory and autonomic deficits, then the lesion is presumably distal to the nerve roots and is thus located either in the nerve plexus or in the peripheral nerve. Flaccid paralysis is only rarely due to a cortical lesion (cf. p. 64); in such cases, the reflexes are preserved or even exaggerated, and the muscle tone is normal or increased.

Complex Clinical Syndromes due to Lesions of Specific Components of the Nervous System

Damage to individual components of the nervous system generally does not cause an isolated motor deficit of the kind described up to this point. Rather, motor deficits are usually accompanied by somatosensory, special sensory, autonomic, cognitive, and/or neuropsychological deficits of variable type and extent depending on the site and extent of the lesion. The complex clinical syndromes due to lesions in specific regions of the brain (telencephalon, diencephalon, basal ganglia, limbic system, cerebellum, and brainstem) will be described in the corresponding chapters. In this section, we will present the typical syndromes arising from lesions of the spinal cord, nerve roots, plexuses, peripheral nerves, motor end plates, and musculature.

Spinal Cord Syndromes

Because the spinal cord contains motor, sensory, and autonomic fibers and nuclei in a tight spatial relationship with one another, lesions of the spinal cord can cause a wide variety of neurological deficits, which can be combined with each other in many different ways. Careful clinical examination usually enables highly precise localization of the lesion, but only if the examiner possesses adequate knowledge of the anatomy of the relevant motor, sensory, and autonomic pathways. Thus, this section will begin with a brief discussion of clinical anatomy. The individual spinal pathways have already been discussed on pp. 39 ff. (afferent pathways) and 59 ff. (efferent pathways).

General anatomical preliminaries. The spinal cord, like the brain, is composed of gray matter and white matter. The white matter contains ascending and descending fiber tracts, while the gray matter contains neurons of different kinds: the anterior horns contain mostly motor neurons (see above), the lateral horns mostly autonomic neurons, and the posterior horns mostly somatosensory neurons participating in a number of different afferent pathways (see below and Chapter 2). In addition, the spinal cord contains an intrinsic neuronal apparatus consisting of interneurons, association neurons, and commissural neurons, whose processes ascend and descend in the fasciculus proprius (Fig. 2.**9**, p. 31).

In the adult, the spinal cord is shorter than the vertebral column: it extends from the craniocervical junction to about the level of the intervertebral disk between the first and second lumbar vertebrae (L1-2) (Fig. 2.**4**, p. 23; this must be borne in mind when localizing the level of a spinal process). The segments of the neural tube (primitive spinal cord) correspond to those of the vertebral column only up to the third month of gestation, after which the growth of the spine progressively outstrips that of the spinal cord. The nerve roots, however, still exit from the spinal canal at the numerically corresponding levels, so that the lower thoracic and lumbar roots must travel an increasingly long distance through the subarachnoid space to reach the intervertebral foramina through which they exit. The spinal cord ends as the **conus medullaris** (or conus terminalis) at the L1 or L2 level (rarely at L3). Below this level, the lumbar sac (theca) contains only nerve root filaments, the so-called **cauda equina** ("horse's tail"; Fig. 3.**22**).

The fanlike filaments of the nerve roots still display the original metameric structure of the spinal cord, but the cord itself shows no segmental division. At two sites, however, the spinal cord is somewhat swollen, namely at the **cervical** and **lumbar enlargements**. The former contains the segments corresponding to the upper limbs (C4-T1), which form the brachial plexus; the latter contains the ones for the lower limbs (L2-S3), which form the lumbosacral plexus (Fig. 2.**4**, p. 23).

Spinal cord lesions occasionally affect only the white matter (e. g., posterior column lesions) or only the gray matter (e. g., acute poliomyelitis), but more often affect both. In the following paragraphs, the manifestations of typical spinal cord syndromes will be presented from a topical point of view. For completeness, a number of syndromes characterized primarily or exclusively by somatosensory deficits will also be presented here.

Syndromes due to Lesions of Individual Spinal Tracts and Nuclear Areas and the Associated Peripheral Nerves

Syndrome of the dorsal root ganglion (Fig. 3.**8**). Infection of one or more spinal ganglia by a neurotropic virus occurs most commonly in the thoracic region and causes painful erythema of the corresponding dermatome(s), followed by the formation of a variable number of cutaneous vesicles. This clinical picture, called **herpes zoster**, is associated with very unpleasant, stabbing pain and paresthesiae in the affected area. The infection may pass from the spinal ganglia into the spinal cord itself, but, if it does, it usually remains confined to a

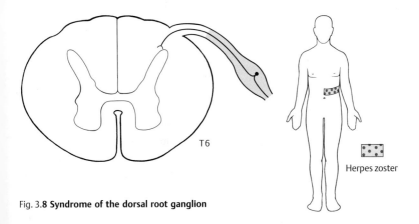

T6

Herpes zoster

Fig. 3.**8 Syndrome of the dorsal root ganglion**

small area within the cord. Involvement of the anterior horns causing flaccid paresis is rare, and hemiparesis or paraparesis is even rarer. Electromyography can demonstrate a segmental motor deficit in up to 2/3 of all cases, but, because herpes zoster is usually found in the thoracic area, the deficit tends to be functionally insignificant, and may escape the patient's notice. In some cases, the cutaneous lesion is absent (herpes sine herpete). Herpes zoster is relatively common, with an incidence of 3-5 cases per 1000 persons per year; immunocompromised individuals (e. g., with AIDS, malignancy, or immunosuppression) are at elevated risk. Treatment with topical dermatological medication as well as aciclovir, or another specific virustatic agent, is recommended. Even with appropriate treatment, postherpetic neuralgia in the affected area is a not uncommon complication. It can be treated symptomatically with various medications, including carbamazepine and gabapentin.

Posterior root syndrome (Fig. 3.**9**). If two or more adjacent posterior roots are completely divided, sensation in the corresponding dermatomes is partially or totally lost. Incomplete posterior root lesions affect different sensory modalities to variable extents, with pain sensation usually being most strongly affected. Because the lesion interrupts the peripheral reflex arc, the sensory deficit is accompanied by hypotonia and hyporeflexia or areflexia in the muscles supplied by the affected roots. These typical deficits are produced only if multiple adjacent roots are affected.

Posterior column syndrome (Fig. 3.**10**). The posterior columns can be secondarily involved by pathological processes affecting the dorsal root ganglion cells and the posterior roots. Lesions of the posterior columns typically impair position and vibration sense, discrimination, and stereognosis; they also produce a positive Romberg sign, as well as gait ataxia that worsens significantly when the eyes are closed (unlike cerebellar ataxia, which does not). Posterior column lesions also often produce hypersensitivity to pain. Possible causes include vitamin B_{12} deficiency (e. g., in "funicular myelosis"; see below), AIDS-associated vacuolar myelopathy, and spinal cord compression (e. g., in cervical spinal stenosis). Tabes dorsalis due to syphilis is rare in North America and Western Europe but is an increasingly common type of posterior column disturbance in other parts of the world.

Posterior horn syndrome (Fig. 3.**11**) can be a clinical manifestation of syringomyelia, hematomyelia, and some intramedullary spinal cord tumors, among other conditions. Like posterior root lesions, posterior horn lesions produce a segmental somatosensory deficit; yet, rather than impairing all sensory modalities like posterior root lesions, posterior horn lesions spare the modalities

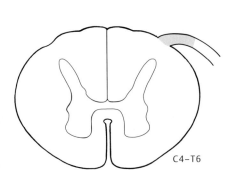

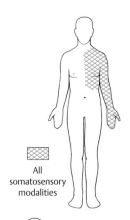

All somatosensory modalities

Fig. 3.9 Posterior root syndrome

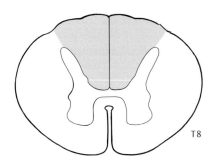

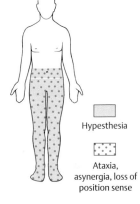

Hypesthesia

Ataxia, asynergia, loss of position sense

Fig. 3.10 Posterior column syndrome

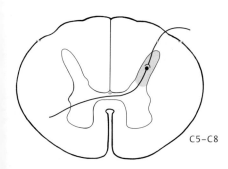

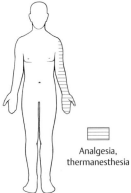

Analgesia, thermanesthesia

Fig. 3.11 Posterior horn syndrome

subserved by the posterior columns, i.e., epicritic and proprioceptive sense. "Only" pain and temperature sensation are lost in the corresponding ipsilateral segments, because these modalities are conducted centrally through a second neuron in the posterior horn (whose axon ascends in the lateral spinothalamic tract). Loss of pain and temperature sensation with sparing of posterior column sense is called a *dissociated somatosensory deficit.* There may be spontaneous pain (deafferentation pain) in the analgesic area.

Pain and temperature sensation are intact below the level of the lesion, as the lateral spinothalamic tract, lying in the anterolateral funiculus, is undamaged and continues to conduct these modalities centrally.

Gray matter syndrome (Fig. 3.**12**). Damage to the central gray matter of the spinal cord by syringomyelia, hematomyelia, intramedullary spinal cord tumors, or other processes interrupts all of the fiber pathways passing through the gray matter. The most prominently affected fibers are those that originate in posterior horn cells and conduct coarse pressure, touch, pain, and temperature sensation; these fibers decussate in the central gray matter and then ascend in the anterior and lateral spinothalamic tracts. A lesion affecting them produces a bilateral dissociated sensory deficit in the cutaneous area supplied by the damaged fibers.

Syringomyelia is characterized by the formation of one or more fluid-filled cavities in the spinal cord; the analogous disease in the brainstem is called syringobulbia. The cavities, called *syringes,* can be formed by a number of different mechanisms and are distributed in different characteristic patterns depending on their mechanism of formation. Some syringes are an expansion of the central canal of the spinal cord, which may or may not communicate with the fourth ventricle; others are a hollowing-out of the parenchyma and are separate from the central canal. The term "hydromyelia" is sometimes used loosely for communicating syringes of the central canal, but it properly refers to an idiopathic, congenital variant of syringomyelia in which the syrinx communicates with the subarachnoid space, and should only be used in this sense. Syringomyelia most commonly affects the cervical spinal cord, typically producing loss of pain and temperature sensation in the shoulders and upper limbs. A progressively expanding syrinx can damage the long tracts of the spinal cord, producing spastic (para)paresis and disturbances of bladder, bowel, and sexual function. Syringobulbia often causes unilateral atrophy of the tongue, hypalgesia or analgesia of the face, and various types of nystagmus depending on the site and configuration of the syrinx.

The syndrome of combined lesions of the posterior columns and corticospinal tracts (funicular myelosis) (Fig. 3.**13**) is most commonly produced by vitamin

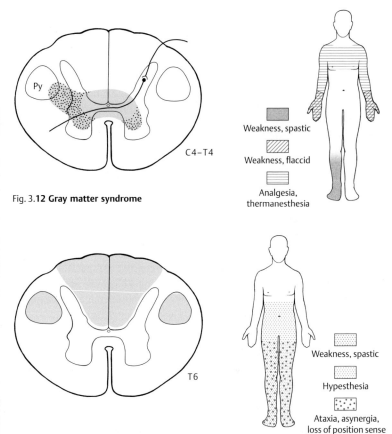

Fig. 3.**12 Gray matter syndrome**

Weakness, spastic

Weakness, flaccid

Analgesia, thermanesthesia

C4–T4

Weakness, spastic

Hypesthesia

Ataxia, asynergia, loss of position sense

T6

Fig. 3.**13 Combined posterior column and corticospinal tract syndrome** (funicular myelosis)

B_{12} deficiency due to a lack of gastric intrinsic factor (e. g., in atrophic gastritis), and is known in such cases as "subacute combined degeneration," or SCD. Foci of demyelination are found in the cervical and thoracic regions in the posterior columns (70–80%), and somewhat less commonly in the pyramidal tracts (40–50%), while the gray matter is usually spared. Posterior column damage causes loss of position and vibration sense in the lower limbs, resulting in spinal ataxia and a positive Romberg sign (unstable stance with eyes closed). The accompanying pyramidal tract damage causes spastic paraparesis with hyperreflexia and bilateral Babinski signs.

Anterior horn syndrome (Fig. 3.**14**). Both acute poliomyelitis and spinal muscle atrophy of various types specifically affect the anterior horn cells, particularly in the cervical and lumbar enlargements of the spinal cord.

In **poliomyelitis** (a viral infection), a variable number of anterior horn cells are acutely and irreversibly lost, mainly in the lumbar region, causing flaccid paresis of the muscles in the corresponding segments. Proximal muscles tend to be more strongly affected than distal ones. The muscles become atrophic and, in severe cases, may be completely replaced by connective tissue and fat. It is rare for all of the muscles of a limb to be affected, because the anterior horn cells are arranged in long vertical columns within the spinal cord (Fig. 2.**10**).

Combined anterior horn and pyramidal tract syndrome (Fig. 3.**15**) is seen in **amyotrophic lateral sclerosis** as the result of degeneration of both cortical and spinal motor neurons. The clinical picture is a combination of flaccid and spastic paresis. Muscle atrophy, appearing early in the course of the disease, is generally so severe that the deep tendon reflexes would ordinarily be absent, if only the lower motor neurons were affected. Yet, because of the simultaneous damage of the upper motor neurons (with consequent pyramidal tract degeneration and spasticity), the reflexes often remain elicitable and may even be exaggerated. Accompanying degeneration of the motor cranial nerve nuclei can cause dysarthria and dysphagia (progressive bulbar palsy).

Syndrome of the corticospinal tracts (Fig. 3.**16**). Loss of cortical motor neurons is followed by degeneration of the corticospinal tracts in a number of different diseases, including **primary lateral sclerosis** (a variant of amyotrophic lateral sclerosis) and the rarer form of hereditary **spastic spinal paralysis**. The most common subform of this disease is due to a mutation of the gene for an ATPase of the AAA family on chromosome 2; the disease appears in childhood and progresses slowly thereafter. Patients complain initially of a feeling of heaviness, then of weakness in the lower limbs. Spastic paraparesis with a spastic gait disturbance gradually develops and worsens. The reflexes are brisker than normal. Spastic paresis of the upper limbs does not develop until much later.

Syndrome of combined involvement of the posterior columns, spinocerebellar tracts, and (possibly) pyramidal tracts (Fig. 3.**17**). When the pathological process affects all of these systems, the differential diagnosis should include spinocerebellar ataxia of Friedreich type, the axonal form of a hereditary neuropathy (HSMN II), and other ataxias.

Characteristic clinical manifestations are produced by the lesions in each of the involved systems. **Friedreich ataxia** begins before age 20 with loss of dorsal root ganglion cells, leading to posterior column degeneration. The clinical re-

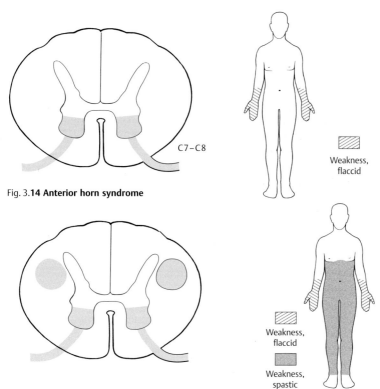

Fig. 3.**14 Anterior horn syndrome**

Fig. 3.**15 Combined anterior horn and pyramidal tract syndrome** (amyotrophic lateral sclerosis)

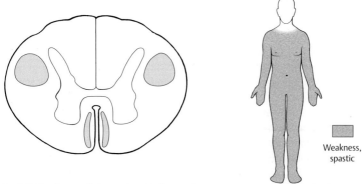

Fig. 3.**16 Syndrome of the corticospinal tracts** (progressive spastic spinal paralysis)

sult is an impairment of position sense, two-point discrimination, and stereognosis, with spinal ataxia and a positive Romberg sign. Pain and temperature sense are largely or completely spared. The ataxia is severe, because both the posterior columns and the spinocerebellar tracts are involved; it is evident when the patient tries to walk, stand, or sit, as well as in the finger-nose-finger and heel-knee-shin tests. The patient's gait is uncoordinated, with festination, and also becomes spastic over time as the pyramidal tracts progressively degenerate. About half of all patients manifest skeletal deformities such as scoliosis or pes cavus (the so-called "Friedreich foot").

According to Harding, Friedreich ataxia can be diagnosed when the following clinical criteria are met:

- Progressive ataxia of no other known cause, beginning before age 25 years
- Autosomal recessive inheritance
- Absent deep tendon reflexes in the lower limbs
- Posterior column disturbance
- Dysarthria within five years of onset

The diagnosis can be definitively established by molecular genetic testing to reveal the underlying genetic defect, a trinucleotide expansion on chromosome 9.

The spinal cord hemisection syndrome (Brown-Séquard syndrome, Fig. 3.**18**) is rare and usually incomplete; its most common causes are spinal trauma and cervical disk herniation. Interruption of the descending motor pathways on one side of the spinal cord causes an initially flaccid, ipsilateral paresis below the level of the lesion (spinal shock), which later becomes spastic and is accompanied by hyperreflexia, Babinski signs, and vasomotor disturbances. At the same time, the interruption of the posterior columns on one side of the spinal cord causes ipsilateral loss of position sense, vibration sense, and tactile discrimination below the level of the lesion. The ataxia that would normally be caused by the posterior column lesion cannot be demonstrated because of the coexisting ipsilateral paresis. Pain and temperature sensation are spared on the side of the lesion, because the fibers subserving these modalities have already crossed to the other side to ascend in the lateral spinothalamic tract, but pain and temperature sensation are lost *contralaterally* below the level of the lesion, because the ipsilateral (crossed) spinothalamic tracts are interrupted.

Simple tactile sensation is not impaired, as this modality is subserved by two different fiber pathways: the posterior columns (uncrossed) and the anterior spinothalamic tract (crossed). Hemisection of the cord leaves one of these two pathways intact for tactile sensation on either side of the body—the contralateral posterior columns for the side contralateral to the lesion, and the contralateral anterior spinothalamic tract for the side ipsilateral to it.

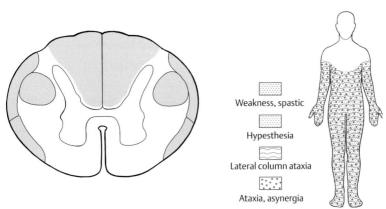

Weakness, spastic

Hypesthesia

Lateral column ataxia

Ataxia, asynergia

Fig. 3.**17 Syndrome of combined involvement of the posterior columns, spinocerebellar tracts, and (possibly) pyramidal tracts**

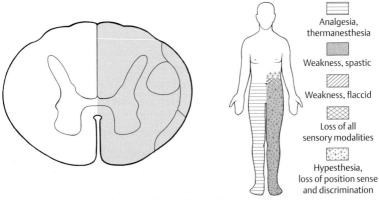

Analgesia, thermanesthesia

Weakness, spastic

Weakness, flaccid

Loss of all sensory modalities

Hypesthesia, loss of position sense and discrimination

Fig. 3.**18 Spinal cord hemisection syndrome** (Brown–Séquard syndrome)

Aside from the interruption of the long tracts, the anterior horn cells may be damaged to a variable extent at the level of the lesion, possibly causing flaccid paresis. Irritation of the posterior roots may also cause paresthesiae or radicular pain in the corresponding dermatomes at the upper border of the sensory disturbance.

Spinal Cord Transection Syndromes

General Symptomatology and Clinical Course of Transection Syndromes

Acute spinal cord transection syndrome (Fig. 3.**19**). The complete spinal cord transection syndrome is most commonly caused by trauma, less commonly by inflammation or infection (transverse myelitis). Acute spinal cord trauma initially produces so-called **spinal shock**, a clinical picture whose pathophysiology is incompletely understood. Below the level of the lesion there is complete, flaccid paralysis, and all modalities of sensation are lost. Bladder, bowel, and sexual function are lost as well. Only the bulbocavernosus reflex is preserved—an important point for the diagnostic differentiation of this condition from polyradiculitis, in which it is typically absent. There are also trophic changes below the level of the lesion, in particular, diminished sweating and disturbed thermoregulation. There is a marked tendency to develop decubitus ulcers. The upper border of the sensory deficit (the "sensory level") is often demarcated by a zone of hyperalgesia.

In the days and weeks after the causative event, the spinal neurons gradually regain their function, at least in part, but remain cut off from most of the centrally derived neural impulses that normally regulate them. They thus become "autonomous," and so-called **spinal automatisms** appear. In many cases, a stimulus below the level of the lesion induces sudden flexion of the hip, knee, and ankle (flexor reflex); if the spinal cord transection syndrome is complete, the limbs retain the flexed position for a long time after the stimulus because of a spastic elevation of muscle tone. (In incomplete spinal cord transection syndrome, on the other hand, the legs are initially flexed upon stimulation, but then return to their original position.) Defecation and urination gradually function again, but are no longer under voluntary control; instead, the bladder and bowel are emptied reflexively once they are filled to a certain point. Detrusor-sphincter dyssynergia causes urinary retention and frequent, reflexive micturition (p. 302). The deep tendon reflexes and muscle tone gradually return and can become pathologically elevated. Sexual potency, however, does not return.

Progressive spinal cord transection syndrome. When spinal cord transection syndrome arises gradually rather than suddenly, e. g., because of a slowly growing tumor, spinal shock does not arise. The transection syndrome in such cases is usually partial, rather than complete. Progressively severe spastic paraparesis develops below the level of the lesion, accompanied by a sensory deficit, bowel, bladder, and sexual dysfunction, and autonomic manifestations (abnormal vasomotor regulation and sweating, tendency to decubitus ulcers).

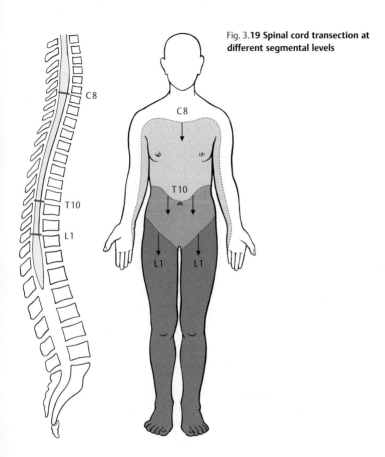

Fig. 3.**19 Spinal cord transection at different segmental levels**

Spinal Cord Transection Syndromes at Different Levels

Cervical spinal cord transection syndrome. Spinal cord transection above the level of the third cervical vertebra is fatal, as it abolishes breathing (total loss of function of the phrenic and intercostal nerves). Such patients can survive only if they can be artificially ventilated within a few minutes of the causative injury, which is very rarely the case. Transection at lower cervical levels produces quadriparesis with involvement of the intercostal muscles; breathing may be dangerously impaired. The upper limbs are affected to a variable extent depending on the level of the lesion. The level can be determined fairly precisely from the sensory deficit found on clinical examination.

Case Presentation 1: *Incomplete Spinal Cord Transection Syndrome due to Parainfectious Myelitis*

The patient, a 33-year-old architect, was sent to the hospital by her family physician after complaining of ascending pins-and-needles paresthesiae in the lower limbs and trunk. She had had a febrile "cold" two weeks earlier. There was no weakness or disturbance of bladder or bowel function.

Clinical examination revealed impairment of epicritic sensation below the C5 level, but no paresis or other neurological abnormalities. CSF

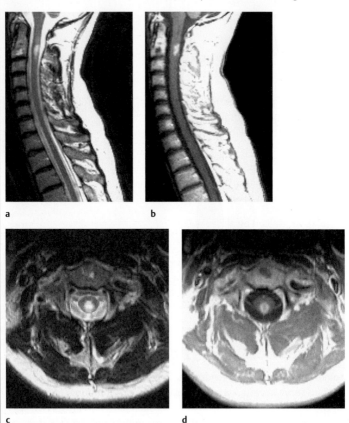

a   b

c   d

Fig. 3.**20 Parainfectious myelitis. a** The sagittal T2-weighted image reveals a lesion with hyperintense signal in the spinal cord at the level of the C2 vertebral body. **b** The T1-weighted sequence after the administration of contrast medium reveals marked enhancement of the lesion. **c** In the axial T2-weighted image, the lesion is seen to occupy the central portion of the cord. **d** Contrast enhancement in the lesion is seen again in the axial T1-weighted image after the administration of contrast medium.

examination yielded an inflammatory picture, with no evidence of chronic CNS inflammation (CSF electrophoresis revealed no oligoclonal bands). MRI of the cervical spinal cord revealed a signal abnormality in the cord at the level of the C2 vertebral body. The rest of the MRI examination was normal. The clinical diagnosis was para-infectious myelitis following a viral upper respiratory tract infection, causing incomplete spinal cord transection syndrome.

The signs and symptoms regressed completely under treatment with cortisone. To date, no other lesions have developed elsewhere in the CNS.

The MRI abnormality in this case would also have been consistent with a diagnosis of multiple sclerosis, which could be excluded only on the basis of the CSF findings and the further course of illness.

Thoracic spinal cord transection syndrome. Transection of the upper thoracic cord spares the upper limbs but impairs breathing and may also cause paralytic ileus through involvement of the splanchnic nerves. Transection of the lower thoracic cord spares the abdominal muscles and does not impair breathing.

Lumbar spinal cord transection syndrome. Traumatic transection of the spinal cord at lumbar levels often causes especially severe disturbances because of concomitant damage of the major supplying artery of the lower spinal cord, the great radicular artery (of Adamkiewicz). The result is infarction of the entire lumbar *and* sacral spinal cord (cf. Case Presentation 3).

Epiconus syndrome, caused by a spinal cord lesion at the L4 to S2 level, is relatively rare (Fig. 3.**22a** and **b**). Unlike conus syndrome (see below), it is associated with spastic or flaccid paresis of the lower limbs, depending on the precise level of the lesion. There is weakness or total paralysis of hip external rotation (L4-S1) and extension (L4-L5), and possibly also of knee flexion (L4-S2) and flexion and extension of the ankles and toes (L4-S2). The Achilles reflex is absent, while the knee-jerk reflex is preserved. The sensory deficit extends from L4 to S5. The bladder and bowel empty only reflexively; sexual potency is lost, and male patients often have priapism. There is transient vasomotor paralysis, as well as a transient loss of sweating.

Conus syndrome, due to a spinal cord lesion at or below S3 (Fig. 3.**22**), is also rare. It can be caused by spinal tumors, ischemia, or a massive lumbar disk herniation.

Case Presentation 2: *Paraparesis due to Spinal Cord Compression by an Epidural Tumor (Lymphoma)*

The patient, a 34-year-old office worker, was in the 34th week of pregnancy when she noted increasing weakness of both lower limbs and impaired sensation on the lower half of the body.

She said the sensory disturbance had begun on the inner surface of the thighs and then spread along the legs and, finally, upward onto the trunk. She had had increasing difficulty with uri-

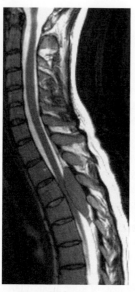 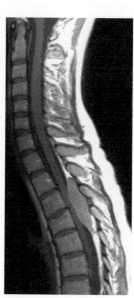

a   b

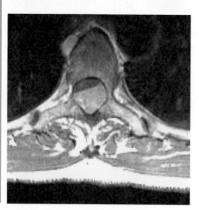

c

Fig. 3.**21 Epidural lymphoma compressing the spinal cord. a** The sagittal T2-weighted image reveals severe spinal cord compression due to a mass displacing the dura mater and the cord ventrally. **b** A moderate degree of homogeneous contrast enhancement in the tumor is seen in the sagittal T1-weighted image after the administration of contrast medium; the tumor has not spread intradurally. **c** Axial T1-weighted image after the administration of contrast medium. The lymphoma fills most of the spinal canal and displaces the spinal cord ventrally and to the right. The cord is significantly darker than the contrast-enhancing tumor.

nation for several weeks, but had attributed this to pregnancy.

Clinical examination revealed spastic paraparesis with bilateral Babinski signs and a sensory deficit below T10 affecting touch and position sense and, to a lesser extent, the protopathic modalities as well. MRI revealed a large mass in the thoracic spinal canal, compressing the spinal cord and displacing it anteriorly.

An emergency cesarean section was performed, and the tumor was neurosurgically removed immediately afterward. Histopathological examination revealed lymphoma. The neurological deficits resolved completely, and no other manifestations of lymphoma were found.

An isolated lesion of the conus medullaris produces the following neurological deficits:

- Detrusor areflexia with urinary retention and overflow incontinence (continual dripping, p. 302)
- Fecal incontinence
- Impotence
- Saddle anesthesia (S3-S5)
- Loss of the anal reflex

The lower limbs are not paretic, and the Achilles reflex is preserved (L5-S2).

If conus syndrome is produced by a tumor, the lumbar and sacral roots descending alongside the conus will be affected sooner or later (Fig. 3.**22**). In such cases, the manifestations of conus syndrome are accompanied by deficits due to involvement of the cauda equina: weakness of the lower limbs, and more extensive sensory deficits than are seen in pure conus syndrome.

Cauda equina syndrome involves the lumbar and sacral nerve roots, which descend alongside and below the conus medullaris, and through the lumbosacral subarachnoid space, to their exit foramina; a tumor (e. g., ependymoma or lipoma) is the usual cause. Patients initially complain of radicular pain in a sciatic distribution, and of severe bladder pain that worsens with coughing or sneezing. Later, variably severe radicular sensory deficits, affecting all sensory modalities, arise at L4 or lower levels. Lesions affecting the upper portion of the cauda equina produce a sensory deficit in the legs and in the saddle area. There may be flaccid paresis of the lower limbs with areflexia; urinary and fecal incontinence also develop, along with impaired sexual function. With lesions of the lower portion of the cauda equina, the sensory deficit is exclusively in the saddle area (S3-S5), and there is no lower limb weakness, but urination, defecation, and sexual function are impaired. Tumors affecting the cauda equina, unlike conus tumors, produce slowly and irregularly progressive clinical manifestations, as the individual nerve roots are affected with variable rapidity, and some of them may be spared until late in the course of the illness.

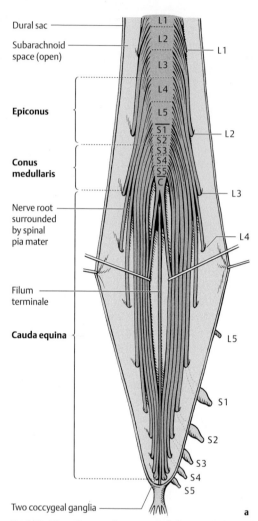

Dural sac

Subarachnoid space (open)

Epiconus

Conus medullaris

Nerve root surrounded by spinal pia mater

Filum terminale

Cauda equina

Two coccygeal ganglia

L1
L2
L3
L4
L5
S1
S2
S3
S4
S5
C

L1
L2
L3
L4
L5
S1
S2
S3
S4
S5

a

Fig. 3.**22a The epiconus, the conus medullaris, and the cauda equina, with the topographical relationships of the nerve roots to the vertebral bodies and intervertebral disks.**
a Posterior view, after opening of the dural sac (theca) and the spinal arachnoid. For the typical syndromes produced by lesions affecting the epiconus, conus medullaris, and cauda equina, see text.

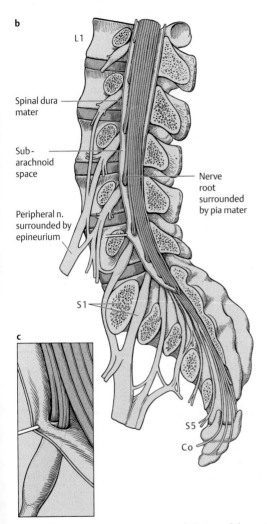

Fig. 3.**22 b, c The epiconus, the conus medullaris, and the cauda equina, with the topographical relationships of the nerve roots to the vertebral bodies and intervertebral disks.**
b Lateral view, after removal of the lateral arches of the vertebrae and opening of the dural sac, revealing the topography of the spine, disks, and nerve roots.
c A funnel-shaped outpouching of the dura mater with openings for the anterior (ventral) and posterior (dorsal) roots.

Case Presentation 3: Lumbosacral Spinal Cord Infarction due to Acute Ischemia in the Territory of the Anterior Spinal Artery (Anterior Spinal Artery Syndrome)

This retired 81-year-old woman stated that she had fallen on the morning of admission because of sudden weakness in both lower limbs. She had intense back pain immediately thereafter, which she attributed to the fall. The lower limbs remained weak, and she became incontinent of urine and stool. She had previously suffered from "decalcified bones" with occasional painful fractures, but there had never before been any weakness. Examination on admission revealed flaccid paraplegia, vesical and anal sphincter dysfunction, and a sensory deficit on the lower limbs and lower portion of the trunk. Pain and temperature sensation were more severely impaired than touch and position sense.

MRI revealed an area of signal abnormality in the lower portion of the spinal cord, epiconus, and conus medullaris. At the level of the conus, the signal abnormality encompassed nearly the entire cross-sectional area of the cord. These findings and the clinical manifestations are consistent with spinal cord infarction due to acute ischemia in the territory of the anterior spinal artery.

On further follow-up, the neurological deficits remained stable, without any worsening or improvement over time.

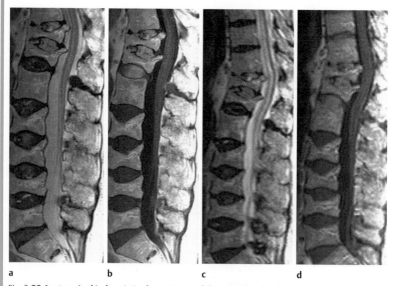

a   b   c   d

Fig. 3.**23 Acute spinal ischemia in the territory of the anterior spinal artery.** Images obtained 12 hours (**a, b, e**) and 3 days (**c, d, f, g**) after the onset of symptoms. The osteoporotic vertebral body fractures seen on these images were old and bore no relation to the acute neurological syndrome. **a** The sagittal T2-weighted image reveals central hyperintensity of the spinal cord in and above the conus medullaris. **b** The T1-weighted image reveals mild contrast enhancement. **c** Three days later, marked hyperintensity can be seen in the spinal cord on the T2-weighted image. **d** The contrast enhancement has not increased.

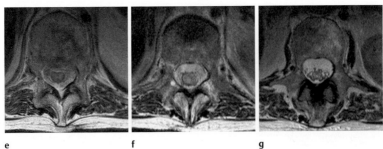

e   f   g

(**e**, **f**, **g**) Axial T2-weighted images. **e** At first, only the spinal gray matter is hyperintense. **f** Three days later, most of the spinal cord is hyperintense; only the dorsal portion of the cord, supplied by the posterolateral vessels, is still of normal signal intensity. Thus, the neural pathway for epicritic sensation is less affected than the pathways for protopathic sensation and motor function. **g** These changes can be followed downward into the conus medullaris.

Vascular Spinal Cord Syndromes

The blood supply of the spinal cord and the clinical syndromes resulting from lesions of individual spinal cord vessels are described in Chapter 11, on p. 439 ff. and p. 489 ff.

Spinal Cord Tumors

Complete or partial spinal cord transection syndrome (including conus syndrome and cauda equina syndrome) is often caused by a tumor. Spinal cord tumors are classified into three types, based on their localization (Fig. 3.**24**):

- Extradural tumors (metastasis, lymphoma, plasmacytoma)
- Intradural extramedullary tumors (meningioma, neurinoma)
- Intradural intramedullary tumors (glioma, ependymoma)

Extradural neoplasms (Fig. 3.**24a** and **b**) tend to grow rapidly, often producing progressively severe manifestations of spinal cord compression: spastic paresis of the parts of the body supplied by the spinal cord below the level of the lesion, and, later, bladder and bowel dysfunction. Pain is a common feature. Dorsally situated tumors mainly cause sensory disturbances; lateral compression of the spinal cord can produce Brown-Séquard syndrome (p. 78).

Intradural extramedullary tumors most commonly arise from the vicinity of the posterior roots (Fig. 3.**24 c**). They initially produce radicular pain and paresthesiae. Later, as they grow, they cause increasing compression of the posterior roots and the spinal cord, first the posterior columns and then the pyramidal

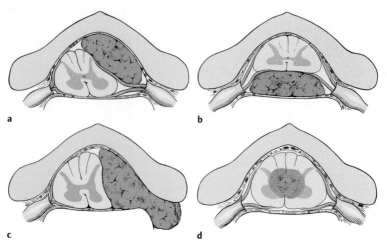

Fig. 3.**24 Spinal cord tumors. (a, b)** Extradural tumor; **a** dorsal to the spinal cord, **b** ventral to the spinal cord. **c** Intradural extramedullary tumor (dumbbell tumor with intraspinal, intraforaminal, and extraforaminal portions). **d** Intradural intramedullary tumor.

tract in the lateral funiculus. The result is a progressively severe spastic paresis of the lower limb, and paresthesiae (particularly cold paresthesiae) in both lower limbs, accompanied by a disturbance of both epicritic and proprioceptive sensation, at first ipsilaterally and then bilaterally. The sensory disturbance usually ascends from caudal to cranial until it reaches the level of the lesion. The spine is tender to percussion at the level of the damaged nerve roots, and the pain is markedly exacerbated by coughing or sneezing. The pain caused by posterior column involvement is of "rheumatic" quality and initially arises at the distal ends of the limbs. Hyperesthesia is not uncommon in the dermatomes supplied by the affected nerve roots; this may be useful for clinical localization of the level of the lesion. As the spinal cord compression progresses, it eventually leads to bladder and bowel dysfunction.

Ventrally situated tumors (Fig. 3.24 c) can involve the anterior nerve roots on one or both sides, causing flaccid paresis, e. g., of the hands (when the tumor is in the cervical region). As the tumor grows, it compresses the pyramidal tract, causing spastic paresis of the ipsilateral lower limb at first, and later of both lower limbs. Traction on the spinal cord due to stretching of the denticulate ligaments may further damage the pyramidal tract. If the compressive lesion is anterolateral to the cord, contralateral pain and temperature sensation may be affected. With ventral as with dorsal tumors, progressive spinal cord compression eventually leads to bladder and bowel dysfunction.

Intradural intramedullary spinal cord tumors (Fig. 3.**24 d**) can be distinguished from extramedullary tumors by the following clinical features:

- They rarely cause radicular pain, instead causing atypical (burning, dull) pain of diffuse localization.
- Dissociated sensory deficits can be an early finding.
- Bladder and bowel dysfunction appear early in the course of tumor growth.
- The sensory level (upper border of the sensory deficit) may ascend, because of longitudinal growth of the tumor, while the sensory level associated with extramedullary tumors generally remains constant, because of transverse growth.
- Muscle atrophy due to involvement of the anterior horns is more common than with extramedullary tumors.
- Spasticity is only rarely as severe as that produced by extramedullary tumors.

High cervical tumors can produce bulbar manifestations as well as fasciculations and fibrillations in the affected limb. Extramedullary tumors are much more common overall than intramedullary tumors.

Tumors at the level of the foramen magnum (meningioma, neurinoma) often initially manifest themselves with pain, paresthesia, and hypesthesia in the C2 region (occipital and great auricular nerves). They can also cause weakness of the sternocleidomastoid and trapezius muscles (accessory nerve).

Dumbbell tumors (or hourglass tumors) are so called because of their unique anatomical configuration (Fig. 3.**24c**). These are mostly neurinomas that arise in the intervertebral foramen and then grow in two directions: into the spinal canal and outward into the paravertebral space. They compress the spinal cord laterally, eventually producing a partial or complete Brown-Séquard syndrome.

Nerve Root Syndromes (Radicular Syndromes)

Preliminary remarks on anatomy. As discussed in the last chapter, the spinal nerves are formed by the union of the posterior and anterior roots.

After exiting from the spinal canal, the fibers of the spinal nerves at different segmental levels regroup to form the three plexuses (Fig. 2.**5**, p. 25)—cervical, brachial, and lumbosacral (see p. 100 ff.). The peripheral nerves emerging from these plexuses each contain fibers from multiple nerve roots. This redistribution of nerve fibers in the plexuses is the reason why the territories innervated by the nerve roots differ from those innervated by the peripheral nerves. Each nerve root supplies a characteristic area of the skin (dermatome) and innervates a characteristic group of muscles (myotome). Most muscles receive nerve

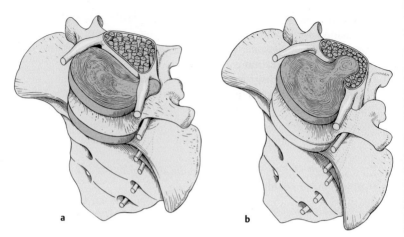

a   b

Fig. 3.**25 a Posterolateral disk herniation** at the L4–5 level. The injured root is *not* the L4 root, which exits through the L4–5 intervertebral foramen, but rather the L5 root, which is medial to it and passes behind the L4–5 intervertebral disk. **b Central disk herniation** at L4–5 with compression of the cauda equina.

fibers from more than one nerve root (polyradicular innervation). The few muscles receiving most or all of their innervation from a single nerve root are called segment-indicating muscles. These matters are discussed more fully in Chapter 2 on p. 24 ff.

Syndrome of nerve root involvement (radicular syndrome). The nerve roots are particularly vulnerable to damage at or near their passage through the intervertebral foramina. Common causes include **stenosing processes** (narrowing of the foramina, e. g., due to bony overgrowth), **disk protrusion**, and **disk herniation** compressing the exiting nerve root (Fig. 3.**25**). Other processes, such as infectious diseases of the vertebral bodies, tumors, and trauma, can also damage the spinal nerve roots as they emerge from the spinal canal.

Radicular lesions produce the following **characteristic manifestations:**

- Pain and sensory deficit in the corresponding dermatome
- Greater impairment of pain sensation than of the other sensory modalities
- Reduced strength in segment-indicating muscles and, rarely and in severe cases, muscle atrophy
- Reflex deficits corresponding to the damaged root(s) (Fig. 2.**13**, p. 36)
- Absence of autonomic deficits (of sweating, piloerection, and vasomotor function) in the limbs, because the sympathetic and parasympathetic fibers

join the peripheral nerves distal to the nerve roots and are thus spared by radicular lesions

Motor deficits in the **segment-indicating muscles** of the individual motor roots are useful for the clinical and electromyographic localization of radicular lesions at cervical and lumbar levels. The more important segment-indicating muscles are listed in Fig. 3.**27** and Fig. 3.**29**.

Radicular Syndromes in Osteochondrosis and Disk Degeneration

Degenerative disorders of the vertebrae and intervertebral disks are the most common cause of radicular lesions.

The intervertebral disks are composed of a pulpy inner portion (nucleus pulposus) surrounded by a fibrous ring (annulus fibrosus). The disks are no longer supplied by blood vessels once the development of the spine is complete. Therefore, as the individual ages, the disks gradually lose their elasticity and turgor and are less able to serve as shock absorbers for the spine. This causes difficulties primarily in the more mobile portions of the spine, i.e., the cervical and lumbar regions.

Osteochondrosis involves degeneration of the disk and of the cartilaginous base and end plates of the vertebral bodies. This results in sclerosis of the cartilaginous tissue and in deformation of the vertebral bodies. The intervertebral disks lose height, and the vertebral bodies on either side are brought closer together. There is also bony overgrowth of the facet joints (**spondylarthrosis**) and of the vertebral bodies themselves (mainly in the cervical region, **uncovertebral arthrosis**). These processes cause stenosis of the intervertebral foramina, with compression of the tissues within them, including the nerve roots (Figs. 3.**26** and 3.**28**).

Cervical Root Lesions of Degenerative Origin

Cervical radicular syndromes are nearly always due to foraminal stenosis of this type, caused by osteochondrosis. The end plates of the cervical vertebrae are normally somewhat elevated on either side of the vertebral body, where they form the uncinate processes, creating a saddlelike structure. When a cervical intervertebral disk degenerates, the vertebral body above sinks like a wedge into the saddlelike depression of the one below, causing increasing pressure on the uncinate processes. Bone remodeling occurs, through which the uncinate processes are gradually displaced laterally and dorsally, and the intervertebral foramina gradually become narrower (Fig. 3.**26**).

Cervical osteochondrosis is most commonly found at C5-6 and C6-7, and often also at C3-4 and C7-T1. Stenosis can affect one or more foramina to a vari-

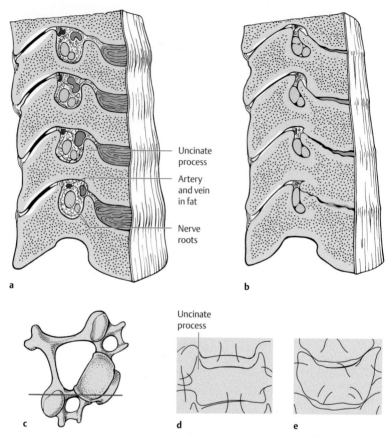

Fig. 3.**26 Intervertebral foramina of the cervical spine** from C3 to C7. **a** Normal width of the foramina. **b** Foraminal stenosis caused by disk degeneration (drawn from a dissected anatomical specimen). **c** Plane of section of **d** and **e**. **d** Normal uncinate processes. **e** Uncinate processes deformed by intervertebral disk generation.

able extent, either unilaterally or bilaterally. Thus, either monosegmental or plurisegmental radicular manifestations may be produced. The most common symptoms are segmental pain and paresthesiae, which are attributable to nerve root irritation. More severe root involvement manifests itself as sensory, motor, and reflex deficits in the corresponding segment(s). In addition to disk degeneration, there may be concomitant arthrotic changes of the facet joints that restrict the mobility of the cervical spine in the involved segments.

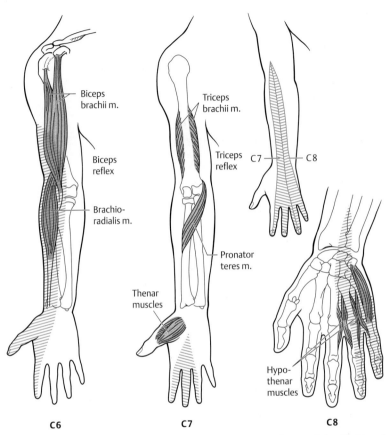

Fig. 3.**27** **Segment-indicating muscles and cutaneous sensory distribution of the C6, C7, and C8 nerve roots** (after Mumenthaler and Schliack).

Individual cervical radicular syndromes (Fig. 3.**27**) are characterized by the following deficits:

- **C3**, **C4:** pain in the neck and shoulder; rarely, partial diaphragmatic palsy
- **C5:** pain with or without hypalgesia in the C5 dermatome; deltoid and biceps weakness
- **C6:** pain with or without hypalgesia in the C6 dermatome; biceps and brachioradialis weakness; diminished biceps reflex

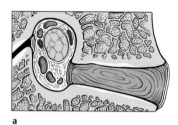
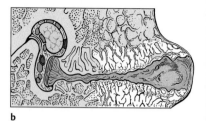

a   b

Fig. 3.**28 a Intervertebral foramen of normal width** between L5 and S1, with dorsal root ganglion. **b Stenotic intervertebral foramen** with deformation of the dorsal root ganglion by the superiorly displaced inferior articular process (drawn from a dissected anatomical specimen).

- **C7:** pain with or without paresthesia or hypalgesia in the C7 dermatome; triceps and pronator teres weakness; possible thenar atrophy; diminished triceps reflex
- **C8:** pain with or without paresthesia or hypalgesia in the C8 dermatome; weakness and possibly atrophy of the hypothenar muscles; diminished triceps and Trömner reflexes

Lumbar Root Lesions of Degenerative Origin

In the lumbar region, the intervertebral disks are thick, and the base and end plates are flat; degenerative disease can cause protrusion or herniation (prolapse) of one or more disks, and the displaced disk tissue can then directly compress the nerve roots and spinal ganglia. In addition, whenever a disk space is narrowed by osteochondrosis, the intervertebral foramina become narrower, which can also cause nerve root compression and radicular pain (Fig. 3.**28**).

Disk degeneration most commonly affects the lowest two lumbar disks, L5-S1 and L4-5, and less commonly the L3-4 disk.

Figure 3.**22b** shows the intimate spatial relationship of the lumbar vertebral bodies, intervertebral disks, and nerve roots. The nerve root exits the lumbar spinal canal in its dural sleeve roughly at the level of the upper third of the vertebral body, proceeding obliquely in a ventrocaudal direction to the intervertebral foramen, the upper portion of which contains the dorsal root ganglion. Thus, a dorsolateral disk protrusion does not directly affect the nerve root exiting at the correspondingly numbered level; rather, it impinges on the nerve root of the next segment below, which passes behind the disk at this level, on its way to its own, lower-lying foramen (Fig. 3.**25**). Only a far lateral disk prolapse can directly compress the correspondingly numbered nerve root.

The L5-S1 intervertebral disk is often somewhat narrower than the others, because the lumbar lordosis is most pronounced at this level. As a result, an L5-S1 disk herniation can impinge on both the L5 and S1 nerve roots, causing a combined L5 and S1 syndrome.

In the lumbar region as in the cervical region, disk herniation most commonly manifests itself with symptoms of radicular irritation (pain and paresthesia) in the affected segments. More severe radicular damage produces segmental sensory and motor deficits.

A patient suffering from lumbar radicular irritation syndrome may report the abrupt cessation of sciatic pain and the simultaneous appearance of weakness or a sensory deficit. This situation arises when the nerve root fibers suddenly cease conducting impulses, implying the impending death of the nerve root. Emergency neurosurgical decompression of the affected root is indicated.

A large disk prolapse can also, in rare cases, penetrate the posterior longitudinal ligament in a dorsomedial position and pass into the lumbar spinal canal, causing cauda equina syndrome ("massive prolapse"; Fig. 3.**25b** and Fig. 3.**30**).

Acute sciatica ("charley-horse") is not necessarily the result of radicular irritation or injury. Another very common cause is the entrapment of parts of the joint capsule in the intervertebral joint. Degenerative disease of the spine is the most important predisposing factor for this condition as well. When the intervertebral disk is narrowed, the intervertebral joint facets are displaced in such a way as to narrow the neural foramina (Fig. 3.**28**). The spine loses height and the joint capsules slacken, so that certain movements can induce entrapment of part of the capsule inside the joint. Chiropractic manipulation can bring rapid relief in such cases.

Individual lumbar radicular syndromes (Fig. 3.**29**) are characterized by the following deficits:

- **L3:** pain with or without paresthesia in the L3 dermatome; quadriceps weakness; diminished or absent quadriceps reflex (patellar or knee-jerk reflex)
- **L4:** pain with or without paresthesia or hypalgesia in the L4 dermatome; quadriceps weakness; diminished quadriceps reflex
- **L5:** pain with or without paresthesia or hypalgesia in the L5 dermatome; weakness of the extensor hallucis longus and often also of the extensor digitorum brevis; loss of the tibialis posterior reflex
- **S1:** pain with or without paresthesia or hypalgesia in the S1 dermatome; weakness of the peronei, gastrocnemius, and soleus muscles; loss of the gastrocnemius reflex (Achilles or ankle-jerk reflex).

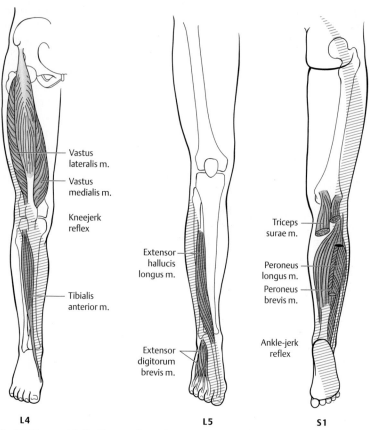

L4   L5   S1

Fig. 3.**29 Segment-indicating muscles and cutaneous sensory distribution of the L4, L5, and S1 nerve roots** (after Mumenthaler and Schliack).

Case Presentation 4: *Massive L4/5 Disk Herniation with Upwardly Displaced Fragment*

This 37-year-old engineer suddenly felt severe pain in the low back while lifting weights in a fitness studio. Shortly afterward, he noted a sensory abnormality in the right thigh and weakness in the right knee, but nonetheless continued with his exercise routine. A few hours later, he had more severe pain and numbness in the right lower limb, and the sensory abnormality was present in the left lower limb also, as well as in the perianal region. He could no longer empty his bladder.

He sought emergency medical attention. Examination on admission to the hospital revealed severe weakness of the lower limb musculature from L4 downward on the right, and from L5 downward on the left. There was markedly diminished sensation in all modalities in a saddle distribution, as well as flaccid bladder paralysis with incipient overflow incontinence.

MRI revealed a large disk herniation originating at the L4–5 level, with a cranially displaced free intraspinal fragment compressing nearly the entire cauda equina (acute cauda equina syndrome).

The patient was immediately transferred to the neurosurgical service for an emergency procedure. The herniated disk tissue was surgically removed the same evening, and the neurological deficits resolved completely thereafter.

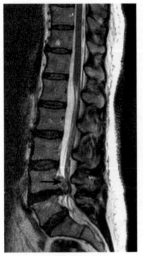
a

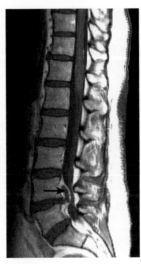
b

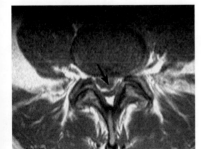
c

Fig. 3.**30 L4/5 disk herniation with upwardly displaced fragment. a** The sagittal T2-weighted image reveals compression of the rootlets of the cauda equina, which are seen as dark filaments surrounded by bright cerebrospinal fluid. The conus medullaris lies at L1. **b** The large disk herniation is seen equally well on the T1-weighted image. It evidently originates in the L4–5 disk space. **c** In the axial T1-weighted image, the lumen of the spinal canal is seen to be nearly entirely filled with prolapsed disk tissue. The herniation is ventral and on the right side (arrow).

Plexus Syndromes

The **cervical plexus** is formed by nerve roots C2-C4, the **brachial plexus** by nerve roots C5-T1, and the **lumbosacral plexus** by nerve roots L1-S3.

Lesions of the Cervical Plexus

The cervical plexus (Fig. 3.31) occupies a relatively sheltered position and is thus rarely injured. Unilateral or bilateral phrenic nerve dysfunction (C3, C4, and C5) is more commonly caused by a mediastinal process than by a cervical plexus lesion.

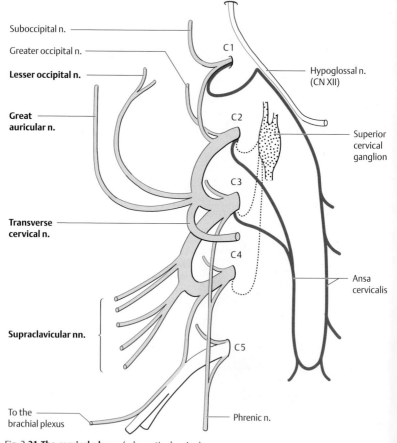

Fig. 3.**31 The cervical plexus** (schematic drawing)

Lesions of the Brachial Plexus

Brachial plexus lesions are classified into two types, upper and lower, on clinical and pragmatic grounds. The anatomy of the brachial plexus is shown in Fig. 3.**32**.

In upper brachial plexus palsy (Duchenne-Erb palsy), due to a lesion of the C5 and C6 nerve roots, the deltoid, biceps, brachialis, and brachioradialis muscles are paretic. There is a sensory deficit overlying the deltoid muscle and on the radial side of the arm and hand.

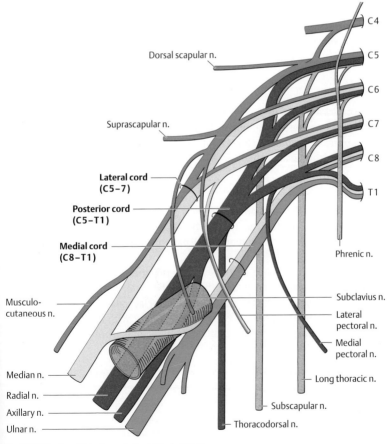

Fig. 3.**32 The brachial plexus** (schematic drawing)

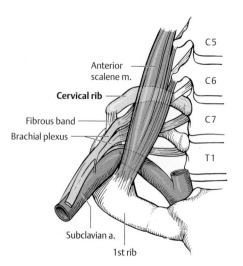

Fig. 3.**33 Scalene syndrome** (thoracic outlet syndrome) due to a cervical rib.

In lower brachial plexus palsy (Klumpke palsy), due to a lesion of the C8 and T1 nerve roots, the wrist and finger flexors and the intrinsic muscles of the hand are paretic. Occasionally, Horner syndrome is present in addition. There are prominent trophic abnormalities of the hand and fingers.

Causes of Brachial Plexus Lesions

Trauma, usually due to road accidents or sporting injuries, is by far the most common cause of damage to the brachial plexus. Men are much more frequently affected than women. Most patients are between 20 and 30 years old.

Brachial plexus damage also has many etiologies other than trauma: *compression syndromes* in the area of the shoulder (scalene syndrome; compression by safety belts, rucksack straps, etc.; costoclavicular syndrome; hyperabduction syndrome); *tumors* (e. g., apical lung tumor with Pancoast syndrome); *inflammatory-allergic lesions* (neuralgic shoulder amyotrophy); and *birth injuries.*

Scalene syndrome (Fig. 3.**33**). The cords of the brachial plexus pass through the so-called scalene hiatus, which is delimited by the anterior and middle scalene muscles and the first rib. The hiatus normally has enough room for the cords of the brachial plexus and the subclavian artery, which accompanies them, but pathological abnormalities such as those associated with a cervical rib can critically narrow the hiatus. In such cases, the cords of the brachial plexus and the subclavian artery must pass over the attachment of the cervical rib to the first (thoracic) rib and are vulnerable to compression at this site. The most prominent symptom of scalene syndrome (a type of thoracic outlet syndrome) is position-dependent pain radiating into the upper limb. Paresthesia and hypesthesia are often present, especially on the ulnar side of the hand. In severe, longstanding cases, there may be weakness of Klumpke type (see above). Damage to the sympathetic nerve fibers traveling with the subclavian artery frequently causes vasomotor disturbances as well.

Lesions of the Lumbosacral Plexus

Here, too, lesions may be classified into two types: lumbar plexus lesions and sacral plexus lesions. The anatomy of the lumbosacral plexus is shown in Fig. 3.**34**.

Lumbar plexus lesions (L1, L2, and L3) are less common than brachial plexus lesions, because of the sheltered location of the lumbar plexus. The causes of damage to both plexuses are largely the same. There are, however, practically no cases of inflammatory-allergic dysfunction of the lumbar plexus (which would be analogous to neuralgic shoulder amyotrophy). On the other hand, metabolic disturbances such as diabetes mellitus are more likely to affect the lumbar plexus than the brachial plexus.

Sacral plexus lesions. The sacral plexus is formed by nerve roots L4, L5, and S1 through S3. The most important nerves emerging from the sacral plexus are the common peroneal and tibial nerves, which are joined together as the sciatic nerve in its course down the posterior thigh. The two nerves separate from one another just above the knee and then follow their individual paths further down the leg (Fig. 3.**35**).

The common peroneal nerve mainly innervates the extensors of the foot and toe, while the tibial nerve innervates the plantar flexors and most of the intrinsic muscles of the foot. A lesion of the common peroneal nerve, or of the common peroneal portion of the sciatic nerve, weakens the extensors, causing a foot drop (steppage gait); a lesion of the tibial nerve weakens the plantar flexors, making toe-walking impossible. Peroneal nerve palsy is more frequent than tibial nerve palsy, because the course of the tibial nerve is relatively sheltered. Peroneal nerve palsy impairs sensation on the lateral surface of the leg and the dorsum of the foot, while tibial nerve palsy impairs sensation on the sole.

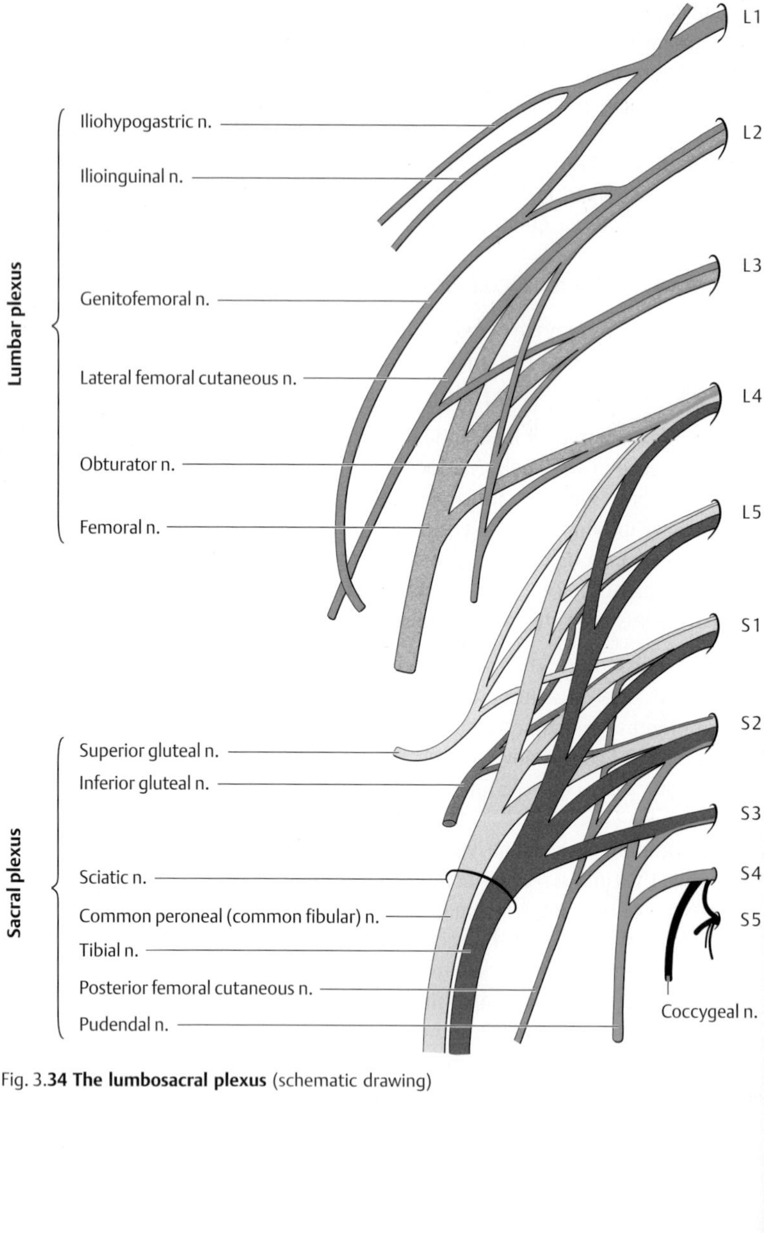

Fig. 3.**34 The lumbosacral plexus** (schematic drawing)

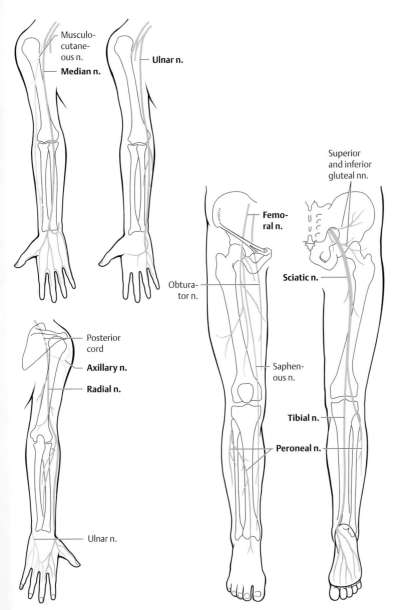

Fig. 3.**35 The course of selected important peripheral nerves**

Peripheral Nerve Syndromes

Transection of a mixed peripheral nerve causes *flaccid paresis* of the muscle(s) supplied by the nerve, a *sensory deficit* in the distribution of the interrupted afferent fibers of the nerve, and *autonomic deficits.*

When the continuity of an axon is disrupted, degeneration of the axon as well as of its myelin sheath begins within hours or days at the site of the injury, travels distally down the axon, and is usually complete within 15-20 days (so-called secondary or *wallerian degeneration*).

Damaged axons in the central nervous system lack the ability to regenerate, but damaged axons in peripheral nerves can do so, as long as their myelin sheaths remain intact to serve as a template for the regrowing axons. Even when a nerve is completely transected, resuturing of the sundered ends can be followed by near-complete regeneration of axons and restoration of functional activity. Electromyography (EMG) and nerve conduction studies are often very helpful in assessing the severity of a peripheral nerve injury and the chances for a good recovery.

Figure 3.**35** illustrates the anatomical course of a number of important peripheral nerves that are commonly injured. Figure 3.**36** shows typical clinical pictures of radial, median, and ulnar nerve palsies.

The more common causes of isolated peripheral nerve palsies are: *compression* of a nerve at an anatomically vulnerable point or bottleneck (scalene syndrome, cubital tunnel syndrome, carpal tunnel syndrome, peroneal nerve injury at the fibular head, tarsal tunnel syndrome); *traumatic injury* (including iatrogenic lesions, e. g., puncture and injection injuries); and *ischemia* (e. g., in compartment syndrome and, less commonly, in infectious/inflammatory processes).

Carpal Tunnel Syndrome

Carpal tunnel syndrome (Fig. 3.**37a**) is caused by median nerve damage in the carpal tunnel, which can be narrowed at the site where the nerve passes under the transverse carpal ligament (flexor retinaculum). Patients typically complain of pain and paresthesiae in the affected hand, which are especially severe at night and may be felt in the entire upper limb (brachialgia paresthetica nocturna), as well as of a feeling of swelling in the wrist or the entire hand. Trophic abnormalities and atrophy of the lateral thenar muscles (abductor pollicis brevis and opponens pollicis) are common in advanced cases. The median nerve contains an unusually large proportion of autonomic fibers; thus, median nerve lesions are a frequent cause of complex regional pain syndrome (previously called reflex sympathetic dystrophy, or Sudeck syndrome).

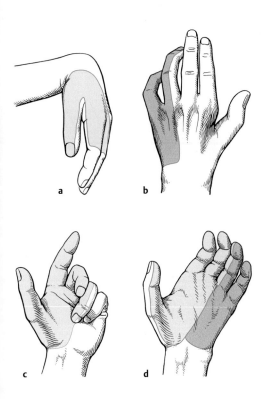

Fig. 3.**36 Typical appearance of peripheral nerve palsies affecting the hand. a** Wrist drop (radial nerve palsy). **b** Claw hand (ulnar nerve palsy). **c** Pope's blessing (median nerve palsy). **d** Monkey hand (combined median and ulnar nerve palsy). The areas of sensory deficit are shaded blue.

Ulnar Nerve Lesions—Cubital Tunnel Syndrome

Ulnar nerve palsy is the second most common peripheral nerve condition, after median nerve palsy. The ulnar nerve is particularly vulnerable to injury at the site of its passage through the cubital tunnel, on the medial side of the extensor aspect of the elbow (Fig. 3.**37b**). It can be damaged here by acute trauma or, even more commonly, by chronic pressure, e. g., by habitually propping up the arm on a hard surface, which may be an unavoidable posture in certain occupations. Paresthesia and hypesthesia in the ulnar portion of the hand are accompanied, in advanced cases, by atrophy of the hypothenar muscles and of the adductor pollicis (ulnar nerve palsy with claw hand).

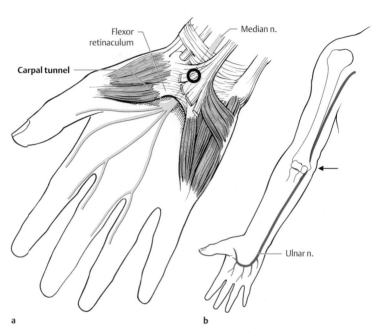

Fig. 3.**37 a Carpal tunnel with median nerve** (carpal tunnel syndrome). **b Cubital tunnel syndrome**: pressure palsy of the ulnar nerve due to external compression or dislocation.

Polyneuropathies

A pathological process affecting multiple peripheral nerves is called polyneuropathy, and an infectious or inflammatory process affecting multiple peripheral nerves is called polyneuritis. Polyneuropathies can be classified by histological-structural criteria (axonal, demyelinating, vascular-ischemic), by the systems they affect (sensory, motor, autonomic), or by the distribution of neurological deficits (mononeuropathy multiplex, distal-symmetric, proximal). Polyneuropathies and polyneuritides have many causes, and their diagnosis and treatment are accordingly complex. A more detailed discussion of these disorders would be beyond the scope of this book.

Differential Diagnosis of Radicular and Peripheral Nerve Lesions

The functions of individual muscles and their radicular (segmental) and peripheral nerve innervation are listed in Table 3.**1**. The information in this table can be used to determine whether muscle weakness in a particular distribution is due to a radicular or a peripheral nerve lesion, and to localize the lesion to the particular root or nerve that is affected.

Table 3.1 Segmental and Peripheral Innervation of Muscles

Function	Muscle	Nerve
I. Cervical plexus, C1–C4		
		Cervical nerves
Flexion, extension, rotation, and lateral flexion of the neck	Deep muscles of the neck (also sternocleidomastoid and trapezius)	C1–C4
Elevation of the upper rib cage, inspiration	Scalene muscles	C3–C5
		Phrenic nerves
Inspiration	Diaphragm	C3, C4, C5
II. Brachial plexus, C5–T1		
		Medial and lateral pectoral nerves
Adduction and internal rotation of the arm and depression of the shoulder from posterior to anterior	Pectoralis major Pectoralis minor	C5–T1
		Long thoracic nerve
Fixation of the scapula on lifting of the arm (protraction of the shoulder)	Serratus anterior	C5–C7
		Dorsal scapular nerve
Elevation and adduction of the scapula toward the spine	Levator scapulae Rhomboids	C4–C5
		Suprascapular nerve
Elevation and external rotation of the arm External rotation of the arm at the shoulder	Supraspinatus Infraspinatus	C4–C6 C4–C6
		Thoracodorsal nerve
Internal rotation of the arm at the shoulder, and adduction from anterior to posterior as well as depression of the elevated arm	Latissimus dorsi Teres major Subscapularis	C5–C8 (from the posterior cord of the brachial plexus)

Table 3.1 (Continued)

Function	Muscle	Nerve
		Axillary nerve
Lateral elevation (abduction) of the arm up to the horizontal position	Deltoid	C5–C6
External rotation of the arm	Teres minor	C4–C5
		Musculocutaneous nerve
Flexion of the arm and forearm, supination	Biceps brachii	C5–C6
Elevation and adduction of the arm	Coracobrachialis	C5–C7
Elbow flexion	Brachialis	C5–C6
		Median nerve
Flexion and radial deviation of the hand	Flexor carpi radialis	C6–C7
Pronation	Pronator teres	C6–C7
Wrist flexion	Palmaris longus	C7–T1
Flexion of the interphalangeal (IP) joint of the thumb	Flexor pollicis longus	C6–C8
Flexion of the proximal IP joints of the 2nd through 5th fingers	Flexor digitorum superficialis	C7–T1
Flexion of the distal IP joints of the 2nd and 3rd fingers	Flexor digitorum profundus (radial part)	C7–T1
Abduction of 1st metacarpal	Abductor pollicis brevis	C7–T1
Flexion of the metacarpophalangeal (MP) joint of the thumb	Flexor pollicis brevis	C7–T1
Opposition of 1st metacarpal	Opponens pollicis brevis	C6–C7
Flexion of MP joints and extension of IP joints of 2nd and 3rd fingers	Lumbricals I, II	C8–T1
		Ulnar nerve
Flexion of MP joints and extension of IP joints of 4th and 5th fingers	Lumbricals III, IV	C8–T1
Flexion and ulnar deviation of the hand	Flexor carpi ulnaris	C7–T1
Flexion of the distal IP joints of the 4th and 5th fingers	Flexor digitorum profundus (ulnar part)	C7–T1
Abduction of 1st metacarpal	Adductor pollicis	C8–T1
Abduction of 5th finger	Abductor digiti quinti	C8–T1
Opposition of 5th finger	Opponens digiti quinti	C7–T1
Flexion of MP joint of 5th finger	Flexor digiti quinti brevis	C7–T1
Flexion of MP and extension of IP joints of 3rd, 4th, and 5th fingers; also ab- and adduction of these fingers	Interossei (palmar and dorsal)	C8–T1

Table 3.1 (Continued)

Function	Muscle	Nerve
		Radial nerve
Elbow extension	Triceps brachii, anconeus	C6–C8
Elbow flexion	Brachioradialis	C5–C6
Extension and radial deviation of hand	Extensor carpi radialis	C6–C8
Extension at MP joints of 2nd through 5th fingers; spreading of the fingers; dorsiflexion of the hand	Extensor digitorum	C6–C8
Extension of 5th finger	Extensor digiti quinti	C6–C8
Extension and ulnar deviation of hand	Extensor carpi ulnaris	C6–C8
Supination	Supinator	C5–C7
Abduction of 1st metacarpal, radial extension of the hand	Abductor pollicis longus	C6–C7
Extension of thumb at MP joint	Extensor pollicis brevis	C7–C8
Extension of thumb at IP joint	Extensor pollicis longus	C7, C8
Extension of 2nd finger at MP joint	Extensor indicis proprius	C6–C8
		Intercostal nerves
Elevation of the ribs, expiration, Valsalva maneuver, anteroflexion and lateral flexion of the trunk	Thoracic and abdominal muscles	

III. Lumbar plexus, T12–L4

Function	Muscle	Nerve
		Femoral nerve
Hip flexion and internal rotation	Iliopsoas	L1–L3
Hip flexion and external rotation; knee flexion and internal rotation	Sartorius	L2–L3
Knee extension	Quadriceps femoris	L2–L4
		Obturator nerve
Thigh adduction	Pectineus	L2–L3
	Adductor longus	L2–L3
	Adductor brevis	L2–L4
	Adductor magnus	L3–L4
	Gracilis	L2–L4
Thigh adduction and external rotation	Obturator externus	L3–L4

IV. Sacral plexus, L5–S1

Function	Muscle	Nerve
		Superior gluteal nerve
Thigh abduction and internal rotation	Gluteus medius	L4–S1
	Gluteus minimus	
Hip flexion; thigh abduction and internal rotation	Tensor fasciae latae	L4–L5
Thigh abduction and external rotation	Piriformis	L5–S1

Table 3.1 (Continued)

Function	Muscle	Nerve
		Inferior gluteal nerve
Hip extension	Gluteus maximus	L4–S2
	Obturator internus	L5–S1
External rotation of the thigh	Gemelli	L4–S1
	Quadratus femoris	L4–S1
		Sciatic nerve
Knee flexion	Biceps femoris	L4–S2
	Semitendinosus	L4–S1
	Semimembranosus	L4–S1
		Deep peroneal nerve
Dorsiflexion and supination of the foot	Tibialis anterior	L4–L5
Extension of toes and foot	Extensor digitorum longus	L4–S1
Extension of 2nd through 5th toes	Extensor digitorum brevis	L4–S1
Extension of great toe	Extensor hallucis longus	L4–S1
	Extensor hallucis brevis	L4–S1
		Superficial peroneal nerve
Dorsiflexion and pronation of the foot	Peroneal muscles	L5–S1
		Tibial nerves
Plantar flexion of the foot in supination	Gastrocnemius	L5–S2
	Soleus	
	(together called triceps surae)	
Supination and plantar flexion of the foot	Tibialis posterior	L4–L5
Flexion of distal IP joints of 2nd through 5th toes; plantar flexion of the foot in supination	Flexor digitorum longus	L5–S2
Flexion of IP joint of great toe	Flexor hallucis longus	L5–S2
Flexion of proximal IP joints of 2nd through 5th toes	Flexor digitorum brevis	S1–S3
Flexion of MP joints of toes, abduction and adduction of toes	Plantar muscles of the foot	S1–S3
		Pudendal nerve
Closure of bladder and bowel	Vesical and anal sphincters	S2–S4

Syndromes of the Neuromuscular Junction and Muscle

Myasthenia

Abnormal fatigability of striated muscle is the cardinal manifestation of disorders of the neuromuscular junction. *Exercise-dependent weakness* often affects the extraocular muscles first, causing ptosis or diplopia, as the motor units of these muscles contain only a small number of muscle fibers. Patients with generalized myasthenia also suffer from dysphagia and exercise-dependent, mainly proximal weakness of skeletal muscle. The most common cause of the myasthenic syndrome is myasthenia gravis (older term: myasthenia gravis pseudoparalytica), an autoimmune disease in which the body forms antibodies against the acetylcholine receptors of the motor end plate. Too few receptors are left for adequate signal transmission, so that the muscles can no longer be sufficiently excited by the nerves that innervate them. The electromyographic correlate is a diminution in size ("decrement") of the muscle action potential on repetitive electrical stimulation of an affected muscle. Myasthenia gravis is diagnosed on the basis of the typical clinical manifestations, the electromyographic decrement, the demonstration of circulating antibodies to the acetylcholine receptor, and the improvement of weakness upon administration of a short-acting acetylcholinesterase inhibitor, such as edrophonium chloride. The disorder can be treated effectively with longer-acting acetylcholinesterase inhibitors, immune suppression, and additionally (in some younger patients) thymectomy.

Myopathy

In contrast to myasthenia, the myopathies (primary disorders of muscle) generally cause slowly progressive, non-exercise-dependent weakness. Myopathic muscle atrophy is less severe than neurogenic muscle atrophy and is partially concealed by fatty replacement of muscle tissue (liposis, also called lipomatosis), so that there may be a discrepancy between the normal or pseudohypertrophic appearance of muscle and the actual degree of weakness. There are no sensory or autonomic deficits, nor are there fasciculations, which would imply a neurogenic lesion. Myalgia and muscle spasms are more common in metabolic than in congenital myopathies.

The many types of myopathy include the muscular dystrophies (X-linked recessive, autosomal dominant, and recessive), metabolic myopathies, myotonic dystrophies (with additional manifestations such as cataract, frontal baldness, and other systemic abnormalities, as in Steinert-Batten-Curschmann dystrophy), and myositides. A systematic discussion of these diseases would be beyond the scope of this book. The most important information for the differential diagnosis of myopathy is derived from a detailed family history, clinical examination, laboratory tests (particularly creatine kinase), and electromyography, as well as from molecular genetic analysis, which has become highly sophisticated in recent years and can now provide an unequivocal diagnosis in many cases. This, in turn, enables a more reliable prognosis and well-founded genetic counseling.

4 Brainstem

4   Brainstem

The brainstem is the most caudally situated and phylogenetically oldest portion of the brain. It is grossly subdivided into the **medulla oblongata** (usually called simply the **medulla**), **pons**, and **midbrain** (or **mesencephalon**). The medulla is the rostral continuation of the spinal cord, while the midbrain lies just below the diencephalon; the pons is the middle portion of the brainstem. Ten of the **12 pairs of cranial nerves** (CN III-XII) exit from the brainstem and are primarily responsible for the innervation of the head and neck. CN I (the olfactory nerve) is the initial segment of the olfactory pathway; CN II (the optic nerve) is, in fact, not a peripheral nerve at all, but rather a tract of the central nervous system.

The brainstem contains a large number of fiber pathways, including all of the **ascending and descending pathways** linking the brain with the periphery. Some of these pathways cross the midline as they pass through the brainstem, and some of them form synapses in it before continuing along their path. The brainstem also contains many **nuclei**, including the **nuclei of cranial nerves III through XII**; the **red nucleus** and **substantia nigra** of the midbrain, the **pontine nuclei**, and the **olivary nuclei** of the medulla, all of which play an important role in motor regulatory circuits; and the nuclei of the **quadrigeminal plate** of the midbrain, which are important relay stations in the visual and auditory pathways. Furthermore, practically the entire brainstem is permeated by a diffuse network of more or less "densely packed" neurons (the **reticular formation**), which contains the essential **autonomic regulatory centers** for many vital bodily functions, including cardiac activity, circulation, and respiration. The reticular formation also sends activating impulses to the cerebral cortex that are necessary for the maintenance of consciousness. Descending pathways from the reticular formation influence the activity of the spinal motor neurons.

Because the brainstem contains so many different nuclei and nerve pathways in such a compact space, even a small lesion within it can produce neurological deficits of several different types occurring simultaneously (as in the various **brainstem vascular syndromes**). A relatively common brainstem finding is so-called crossed paralysis or **alternating hemiplegia**, in which cranial nerve deficits ipsilateral to the lesion are seen in combination with paralysis of the contralateral half of the body.

In general, cranial nerve deficits can be classified as **supranuclear**, i.e., caused by a lesion in a descending pathway from higher centers, usually the cerebral cortex, which terminates in the corresponding cranial nerve nucleus in the brainstem; **nuclear**, if the lesion is in the cranial nerve nucleus itself; **fascicular**, if the lesion involves nerve root fibers before their exit from the brainstem; or **peripheral**, if the lesion involves the cranial nerve proper after its exit from the brainstem. The type of deficit produced depends on the site of the lesion.

Surface Anatomy of the Brainstem

The **three brainstem segments**, i.e., the midbrain, pons, and medulla, have clearly defined borders on the ventral surface of the brainstem (Fig. 4.**1a**).

Medulla

The medulla extends from the site of exit of the roots of the first cervical nerve (C1), at the level of the foramen magnum, to its junction with the pons 2.5-3 cm more rostrally.

Dorsal view. The *gracile tubercles* are seen on either side of the midline, flanked by the *cuneate tubercles* (Fig. 4.**1b**). These small protrusions are produced by the underlying nucleus gracilis and nucleus cuneatus of both sides. These are the relay nuclei in which the posterior column fibers of the spinal cord form synapses onto the second neurons of the afferent pathway, which, in turn, project by way of the medial lemniscus to the thalamus. The rostral border of the medulla is defined by a line drawn through the caudal portion of the middle cerebellar peduncles. The floor of the fourth ventricle, or *rhomboid fossa*, is bounded laterally by the inferior and superior cerebellar peduncles and divided into rostral and caudal portions by the striae medullares, which contain fibers running from the arcuate nuclei to the cerebellum. The caudal part of the floor contains a number of protrusions (tubercles) produced by the underlying cranial nerve nuclei, including the *vagal triangle* (or "trigone"; dorsal nucleus of the vagus nerve), the *hypoglossal triangle* (nucleus of the hypoglossal nerve), and the *vestibular area* (vestibular and cochlear nuclei), while the rostral part contains the facial tubercle, which is produced by the fibers of the facial nerve as they course around the abducens nucleus. The roof of the fourth ventricle is made up of the superior medullary velum, the cerebellar peduncles, and the cerebellum itself.

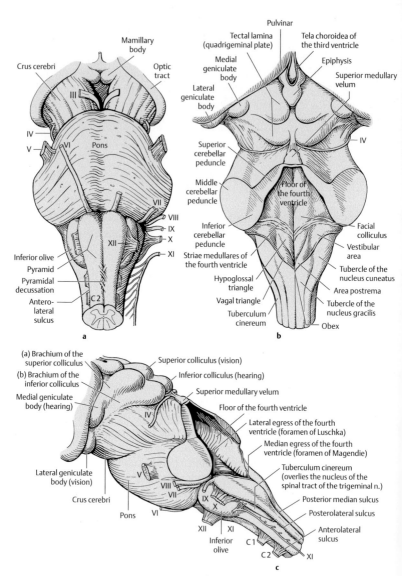

Fig. 4.**1 Brainstem. a** Ventral view. **b** Dorsal view. **c** Lateral view.

Ventral and lateral views. A ventral view of the medulla (Fig. 4.**1a**) reveals the *pyramids*, which lend their names to the pyramidal tracts, whose fibers course through them. The *pyramidal decussation* can also be seen here. Lateral to the pyramid on either side is another protrusion called the olive, which contains the *inferior olivary nucleus.*

The *hypoglossal nerve* (XII) emerges from the brainstem in the ventrolateral sulcus between the pyramid and the olive. The nuclei of the hypoglossal nerve, like those of the nerves to the extraocular muscles, are located near the midline in the brainstem, in the so-called basal lamina. Dorsal to the olive, the roots of the *accessory* (XI), *vagus* (X), and *glossopharyngeal* (IX) *nerves* emerge from the brainstem in a vertically oriented row (Fig. 4.**1a** and **c**). Further dorsally, between the exit of these nerves and the dorsolateral sulcus, lies the *tuberculum cinereum*, formed by the nucleus of the spinal tract of the trigeminal nerve. This is also the site of the posterior spinocerebellar tract, which ascends to the cerebellum by way of the inferior cerebellar peduncle (restiform body).

Pons

Ventral view. The pons ("bridge") is so called because, when viewed from the front, it appears to connect the two cerebellar hemispheres to each other with a broad band of horizontally disposed fibers, which is bounded caudally by the medulla and rostrally by the cerebral peduncles (crura cerebri) of the midbrain. The descending *corticopontine fibers* form a synapse with their second neurons on the ipsilateral side of the pons, which give rise to these horizontally disposed pontocerebellar fibers, which then, in turn, cross the midline and travel by way of the middle cerebellar peduncle to the cerebellum. A shallow groove in the midline of the ventral aspect of the pons contains the vertically coursing basilar artery. The groove is not caused by the artery, but rather by the bulges on either side produced by the pyramidal tracts as they descend through the basis pontis.

Lateral view. The lateral view (Fig. 4.**1c**) reveals the horizontally disposed pontine fibers coming together to form the *middle cerebellar peduncle* (brachium pontis). The *trigeminal nerve* (CN V) emerges from the pons just medial to the origin of the middle cerebellar peduncle.

Dorsal view. The dorsal aspect of the pons forms the superior portion of the floor of the fourth ventricle. It takes the form of a triangle whose base is a horizontal line defining the border between the dorsal aspects of the pons and the medulla. At either end of this line, the fourth ventricle opens into the subarachnoid space through a *lateral aperture* (*foramen of Luschka*). The unpaired *median aperture* of the fourth ventricle (*foramen of Magendie*) is seen at the caudal end of the ventricle (Fig. **4.1c**). The roof of the fourth ventricle is formed by the superior cerebellar peduncles (brachia conjunctiva) and the superior medullary velum.

Midbrain

The midbrain (mesencephalon) lies between the pons and the diencephalon.

Ventral view. The ventral view reveals two prominent bundles of fibers converging onto the pons. These are the *cerebral peduncles*, or, as they are alternatively called, the *crura cerebri* (singular: *crus cerebri*). The groove between the peduncles, known as the interpeduncular fossa, is the site of emergence of the two *oculomotor nerves* (CN III) from the brainstem. The cerebral peduncles disappear caudally as they enter the pons; rostrally, they are encircled by the *optic tracts* before entering the cerebral hemispheres (Fig. **4.1a**).

Dorsal view. The dorsal aspect of the midbrain (the midbrain *tectum*, i.e., "roof") contains four protrusions collectively termed the *quadrigeminal plate*. Visual information is processed in the upper two protrusions (the *superior colliculi*), while auditory information is processed in the lower two protrusions (the *inferior colliculi*), which are somewhat smaller. The *trochlear nerve* (CN IV) emerges from the brainstem just below the inferior colliculus on either side and then courses ventrally around the cerebral peduncle. It is the only cranial nerve that emerges from the dorsal aspect of the brainstem.

Lateral view. The two small protrusions lying lateral to the quadrigeminal plate are the *medial geniculate body* (an auditory relay area) and the *lateral geniculate body* (a visual relay area). The geniculate bodies are components of the thalamus and thus belong not to the brainstem but to the diencephalon.

For didactic reasons, the internal structure of the brainstem will be presented after the cranial nerves have been discussed.

Cranial Nerves

Origin, Components, and Functions

Figure **4.2** is a schematic dorsal view of the brainstem, in which the motor and parasympathetic cranial nerve nuclei are shown on the right and the somatosensory and special sensory nuclei are shown on the left. Lateral views showing the anatomical relations of the motor and parasympathetic nuclei, and of

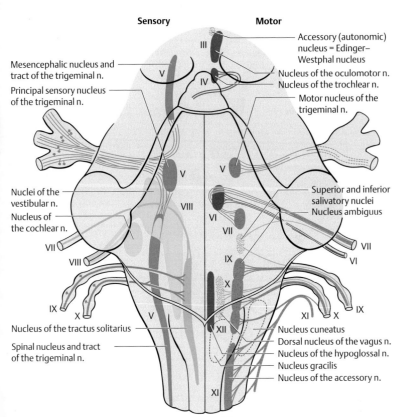

Fig. 4.**2 Cranial nerve nuclei, dorsal view** (schematic drawing). The somatosensory and special sensory nuclei are shown on the left side of the figure, the motor and parasympathetic nuclei on the right.

the somatosensory and special sensory nuclei, are found in Figures 4.**3** and 4.**4**, respectively.

The origin, components, and function of the individual cranial nerves are listed in Table 4.**1**. Figure 4.**5** provides a synoptic view of the sites of emergence of all 12 cranial nerves from the brainstem, their functional components, and their peripheral sites of origin and termination. All 12 cranial nerves are seen in the figure, from I (olfactory nerve) to XII (hypoglossal nerve); it should be borne in mind, however, that the second cranial "nerve"—the optic nerve—is actually not a peripheral nerve at all, but rather a tract of the central nervous system.

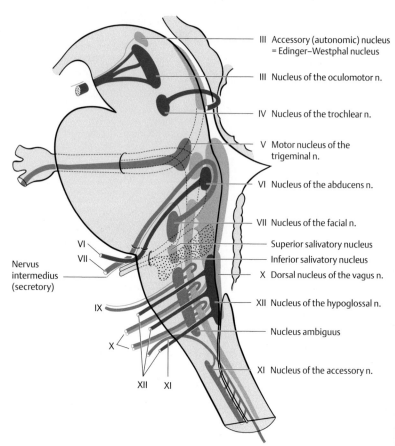

III Accessory (autonomic) nucleus
= Edinger–Westphal nucleus

III Nucleus of the oculomotor n.

IV Nucleus of the trochlear n.

V Motor nucleus of the
trigeminal n.

VI Nucleus of the abducens n.

VII Nucleus of the facial n.

Superior salivatory nucleus

Inferior salivatory nucleus

X Dorsal nucleus of the vagus n.

XII Nucleus of the hypoglossal n.

Nucleus ambiguus

XI Nucleus of the accessory n.

VI

VII

Nervus
intermedius
(secretory)

IX

X

XII   XI

Fig. 4.**3 Motor and parasympathetic cranial nerve nuclei, lateral view** (schematic drawing)

Recall that spinal nerve fibers can be classified as somatic afferent, somatic efferent, vegetative afferent, and vegetative efferent. The classification
of cranial nerve fibers is a little more complicated, for two reasons. Some of
the cranial nerve fibers are special sensory fibers arising from the sense organs of the head (vision, hearing, taste, smell). Furthermore, some of the
efferent cranial nerve fibers arise in nuclear areas that are embryologically
derived from the branchial arches; these fibers innervate muscles of
branchial origin.

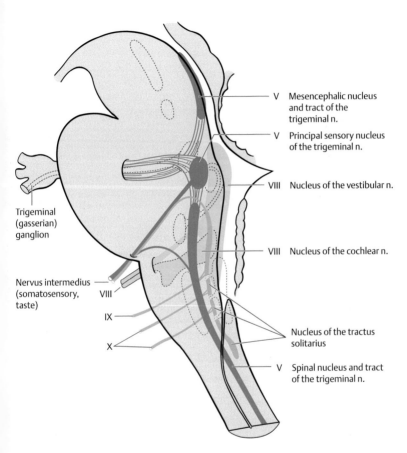

V Mesencephalic nucleus and tract of the trigeminal n.

V Principal sensory nucleus of the trigeminal n.

VIII Nucleus of the vestibular n.

Trigeminal (gasserian) ganglion

VIII Nucleus of the cochlear n.

Nervus intermedius (somatosensory, taste)

VIII

IX

X

Nucleus of the tractus solitarius

V Spinal nucleus and tract of the trigeminal n.

Fig. 4.**4 Somatosensory and special sensory cranial nerve nuclei, lateral view** (schematic drawing)

There results a sevenfold classification of cranial nerve fibers, as follows:

- *Somatic afferent fibers* (pain, temperature, touch, pressure, and proprioceptive sense from receptors in the skin, joints, tendons, etc.)
- *Vegetative afferent fibers* (or, alternatively, *visceral afferent fibers*), which carry impulses (pain) from the internal organs
- *Special somatic afferent fibers* carrying impulses from special receptors (eye, ear)
- *Special visceral afferent fibers* carrying impulses related to taste and smell

Table 4.1 The Cranial Nerves

Name	Components	Origin	Function
I. **Olfactory nerve (or olfactory fasciculus)**	Special visceral afferent	Olfactory cells of the olfactory epithelium	Olfaction
II. **Optic nerve (or optic fasciculus)**	Special somatic afferent	Retina, retinal ganglion cells	Vision
III. **Oculomotor nerve**	(a) Somatic efferent	Nucleus of the oculomotor nerve (midbrain)	Innervates superior, inferior, and medial rectus muscles, inferior oblique muscle, and levator palpebrae muscle
	(b) Visceral efferent (parasympathetic)	Edinger–Westphal nuclei	Sphincter pupillae muscle, ciliary muscle
	(c) Somatic afferent	Proprioceptors in the extraocular muscles	Proprioception
IV. **Trochlear nerve**	(a) Somatic efferent	Nucleus of the trochlear nerve (midbrain)	Superior oblique muscle
	(b) Somatic afferent	Proprioceptors	Proprioception
V. **Trigeminal nerve**	(a) somatic afferent	Bipolar cells in the semilunar ganglion	Sensation on the face and in the nasal and oral cavities
1st branchial arch	(b) Branchial efferent	Motor nucleus of the trigeminal nerve	Muscles of mastication
	(c) Somatic afferent	Proprioception	Proprioception
VI. **Abducens nerve**	Somatic efferent	Nucleus of the abducens nerve	Lateral rectus muscle
VII. **Facial nerve**	(a) Branchial efferent	Nucleus of the facial nerve	Muscles of facial expression, platysma, stylohyoideus muscle, digastric muscle
Nervus inter- medius 2nd branchial arch	(b) Visceral efferent	Superior salivatory nucleus	Nasal and lacrimal glands, salivation, sublingual and submandibular glands
	(c) Special visceral afferent	Geniculate ganglion	Taste (anterior 2/3 of tongue)
	(d) Somatic afferent	Geniculate ganglion	External ear, portions of the auditory canal, external surface of the tympanic membrane (somatosensory)

Table 4.1 The Cranial Nerves (Continued)

Name	Components	Origin	Function
VIII. Vestibulo-cochlear nerve	Special somatic afferent	(a) Vestibular ganglion	Equilibrium, cristae of the semilunar canals, maculae of the utricle and saccule
		(b) Spiral ganglion	Hearing, organ of Corti
IX. Glossopharyn-geal nerve	(a) Branchial efferent	Nucleus ambiguus	Stylopharyngeus muscle, pharyngeal muscles
3rd branchial arch	(b) Visceral efferent (parasympathetic)	Inferior salivatory nucleus	Salivation Parotid gland
	(c) Special visceral afferent	Inferior ganglion	Taste (posterior 1/3 of the tongue)
	(d) Visceral afferent	Superior ganglion	Somatosensory: posterior 1/3 of the tongue and pharynx (gag reflex)
	(e) Somatic afferent	Superior ganglion	Middle ear, eustachian tube (somatosensory)
X. Vagus nerve	(a) Branchial efferent	Nucleus ambiguus	Muscles of the larynx and pharynx
4th branchial arch	(b) Visceral efferent	Dorsal nucleus of the vagus nerve	Thoracic and abdominal viscera (parasympathetic)
	(c) Visceral afferent	Inferior (nodose) ganglion	Abdominal cavity (somatosensory)
	(d) Special visceral afferent		Taste: epiglottis
	(e) Somatic afferent	Superior (jugular) ganglion	Auditory canal, dura mater (somato-sensory)
XI. Accessory nerve	(a) Branchial efferent	Nucleus ambiguus	Muscles of the larynx and pharynx
	(b) Somatic efferent	Anterior horn cells	Sternocleidomastoid and trapezius muscles
XII. Hypoglossal nerve	Somatic efferent	Nucleus of the hypo-glossal nerve	Muscles of the tongue

- *General somatic efferent fibers* carrying motor impulses to the skeletal musculature (oculomotor, trochlear, abducens, and hypoglossal nerves)
- *Visceral efferent fibers* innervating the smooth muscles, the cardiac musculature, and the glands (both sympathetic and parasympathetic)

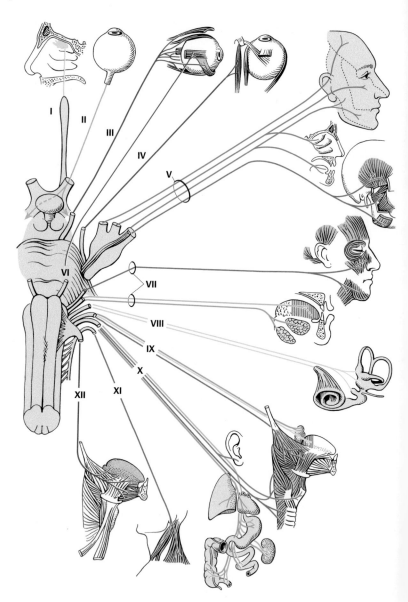

Fig. 4.5 **Cranial nerves: sites of exit from the brainstem, components, and distribution**

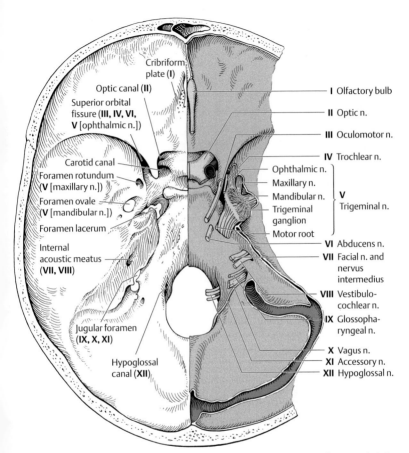

Fig. 4.6 Sites of exit of the cranial nerves from the skull. The exit foramina are shown on the left, the transected cranial nerves on the right.

- *Special branchial efferent fibers* innervating muscles that are derived from the mesodermal branchial arches, i.e., the motor portions of the facial nerve (2nd branchial arch), glossopharyngeal nerve (3rd branchial arch), and vagus nerve (4th branchial arch and below)

The cranial nerves exit from the skull through the openings (foramina, fissures, canals) depicted on the left side in Figure 4.**6**. The cut-off nerve stumps in their corresponding openings are shown on the right.

Olfactory System (CN I)

The olfactory pathway (Figs. **4.7** and 4.**8**) is composed of the olfactory epithelium of the nose, the fila olfactoria (olfactory nerve = CN I), the olfactory bulb and tract, and a cortical area (the paleocortex) extending from the uncus of the temporal lobe across the anterior perforated substance to the medial surface of the frontal lobe under the genu of the corpus callosum.

The olfactory epithelium occupies an area of about 2 cm^2 in the roof of each nasal cavity, overlying portions of the superior nasal concha and of the nasal septum. It contains receptor cells, supportive cells, and glands (Bowman's glands) that secrete a serous fluid, the so-called olfactory mucus, in which aromatic substances are probably dissolved. The *sensory cells* (*olfactory cells*) are bipolar cells whose peripheral processes terminate in the olfactory hairs of the olfactory epithelium.

Fila olfactoria and olfactory bulb. The central processes (neurites) of the olfactory cells coalesce into bundles containing hundreds of unmyelinated fibers surrounded by a Schwann-cell sheath. These fila olfactoria, about 20 on either side, are, in fact, the olfactory nerves (CN I is thus composed of peripheral nerve fibers, but is not a single peripheral nerve in the usual sense). They pass through small holes in the cribriform ("sievelike") plate and enter the olfactory bulb, where they form the first synapse of the olfactory pathway. Although it is not physically located in the cerebral cortex, the olfactory bulb is actually a piece of the telencephalon. Within it, complex synapses are made onto the dendrites of mitral cells, tufted cells, and granule cells.

Olfactory pathway. The first neuron of the olfactory pathway is the *bipolar olfactory cell*; the second neurons are the *mitral* and *tufted cells* of the olfactory bulb. The neurites of these cells form the *olfactory tract* (2nd neuron), which lies adjacent to and just below the frontobasal (orbitofrontal) cortex. The olfactory tract divides into the *lateral* and *medial olfactory striae* in front of the anterior perforated substance; another portion of it terminates in the *olfactory trigone*, which also lies in front of the anterior perforated substance. The fibers of the lateral stria travel by way of the limen insulae to the *amygdala, semilunar gyrus*, and *ambient gyrus* (prepyriform area). This is the site of the 3rd neuron, which projects to the anterior portion of the *parahippocampal gyrus* (*Brodmann area 28*, containing the cortical projection fields and association area of the olfactory system). The fibers of the medial stria terminate on nuclei of the *septal area* below the genu of the corpus callosum (subcallosal area) and in front of the *anterior commissure*. Fibers emerging from these nuclei project, in turn, to the opposite hemisphere and to the limbic system. The olfactory path-

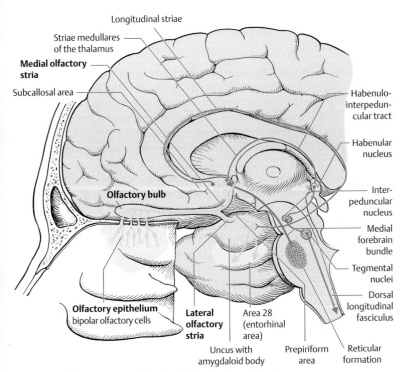

Longitudinal striae

Striae medullares
of the thalamus

**Medial olfactory
stria**

Subcallosal area

Olfactory bulb

Olfactory epithelium
bipolar olfactory cells

**Lateral
olfactory
stria**

Uncus with
amygdaloid body

Area 28
(entorhinal
area)

Prepiriform
area

Habenulo-
interpedun-
cular tract

Habenular
nucleus

Inter-
peduncular
nucleus

Medial
forebrain
bundle

Tegmental
nuclei

Dorsal
longitudinal
fasciculus

Reticular
formation

Fig. 4.**7 The olfactory nerve and tract and the olfactory pathway**

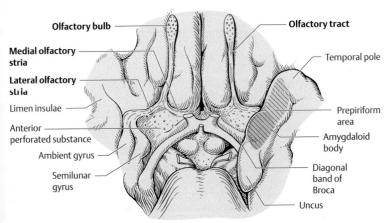

Olfactory bulb

**Medial olfactory
stria**

**Lateral olfactory
stria**

Limen insulae

Anterior
perforated substance

Ambient gyrus

Semilunar
gyrus

Olfactory tract

Temporal pole

Prepiriform
area

Amygdaloid
body

Diagonal
band of
Broca

Uncus

Fig. 4.**8 The olfactory nerve and tract as seen from below**

way is the only sensory pathway that reaches the cerebral cortex without going through a relay in the thalamus. Its central connections are complex and still incompletely known.

Connections of the olfactory system with other brain areas. An appetizing aroma excites the appetite and induces reflex salivation, while a foul smell induces nausea and the urge to vomit, or even actual vomiting. These processes also involve the emotions: some odors are pleasant, others unpleasant. Such emotions probably come about through connections of the olfactory system with the hypothalamus, thalamus, and limbic system. Among its other connections, the septal area sends association fibers to the cingulate gyrus.

The main connections of the olfactory system with autonomic areas are the *medial forebrain bundle* and the *striae medullares thalami* (Fig. 6.**9**, p. 277). The medial forebrain bundle runs laterally through the hypothalamus and gives off branches to hypothalamic nuclei. Some of its fibers continue into the brainstem to terminate in autonomic centers in the reticular formation, the salivatory nuclei, and the dorsal nucleus of the vagus nerve. The striae medullares thalami terminate in the habenular nucleus; this pathway then continues to the interpeduncular nucleus and the brainstem reticular formation (Fig. 6.**9**, p. 277).

Disturbances of smell can be classified as either quantitative or qualitative. Quantitative disturbances of smell include *hyposmia* (diminished smell) and *anosmia* (absence of smell). They are always due either to peripheral damage of the olfactory nerve, that is, of the fila olfactoria (e. g., because of rhinitis, trauma with disruption of the fila in the cribriform plate, or side effects of medication), or to central damage of the second neuron in the olfactory bulb and/or tract (olfactory groove meningioma is a classic cause). Qualitative disturbances of smell, also known as parosmias, may consist of an unpleasant *cacosmia* (e. g., fecal odor) or of *hyperosmia* (abnormally intense smell). They are usually due to central dysfunction, as in temporal lobe epilepsy.

Visual System (CN II)

Visual pathway

The retina (Fig. 4.**9a**) is the receptor surface for visual information. Like the optic nerve, it is a portion of the brain, despite its physical location at the periphery of the central nervous system. Its most important components are the *sensory receptor cells*, or *photoreceptors*, and several types of *neurons* of the visual pathway. The deepest cellular layer of the retina contains the photoreceptors (rods and cones); the two more superficial layers contain the bipolar neurons and the ganglion cells.

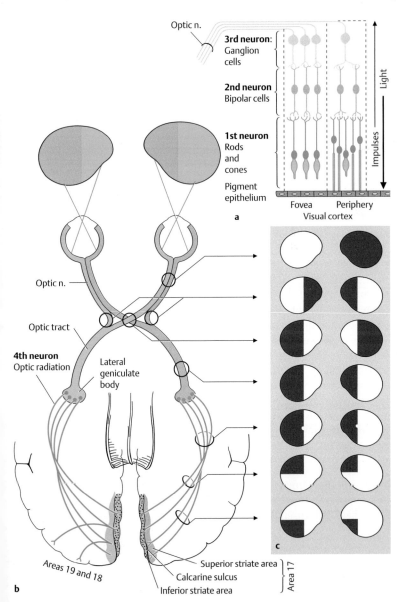

Optic n.

3rd neuron:
Ganglion
cells

2nd neuron
Bipolar cells

1st neuron
Rods
and
cones

Pigment
epithelium

Light

Impulses

Fovea   Periphery

Visual cortex

a

Optic n.

Optic tract

4th neuron
Optic radiation

Lateral
geniculate
body

Areas 19 and 18

Superior striate area
Calcarine sulcus
Inferior striate area

Area 17

b

c

Fig. 4.**9 The optic nerve and the visual pathway. a** Composition of the retina (schematic drawing).
b The visual pathway, with sites of possible lesions. **c** The corresponding visual field deficits.

Rods and cones. When light falls on the retina, it induces a photochemical reaction in the rods and cones, which leads to the generation of impulses that are ultimately propagated to the visual cortex. The rods were long thought to be responsible for the perception of brightness and for vision in dim light, while the cones were thought to subserve color perception and vision in bright light. More recent research, however, has cast doubt on these hypotheses. The underlying mechanisms of these processes are probably much more complex but cannot be discussed here in any further detail.

The *fovea* is the site of sharpest vision in the retina and contains only cones, which project onto the bipolar cells of the next neuronal layer in a one-to-one relationship. The remainder of the retina contains a mixture of rods and cones.

The retinal image of a visually perceived object is upside-down and with left and right inverted, just like the image on the film in a camera.

Optic nerve, chiasm, and tract. The retinal bipolar cells receive input onto their dendrites from the rods and cones and transmit impulses further centrally to the ganglion cell layer. The long axons of the ganglion cells pass through the optic papilla (disk) and leave the eye as the optic nerve, which contains about 1 million fibers. Half of these fibers decussate in the *optic chiasm*: the fibers from the temporal half of each retina remain uncrossed, while those from the nasal half of each retina cross to the opposite side (Fig. 4.**9a**).

Thus, at positions distal (posterior) to the optic chiasm, fibers from the temporal half of the ipsilateral retina and the nasal half of the contralateral retina are united in the *optic tract.*

A small contingent of optic nerve fibers branches off the optic tracts and travels to the superior colliculi and to nuclei in the pretectal area (see Fig. 4.**26**). These fibers constitute the afferent arm of various visual reflexes, and, in particular, of the important *pupillary light reflex*, which will be discussed further below (p. 155).

Lateral geniculate body, optic radiation, and visual cortex. The optic tract terminates in the *lateral geniculate body*, which contains six cellular layers. Most of the optic tract fibers end here, forming synapses with lateral geniculate neurons. These, in turn, emit fibers that run in the hindmost portion of the internal capsule (Fig. 3.**2**, p. 58) and then form a broad band that courses around the temporal and occipital horns of the lateral ventricle, the so-called *optic radiation* (of Gratiolet; see Fig. 4.**10**). The fibers of the optic radiation terminate in the *visual cortex*, which is located on the medial surface of the occipital lobe, within, above, and below the calcarine fissure (*Brodmann area 17*). Fibers derived from the macula occupy the largest area of the visual cortex (Fig. 4.**11**). Area 17 is also known as the *striate cortex* because it contains the stripe of Gen-

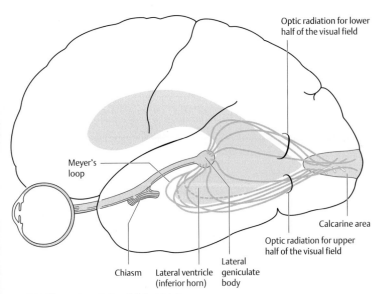

Optic radiation for lower half of the visual field

Meyer's loop

Calcarine area

Optic radiation for upper half of the visual field

Chiasm

Lateral ventricle (inferior horn)

Lateral geniculate body

Fig. 4.**10 The optic radiation** (of Gratriolet)

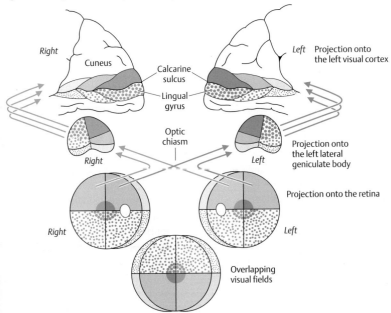

Right

Left Projection onto the left visual cortex

Cuneus

Calcarine sulcus

Lingual gyrus

Optic chiasm

Right

Left Projection onto the left lateral geniculate body

Projection onto the retina

Right

Left

Overlapping visual fields

Fig. 4.**11 Projection of the visual fields onto the retina, lateral geniculate body, and visual cortex**

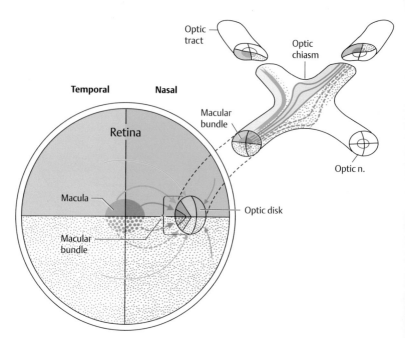

Fig. 4.**12 Position of the macular bundle in the retina, optic nerve, and optic chiasm**

nari, a white band composed of horizontally running fibers, which can be seen with the naked eye in sectioned anatomical specimens.

Somatotopic organization of the visual pathway. Although the fibers of the visual pathway partially decussate in the optic chiasm, a strict point-to-point somatotopic organization of the individual nerve fibers is preserved all the way from the retina to the visual cortex.

Visual information is transmitted centrally as follows. An object located in the left visual field gives rise to images on the nasal half of the left retina and the temporal half of the right retina. Optic nerve fibers derived from the nasal half of the left retina cross to the left side in the optic chiasm to join the fibers from the temporal half of the right retina in the right optic tract. These fibers then pass to a relay station in the right lateral geniculate body, and then by way of the right optic radiation into the right visual cortex. The right visual cortex is thus responsible for the perception of objects in the left visual field; in analogous fashion, all visual impulses relating to the right visual field are transmitted through the left optic tract and radiation into the left visual cortex (Fig. 4.**9b**).

Visual fibers derived from the macula are found in the temporal portion of the optic disk and in the central portion of the optic nerve (Fig. 4.**12**). Damage to these fibers can be seen by ophthalmoscopy as atrophy of the temporal portion of the disk (temporal pallor).

Lesions along the Visual Pathway

Optic nerve lesions. The optic nerve can be damaged at the papilla, in its anterior segment, or in its retrobulbar segment (i.e., behind the eye). **Lesions of the papilla** (e. g., *papilledema*, caused by intracranial hypertension and by a variety of metabolic disorders) can be seen by ophthalmoscopy. **Lesions of the anterior segment of the optic nerve** are often due to vasculitis (e. g., temporal arteritis). **Retrobulbar lesions** are a cardinal finding in multiple sclerosis (retrobulbar neuritis). Lesions at any of these sites can cause long-term impairment or loss of vision in the affected eye. Brief episodes of visual impairment in a single eye, lasting from a few seconds to several minutes ("transient monocular blindness"), are designated **amaurosis fugax** and are generally caused by microembolism into the retina. In such cases, the internal carotid artery is often the source of emboli and should be investigated for a possible stenosis.

Lesions of the optic chiasm, such as those produced by a pituitary tumor, craniopharyngioma, or meningioma of the tuberculum sellae, generally affect the decussating fibers in the central portion of the chiasm. The result is partial blindness for objects in the temporal half of the visual field of either eye, i.e., **bitemporal hemianopsia** (the "blinker phenomenon," where the reference is to a horse's blinkers). Fibers in the lower portion of the chiasm, derived from the lower portion of the chiasm, are commonly affected first by such processes; thus, bitemporal upper quadrantanopsia is a common early finding. Only color vision may be impaired at first.

Less commonly, however, a lesion of the chiasm can cause **binasal hemianopsia**, e. g., when a tumor has grown around the chiasm and compresses it from both sides (thus mainly affecting the laterally located, uncrossed fibers derived from the temporal halves of the two retinas, which are responsible for perception in the nasal hemifield of each eye). Aneurysms of the internal carotid artery and basilar meningitis are further possible causes, but the binasal hemianopsia in such cases is rarely pure.

Bitemporal and binasal hemianopsia are both termed **heteronymous**, because they affect opposite halves of the visual fields of the two eyes: the former affects the right hemifield of the right eye and the left hemifield of the left eye, while the latter affects the left hemifield of the right eye and the right hemifield of the left eye.

Optic tract lesions, on the other hand, cause **homonymous hemianopsia**, in which the hemifield of the same side is affected in each eye. When the fibers of the right optic tract are interrupted, for example, no visual impulses derived from the right side of either retina can reach the visual cortex. The result is blindness in the left half of the visual field of each eye (Figs. 4.**9b** and **c**). Optic tract lesions are usually caused by a tumor or basilar meningitis, less often by trauma.

Because an interruption of the optic tract also affects the optic nerve fibers traveling to the superior colliculi and to the pretectal area (cf. p. 155), it impairs the pupillary light reflex in response to light falling on the side of the retina

Case Presentation 1: *Lesion of the Optic Tract in a Patient with Multiple Sclerosis*

This 19-year-old female high-school senior, previously in excellent health, noted a visual disturbance in which she had blurry vision whenever she looked in certain directions. Within 24 hours, this blurriness spread over the entire right hemifield. She consulted her family doctor, who referred her to the hospital.

The admitting neurologist's visual field examination revealed right homonymous hemianopsia sparing the uppermost portion of the right hemifield. The remainder of the neurological examination was normal, as were the general physical examination and all routine laboratory tests.

Further tests were performed, including an MRI scan of the head, a cerebrospinal fluid examination, and recording of the visual evoked potentials (VEP). All of these tests confirmed the clinical suspicion of an inflammatory disease affecting the CNS (multiple sclerosis) producing a lesion along the course of the left optic tract. The patient was given cortisone-bolus therapy and her symptoms resolved within three days.

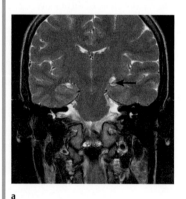
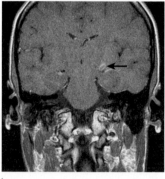

a
b

Fig. 4.**13 Inflammatory lesion of the left optic tract in a patient with multiple sclerosis, as revealed by MRI. a** The T2-weighted coronal image shows a hyperintense lesion along the course of the left optic radiation above the choroidal fissure, sparing only the basal portion of the optic tract (arrow). **b** The T1-weighted coronal image after intravenous administration of contrast material reveals enhancement at this site, indicating a focus of acute inflammation.

ipsilateral to the lesion. In theory, this *hemianopic light reflex test* could be used to distinguish optic tract lesions from lesions located more distally in the visual pathway. In practice, however, it is very difficult to shine a light onto one half of the retina exclusively, and the test is of no use in clinical diagnosis.

Lesions of the optic radiation. A lesion affecting the proximal portion of the optic radiation also causes **homonymous hemianopsia**, which, however, is often *incomplete*, because the fibers of the optic radiation are spread over a broad area (Fig. 4.**9**). Homonymous upper quadrantanopsia implies a lesion in the anterior temporal lobe, affecting the part of the radiation known as Meyer's loop (Fig. 4.**10**). Homonymous lower quadrantanopsia implies a lesion in the parietal or occipital portion of the optic radiation.

Eye Movements (CN III, IV, and VI)

Three cranial nerves innervate the muscles of the eyes: the oculomotor nerve (CN III), the trochlear nerve (CN IV), and the abducens nerve (CN VI) (Figs. 4.**14** and 4.**15**).

The nuclei of the oculomotor and trochlear nerves lie in the midbrain tegmentum, while the nucleus of the abducens nerve lies in the portion of the pontine tegmentum underlying the floor of the fourth ventricle.

The discussion of eye movements in this chapter will begin as simply as possible, i.e., with the movements of a single eye induced by impulses in each of

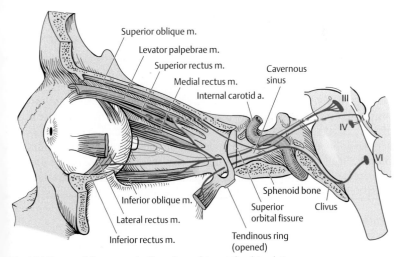

Fig. 4.**14 Course of the nerves to the extraocular muscles**: lateral view

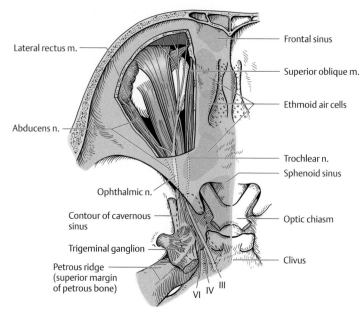

Lateral rectus m.

Frontal sinus

Superior oblique m.

Ethmoid air cells

Abducens n.

Trochlear n.

Sphenoid sinus

Ophthalmic n.

Contour of cavernous sinus

Optic chiasm

Trigeminal ganglion

Petrous ridge (superior margin of petrous bone)

Clivus

VI IV III

Fig. 4.**15 Course of the nerves to the extraocular muscles**: dorsal view

the individual nerves to the eye muscles. It should be borne in mind from the outset, however, that eye movements are usually conjugate, i.e., they usually occur in the same direction (mostly horizontally or vertically) in both eyes at once. Conjugate horizontal movements, in particular, involve simultaneous movement of the two eyes in opposite senses with respect to the midline: one eye moves medially, while the other moves laterally. Conjugate movements thus depend on the precisely coordinated innervation of the two eyes, and of the nuclei of the muscles subserving eye movement on the two sides. The complex central nervous connections enabling such movements will be dealt with later in this chapter. Finally, the nerves innervating the eye muscles also take part in a number of reflexes: accommodation, convergence, the pupillary light reflex, and the visual defense reflex. These reflexes will also be discussed in this chapter.

Oculomotor nerve (CN III)

The **nuclear area** of the oculomotor nerve lies in the periaqueductal gray matter of the midbrain, ventral to the aqueduct, at the level of the superior col-

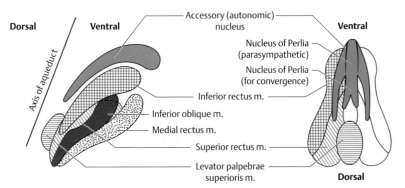

Fig. 4.**16 Oculomotor nucleus complex** (after Warwick).

liculi. It has two major components: (1) a medially situated parasympathetic nucleus, the so-called *Edinger-Westphal nucleus* (or accessory autonomic nucleus), which innervates the intraocular muscles (the sphincter pupillae muscle and the ciliary muscle); and (2) a larger and more laterally situated *nuclear complex for four of the six extraocular muscles* (the superior, inferior, and medial rectus muscles and the inferior oblique muscle). There is also a small *nuclear area for the levator palpebrae muscle* (cf. Warwick's diagram of the simian oculomotor nuclear complex, Fig. 4.**16**).

The motor **radicular fibers** that emerge from these nuclear areas travel ventrally together with the parasympathetic fibers; some of them cross the midline, others do not (all of the fibers for the superior rectus muscle cross the midline). The combined motor and parasympathetic fibers traverse the red nucleus and finally exit the brainstem in the interpeduncular fossa as the oculomotor nerve.

The **oculomotor nerve** first runs posteriorly between the superior cerebellar and posterior cerebral arteries (Fig. 4.**17**), in close apposition to the tentorial edge, then penetrates the dura mater, traverses the cavernous sinus, and enters the orbit through the superior orbital fissure (Figs. 4.**15** and 4.**17**). The parasympathetic portion of the nerve branches off at this point and travels to the ciliary ganglion, where the preganglionic fibers terminate and the ganglion cells give off short postganglionic fibers to innervate the intraocular muscles.

The somatic motor fibers of the oculomotor nerve divide into two branches, a superior branch supplying the levator palpebrae and superior rectus muscles, and an inferior branch supplying the medial and inferior recti and the inferior oblique muscle.

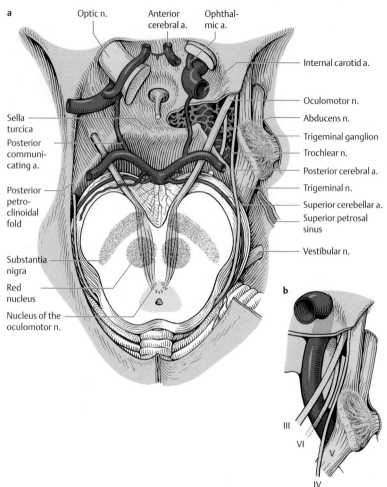

a

Optic n.

Anterior cerebral a.

Ophthalmic a.

Internal carotid a.

Oculomotor n.

Sella turcica

Abducens n.

Trigeminal ganglion

Posterior communicating a.

Trochlear n.

Posterior cerebral a.

Trigeminal n.

Posterior petroclinoidal fold

Superior cerebellar a.

Superior petrosal sinus

Vestibular n.

Substantia nigra

Red nucleus

Nucleus of the oculomotor n.

b

III

VI

V

IV

Fig. 4.**17 a Topographic relationship of the nerves supplying the extraocular muscles to the internal carotid artery and the trigeminal ganglion** with branches of the trigeminal nerve in the cavernous sinus, as viewed from above. **b** Sagittal view.

Trochlear nerve (CN IV)

The **nucleus** of the fourth cranial nerve lies ventral to the periaqueductal gray matter immediately below the oculomotor nuclear complex at the level of the inferior colliculi. Its **radicular fibers** run around the central gray matter and cross to the opposite side within the superior medullary velum. The **trochlear nerve** then exits the *dorsal* surface of the brainstem (it is the only cranial nerve that does this), emerging from the midbrain tectum into the quadrigeminal cistern. Its further course takes it laterally around the cerebral peduncle toward the ventral surface of the brainstem, so that it reaches the orbit through the superior orbital fissure together with the oculomotor nerve. It then passes to the superior oblique muscle, which it innervates. The eye movements subserved by this muscle include depression of the eye, internal rotation (cycloinversion), and slight abduction.

Abducens Nerve (CN VI)

The **nucleus** of the sixth cranial nerve lies in the caudal pontine tegmentum, just beneath the floor of the fourth ventricle. The **radicular fibers** of the seventh cranial nerve (the facial nerve) loop around the nucleus of the abducens nerve at this site. The radicular fibers of the abducens nerve traverse the pons and exit from the brainstem at the pontomedullary junction. The **abducens nerve** then runs along the ventral surface of the pons lateral to the basilar artery, perforates the dura, and joins the other nerves to the eye muscles in the cavernous sinus. Within the sinus, the third, fourth, and sixth cranial nerves are in a close spatial relation with the first and second branches of the trigeminal nerve, as well as with the internal carotid artery (Fig. 4.**17**). Moreover, the nerves in the cavernous sinus lie very near the superior and lateral portions of the sphenoid and ethmoid sinuses (Fig. 4.**15**).

Figure 4.**18** depicts the actions of the individual eye muscles in the six diagnostic directions of gaze. Figure 4.**19** shows the abnormalities of eye position and the types of diplopia that are caused by palsy of each of the three nerves subserving eye movements.

Pareses of the Eye Muscles

Weakness of one or more of the extraocular muscles *impairs movement of the affected eye and restricts its ability to gaze in a particular direction or directions.* The corneal reflex test, in which the examiner notes the position of the light reflex on both corneas from a point source held in front of the eyes in the midline, often reveals a mild asymmetry, indicating a mild *deviation of the visual axis of the eye* at rest. A diplopia test with red-green spectacles, or with a light wand, reveals that the image arising from the affected eye is the one that lies in the direction in which that eye is normally moved by the paretic muscle. The two images are farthest apart when the patient gazes in this direction; the more peripheral image is the one arising from the affected eye (Fig. 4.**19**).

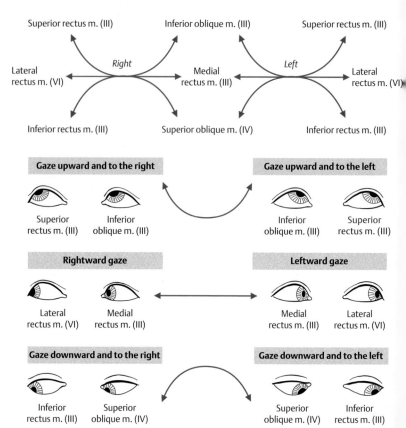

Fig. 4.**18 Diagram of eye position in the six diagnostic positions of gaze**, in which weakness of one or more of the extraocular muscles can be most easily detected

Horizontal deviations of eye position are designated *esotropia* (inward deviation) and *exotropia* (outward deviation), while vertical deviations are designated *hypertropia* and *hypotropia* (upward and downward deviation, respectively).

A lesion in the nucleus of one of the cranial nerves that subserve eye movements causes approximately the same deficit as a lesion of the peripheral nerve itself. Nuclear lesions can usually be clinically distinguished from nerve lesions because of further deficits due to damage of brainstem structures adjacent to the affected nucleus.

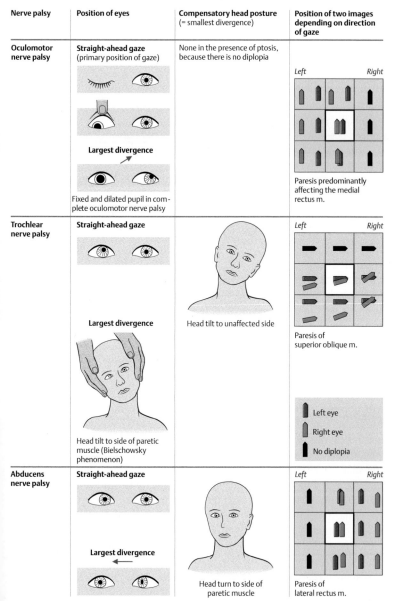

Nerve palsy	Position of eyes	Compensatory head posture (= smallest divergence)	Position of two images depending on direction of gaze
Oculomotor nerve palsy	**Straight-ahead gaze** (primary position of gaze) ... **Largest divergence** ... Fixed and dilated pupil in complete oculomotor nerve palsy	None in the presence of ptosis, because there is no diplopia	*Left* *Right* ... Paresis predominantly affecting the medial rectus m.
Trochlear nerve palsy	**Straight-ahead gaze** ... **Largest divergence** ... Head tilt to side of paretic muscle (Bielschowsky phenomenon)	Head tilt to unaffected side	*Left* *Right* ... Paresis of superior oblique m. ... Left eye / Right eye / No diplopia
Abducens nerve palsy	**Straight-ahead gaze** ... **Largest divergence**	Head turn to side of paretic muscle	*Left* *Right* ... Paresis of lateral rectus m.

Fig. 4.19 Eye position and diplopia in various kinds of extraocular muscle palsy. The clinical effects of right-sided lesions are shown. After Mumenthaler M and Mattle H: Neurology, 4th ed. (transl. E. Taub), Thieme, Stuttgart/New York, 2004.

Oculomotor Nerve Palsy

A complete oculomotor nerve palsy produces the following constellation of findings (Fig. 4.**19**):

- *Ptosis*, caused by paralysis of the levator palpebrae muscle and unopposed contraction of the orbicularis oculi muscle, which is innervated by the facial nerve (the lid space may be slightly open because of contraction of the frontalis muscle).
- *Fixed position of the eye, looking downward and outward,* caused by unopposed contraction of the lateral rectus and superior oblique muscles (innervated by CN VI and IV, respectively).
- *Dilation of the pupil,* caused by loss of contraction of the sphincter pupillae muscle, innervated by the parasympathetic portion of the oculomotor nerve (p. 157); the pupillary light and accommodation reflexes are absent (the latter because of simultaneous loss of contraction of the ciliary muscle).

An isolated paralysis of the intraocular muscles, i.e., the sphincter pupillae muscle and the ciliary muscle, is called internal ophthalmoplegia. The globe remains fully mobile, but there is an absolute paralysis of the pupil, i.e., both the direct and the consensual light reflexes are absent, and loss of accommodation causes blurry vision. Internal ophthalmoplegia is due to selective damage of the parasympathetic fibers of the oculomotor nerve.

External ophthalmoplegia is present when the motility of the globe is restricted but the autonomic (parasympathetic) innervation of the eye is preserved.

Oculomotor nerve palsies account for about 30% of all palsies affecting the muscles of eye movement (abducens nerve palsies are more common, accounting for 40–50% of cases). Ptosis is more common with lesions of the (peripheral) nerve itself, rarer with lesions of its nuclear complex within the brainstem. Once the nerve emerges from the brainstem, the pupillomotor fibers lie in the outer portion of the nerve, directly beneath the epineurium, and are thus more vulnerable than the other fibers of the nerve to compression by trauma, tumors, or aneurysms. For the same reason, the pupillomotor fibers are less commonly damaged by vascular lesions, such as those caused by diabetes. The more common causes of isolated oculomotor nerve palsy are aneurysms (approx. 30%), tumors (approx. 15%), and vascular lesions (including diabetes, approx. 15–20%).

Trochlear Nerve Palsy

Trochlear nerve palsy paralyzes the superior oblique muscle. The affected eye deviates upward and slightly inward, i.e., medially, toward the side of the normal eye (Fig. 4.**19**). The deviation is most evident, and the diplopia most extreme, when the patient looks downward and inward. Another way of bringing out the upward-and-inward deviation of the affected eye and the resulting diplopia is by having the patient tilt the head to the affected side while fixating on an object with the normal eye (*Bielschowsky test*).

The more common causes of trochlear nerve palsy are trauma (30-60% of cases), vascular lesions, and tumors.

Case Presentation 2: *Nuclear Lesion of the Trochlear Nerve due to a Brainstem Infarct*

This 46-year-old male company employee became mildly nauseated one afternoon while at work. His co-workers subsequently recalled that he momentarily seemed strangely "distant," though he had no recollection of this. The nausea resolved after a short while, only to be immediately followed by the onset of diplopia, particularly on downward gaze, of which he became aware while descending a staircase. Concerned about these symptoms, he presented to the hospital for evaluation.

The clinical examination (eye position and movements) indicated paresis of the left super-ior oblique muscle as the cause of diplopia. An MRI scan was obtained to rule out an intracranial mass. The T2-weighted image revealed a midbrain lesion affecting the nucleus of the trochlear nerve on the left (Fig. 4.**20**). There was no evidence of a diffusion abnormality or of contrast enhancement on the corresponding images. The radiological findings and the clinical course (acute onset of nausea followed by sudden diplopia) were considered to be most consistent with an ischemic event (acute lacunar midbrain stroke). There was no evidence of inflammatory disease affecting the CNS.

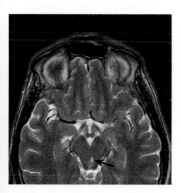

Fig. 4.**20 Nuclear lesion of the left trochlear nerve with paresis of the superior oblique muscle due to an acute midbrain infarct.** This T2-weighted image reveals a hyperintense lesion in the midbrain (arrow).

Abducens Palsy

The affected eye is deviated inward on primary (straight-ahead) gaze and cannot be abducted, because the lateral rectus muscle is paralyzed. The inward squint is also referred to as convergent strabismus. When looking toward the nose, the paretic eye rotates upward and inward because of the predominant action of the inferior oblique muscle.

Abducens palsy is usually an isolated finding and is most commonly caused by tumors or vascular lesions. Among all of the cranial nerves, the abducens nerve has the longest course within the subarachnoid space; thus, abducens palsies can be caused by meningitis and by subarachnoid hemorrhage, as well as by elevated intracranial pressure (intracranial hypertension). Unilateral abducens palsy may accompany generalized intracranial hypertension and is not necessarily a lateralizing sign. Abducens palsy is also occasionally produced by the temporary disturbance of intracranial pressure after a lumbar puncture.

Conjugate Eye Movements

Positioning and stabilizing the image of an object exactly on the fovea of both eyes at the same time requires precisely coordinated activity of the eye muscles. The agonist and antagonist muscles of the two eyes are always simultaneously innervated (*Hering's law*), and each contraction of an agonist occurs in conjunction with relaxation of the corresponding antagonist (*Sherrington's law*). Conjugate movements of both eyes in the same direction are called *versive* movements (from the Latin for "turning"), while movements of the two eyes in opposite directions are *vergence* movements (either *convergence* or *divergence*). Movements of a single eye are called either *duction* or *torsion* (rotatory movement).

Horizontal and Vertical Gaze

Conjugate horizontal gaze. The central relay nucleus of the oculomotor system is found in the **paramedian pontine reticular formation** (PPRF or "pontine gaze center"), which lies adjacent to the nucleus of the abducens nerve. The PPRF is the site of origin of all of the neural connections participating in conjugate horizontal gaze, in particular the fibers that connect the ipsilateral abducens nucleus to the portion of the contralateral oculomotor nucleus innervating the medial rectus muscle. These fibers run in the **medial longitudinal fasciculus** (MLF), a white-matter tract that ascends and descends the brainstem on both sides near the midline. The MLF, which extends from the midbrain all the way to the cervical spinal cord, serves to interconnect all of the individual nuclei innervating the eye muscles (Fig. 4.**21**). It also conveys impulses to and from the

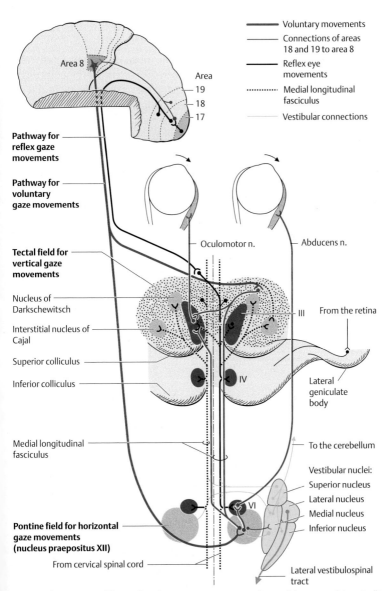

Fig. 4.21 The anatomical basis of conjugate eye movements: the cranial nerve nuclei controlling the extraocular muscles, the medial longitudinal fasciculus, and the vestibular nucleus complex, with the supranuclear and infranuclear pathways for voluntary and reflex conjugate eye movements. (Drawing based partly on Hassler.)

cervical spinal cord (anterior and posterior cervical musculature), the vestibular nuclei, the basal ganglia, and the cerebral cortex.

Disturbances of conjugate horizontal gaze. If the medial longitudinal fasciculus is damaged on the left side (for example), then the patient's left medial rectus muscle is no longer activated on attempted conjugate gaze to the right, and the left eye stays behind, i.e., it comes no further medially than the midline. At the same time, monocular nystagmus is seen in the right eye, whose movement to the right (abduction) is subserved by the right abducens nerve. This combination of findings is called **internuclear ophthalmoplegia** (INO, Fig. 4.**22**). It is important to realize that INO involves neither a nuclear nor a peripheral palsy of the nerves to the eye muscles: in the patient just described, the left medial rectus muscle will contract normally on convergence of the two eyes.

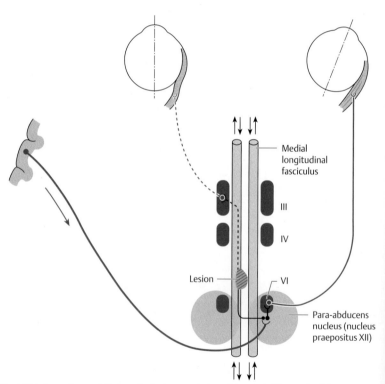

Fig. 4.**22 Internuclear ophthalmoplegia** due to a lesion of the medial longitudinal fasciculus

As mentioned, the MLF lies near the midline; the two medial longitudinal fasciculi in fact lie very near each other, and damage to them is usually bilateral. The above findings of internuclear ophthalmoplegia are thus usually seen on attempted gaze in either direction: the adducting eye comes no further medially than the midline, while the abducting (leading) eye manifests nystagmus. All other eye movements are intact, and the pupillary reflexes are intact.

Multiple sclerosis is the most common cause of internuclear ophthalmoplegia. Others include encephalitis and (in older patients) vascular disturbances.

Conjugate vertical gaze. The vertical gaze center lies in the *rostrodorsal portion of the midbrain reticular formation* (Fig. 4.**21**) and consists of a number of specialized nuclei: the *prestitial nucleus* in the rear wall of the third ventricle

---

Case Presentation 3: **Internuclear Ophthalmoplegia in a Patient with an Acute Brainstem Stroke**

This previously healthy 48-year-old man was admitted to the hospital because of the sudden onset of nausea, vomiting, and diplopia. Neurological examination revealed the typical findings of internuclear ophthalmoplegia (see above) and no other deficits. The internuclear ophthalmoplegia largely resolved over the subsequent course of the patient's illness.

The clinical course and radiological findings pointed to an ischemic event (lacunar brainstem stroke involving the medial longitudinal fasciculus). There was no evidence of a CNS inflammatory process. No embolic source was found.

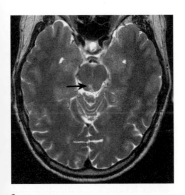
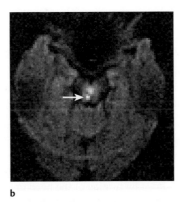

a   b

Fig. 4.**23 Internuclear ophthalmoplegia in a patient with an acute midbrain infarct. a** The thin-section axial T2-weighted image of the midbrain shows a hyperintense right paramedian lesion adjacent to the aqueduct. **b** The axial diffusion-weighted image shows a fresh lesion at this site. The two findings, taken together, indicate an ischemic event.

for upward gaze; the *nucleus of the posterior commissure* for downward gaze; and the *interstitial nucleus of Cajal* and the *nucleus of Darkschewitsch* for conjugate rotatory movements.

Other conjugate gaze centers. Vertical gaze movements can also be generated from neurons lying at the **anterior border of the superior colliculi**. Disturbances affecting this area cause paresis of upward gaze (Parinaud syndrome).

Impulses originating in the **occipital lobes** also travel to the contralateral pontine gaze centers (para-abducens nucleus) to initiate conjugate lateral gaze movements. Experimental stimulation of occipital areas 18 and 19 has been found to provoke conjugate gaze movements that are most often lateral, though sometimes upward or downward (lateral gaze movements are certainly the most important type in human beings, as they are far more frequent than the other two types) (Fig. 4.**21**, p. 147).

Voluntary eye movements are initiated by neurons of the **frontal eye field** in Brodmann area 8 (and perhaps also parts of areas 6 and 9), anterior to the precentral gyrus (Fig. 4.**21**). The most common result of stimulation or irritation in this area, e. g., during an epileptic seizure, is a conjugate lateral gaze movement to the opposite side (*déviation conjuguée*, see below) (Fig. 4.**24**). This eye movement is occasionally accompanied by turning of the head to the opposite side.

The **pathway from the frontal eye field to the brainstem nuclei subserving eye movements** has not yet been fully traced. It is currently thought that fibers of this pathway run in the internal capsule and the cerebral peduncle together with the corticonuclear tract, but then do not terminate directly in the nuclei subserving eye movement, reaching them instead through a number of "way stations" including the superior colliculi, interneurons of the reticular formation, and the medial longitudinal fasciculus (Fig. 4.**21**).

All voluntary movements are under the influence of *reflex arcs*, not only visual, but also auditory, vestibular, and proprioceptive (from the cervical and nuchal musculature to the spinotectal tract and medial longitudinal fasciculus).

Lesions of the gaze centers. **Destruction of area 8** on one side results in a preponderance of impulses coming from the corresponding area of the opposite hemisphere, producing conjugate gaze toward the side of the lesion (i.e., *déviation conjuguée* looking toward the focus). The gaze deviation is occasionally accompanied by turning of the head to the side of the lesion. The patient cannot *voluntarily* look to the other side, but can do so in *reflex* fashion, as when visually pursuing an object that is slowly moved into the contralateral visual field. (The opposite is found in lesions of the occipital lobe, as discussed below.) Gaze deviation due to a lesion of the frontal eye field generally resolves after a brief

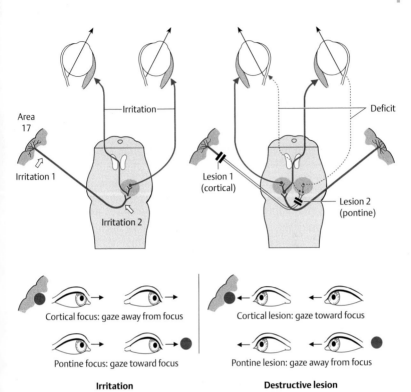

Fig. 4.**24 Conjugate deviation due to cortical and pontine foci** (irritative or destructive)

period. In contrast to a destructive lesion, **stimulation or irritation of area 8** (as in an epileptic seizure) produces conjugate gaze away from the side of the focus.

The situation is different with **pontine lesions** because the corticopontine pathways are crossed (Fig. 4.**24**). Stimulation or irritation of the pontine gaze center produces ipsilateral gaze deviation, while a destructive lesion causes contralateral gaze deviation. Gaze deviation of pontine origin rarely resolves completely.

Reflex Conjugate Gaze Movements

"Fixation reflex." When we direct our gaze onto an object voluntarily, we do so with very fast, abrupt, and precise eye movements, called saccades. Most eye movements, however, occur in reflex fashion: when an object enters our visual field, our attention, and our gaze, are directed to it automatically. If the object moves, the eyes pursue it involuntarily so that its image remains on the fovea, the portion of the retina in which vision is sharpest. This occurs regardless of whether the observer or the object is in motion (or both). All voluntary eye movements thus have involuntary reflex components. In the English-language literature, the quasi-reflex processes that maintain the visual image of an object on the fovea are referred to as the fixation reflex.

The **afferent arm** of the fixation reflex extends from the retina along the visual pathway to the visual cortex (area 17), from which further impulses are sent to areas 18 and 19. The efferent arm returns from these areas to the contralateral mesencephalic and pontine gaze centers, probably by way of the optic radiation (though the exact location of these fibers is still unknown). These gaze centers then project to the cranial nerve nuclei subserving eye movements to complete the reflex arc. Some of the efferent fibers probably run directly to the brainstem gaze centers, while others pass first to the frontal eye field (area 8).

Lesions affecting the fixation reflex. If the occipital areas involved in the fixation reflex are damaged, the reflex no longer functions properly. The patient can look voluntarily in any direction, but can no longer pursue an object visually, keeping its image fixed on the fovea. The object immediately slips out of the zone of sharpest vision, and the patient has to find it again with voluntary eye movements.

Optokinetic nystagmus. When a person looks directly at an object, the image of the object on each retina falls on the fovea, and despite the actual presence of two images—one on each retina—the object is perceived as one (fusion). If the object should then move in any direction, either closer to or farther away from the observer, vertically, or horizontally, *smooth pursuit movements* of the eyes will hold its image on the fovea of each eye (cf. the above discussion of the fixation reflex). As soon as the image of the object moves out of the fovea, impulses travel in a reflex arc from the retina along the visual pathway to the visual cortex, and then through the occipitotectal fibers back to the cranial nerve nuclei that innervate the eye muscles, causing them to contract in such a way as to retrieve the image onto the fovea (this is called the *optokinetic* process). The jerky eye movements produced in this way, known as *optokinetic nystagmus*, can be observed easily in persons watching the passing scenery from a train or car window, for example. It can be reproduced in the clinical setting by having the patient watch a rotating, striped drum: the patient's gaze pursues one of the stripes until it disappears around the side of the drum, then snaps back to catch another stripe, and so on, repeatedly. Thus, optokinetic nystagmus consists of slow and fast phases, i.e., relatively slow pursuit movements in alternation with faster, corrective jumps in the opposite direction. If the reflex arc for optokinetic nystagmus is broken at any point, the reflex is lost. Absence of optokinetic nystagmus is always pathological.

Convergence and Accommodation

These reflexes are evoked by watching an object as it moves closer to the observer in the visual field. The so-called near response actually consists of three processes that occur simultaneously:

- **Convergence:** the medial rectus muscles of the two eyes are activated so that the optical axis of each continues to point directly to the object under observation. This keeps the image of the object on the fovea of each eye.
- **Accommodation:** contraction of the ciliary muscle slackens the suspending apparatus of the lens. Because it is intrinsically elastic, the lens then takes on a more spherical shape, and thus a higher refractive power. This process keeps the retinal image of an object in focus as it is moved closer to the eye. Conversely, when the object is moved farther away or the individual's gaze is redirected onto a more distant point, relaxation of the ciliary muscle allows the suspending apparatus to pull the lens back into a flatter shape, lowering its refractive power and once again bringing the visual image into sharp focus (Fig. 4.**25**).
- **Pupillary constriction:** the pupil constricts to keep the retinal image of the near object as sharp as possible. (A camera shutter functions similarly: the closer the object to be photographed, the narrower the aperture must be to keep it in focus.)

All three of these processes can be brought about voluntarily by fixating on a near object and also occur as reflexes when a distant object moves closer to the observer.

Anatomical substrate of convergence and accommodation (Fig. 4.**25**). The **afferent** impulses travel from the retina to the visual cortex, and the **efferent** impulses from the visual cortex to the pretectal area and then to the parasympathetic *nucleus of Perlia*, which lies medial and ventral to the Edinger-Westphal nucleus (accessory autonomic nucleus). From the nucleus of Perlia on either side, impulses travel to the *nuclear area of the medial rectus muscle* (for ocular convergence) and to the *Edinger-Westphal nucleus*, from which they proceed to the ciliary ganglion and muscle (for accommodation) and to the pupillary sphincter (for pupilloconstriction) (Fig. 4.**26**). The neural pathways to the ciliary muscle and the pupillary sphincter are presumably distinct, because the

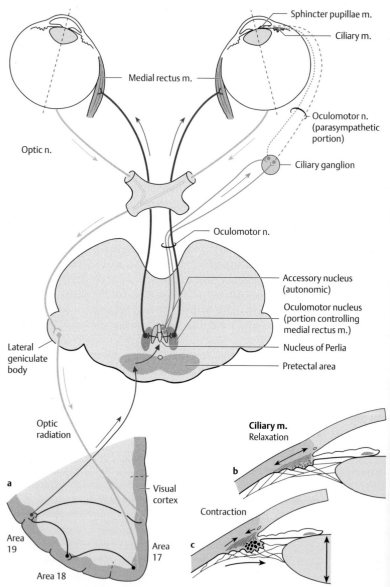

Sphincter pupillae m.

Ciliary m.

Medial rectus m.

Oculomotor n. (parasympathetic portion)

Optic n.

Ciliary ganglion

Oculomotor n.

Accessory nucleus (autonomic)

Oculomotor nucleus (portion controlling medial rectus m.)

Lateral geniculate body

Nucleus of Perlia

Pretectal area

Optic radiation

Ciliary m. Relaxation

b

Contraction

a

Visual cortex

Area 19

Area 17

Area 18

c

Fig. 4.**25 a The anatomical basis of convergence and accommodation**. **b** The ciliary muscle in relaxation (vision at a distance). **c** The ciliary muscle in contraction (near vision).

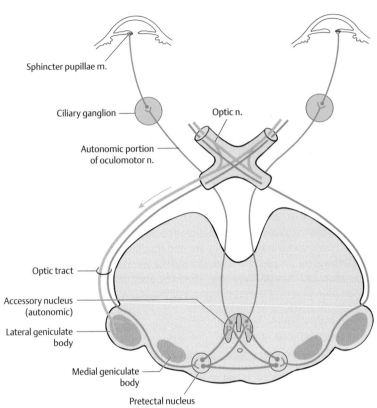

Sphincter pupillae m.

Ciliary ganglion

Optic n.

Autonomic portion
of oculomotor n.

Optic tract

Accessory nucleus
(autonomic)

Lateral geniculate
body

Medial geniculate
body

Pretectal nucleus

Fig. 4.**26 The pupillary light reflex**

accommodation and light reflexes can be differentially affected in various conditions. In neurosyphilis, for example, one can find the phenomenon of the
Argyll Robertson pupil: the light reflex is absent, but convergence and accommodation are preserved.

Regulation of the Pupillary Light Reflex

The width of the pupil varies in relation to the incident light: bright light induces pupillary constriction, and darkness induces pupillary dilation. The
pupillary light reflex serves to modulate the amount of light falling on the retina, both to protect the photoreceptors from potentially damaging, excessive illumination, and to keep the visual images of objects in the best possible focus

on the retina, in analogous fashion to a camera shutter. This reflex is entirely involuntary; the cerebral cortex is not involved in the reflex loop.

Afferent arm of the pupillary light reflex (Fig. 4.**26**). The afferent fibers accompany the visual fibers in the optic nerve and tract nearly to the lateral geniculate body, but, instead of entering the latter, they turn off in the direction of the superior colliculi and terminate in the *nuclei of the pretectal area*. Interneurons located here project further to the parasympathetic *Edinger-Westphal nuclei* (accessory autonomic nuclei) on both sides (Fig. 4.**26**). This bilateral innervation of the Edinger-Westphal nuclei is the anatomical basis of the consensual light response: illumination of one eye induces constriction not just of that pupil, but of the contralateral pupil as well.

Lesions of the afferent pathway. Lesions of the optic radiation, visual cortex, or superior colliculi have no effect on the pupillary light reflex. A lesion of the *pretectal area*, however, abolishes the reflex. This indicates that the former structures do not participate in the reflex arc, and that the afferent arm of the reflex arc must traverse the pretectal area, though the precise anatomical localization of this pathway is not yet fully clear. Similarly, *optic nerve lesions*, which interrupt the afferent arm of the reflex arc at a different site, impair the pupillary response to illumination of the eye on the side of the lesion: neither the ipsilateral nor the contralateral pupil will constrict normally. Illumination of the other eye is followed by normal constriction of both pupils. These findings imply the presence of an *afferent pupillary defect*.

Efferent arm of the pupillary light reflex (Fig. 4.**26**). The efferent fibers originate in the *Edinger-Westphal nucleus* and travel in the *oculomotor nerve* to the orbit. The parasympathetic preganglionic fibers branch off from the oculomotor nerve within the orbit and travel to the *ciliary ganglion*, whose ganglion cells constitute a synaptic relay station. The short postganglionic fibers emerge from the ciliary ganglion and then enter the globe to innervate the sphincter pupillae muscle (Fig. 4.**26**).

Lesions of the efferent pathway. If the oculomotor nerve or ciliary ganglion is damaged, the impulses from the Edinger-Westphal nucleus can no longer reach the sphincter pupillae muscle of the ipsilateral eye. The result is mydriasis with absence of the light reflex.

Other stimuli affecting the width of the pupils. The width of the pupils varies not only in response to the incident light but also in response to various kinds of stimuli arising outside the eye. *Very painful stimuli*, such as a deep pinch of the nuchal musculature, as well as *heightened emotional arousal* can induce pupillary dilatation. The mydriasis seen in these situations was long attributed to increased activity of the sympathetic nervous system, leading to contraction of the dilator pupillae muscle (which is discussed further below). Recent studies have shown, however, that decreased activity of the parasympathetic innervation of the pupil is probably the more important factor.

Anisocoria. The word "anisocoria" comes from the Greek and means, literally, inequality of the pupils (it is thus redundant to state, "The pupils are anisocoric"). A mild disparity of pupillary width is often noted in normal persons (physiological anisocoria), but a larger disparity should provoke suspicion of a (unilateral) intracranial mass compressing the oculomotor nerve. In clinical situations, it is important to remember that anisocoria is often produced by the instillation of dilating or constricting drugs into one eye (which should be avoided, for example, in comatose patients).

Sympathetic and Parasympathetic Innervation of the Eye

Parasympathetic innervation of the eye (Fig. 4.27). The parasympathetic innervation of the sphincter pupillae muscle and of the ciliary muscle was discussed above in connection with the pupillary light reflex and the accommodation reflex (pp. 153 ff.). Activation of the parasympathetic supply to the eye is manifested by pupillary constriction (miosis) and accommodation in response to a near object.

Sympathetic innervation of the eye (Fig. 4.27). The nuclear area from which the sympathetic innervation of the eye arises, the so-called *ciliospinal center*, is located in the lateral horn of the spinal cord from C8 to T2. The preganglionic fibers originate here and ascend to a relay station in the superior cervical ganglion, from which the postganglionic fibers emerge and then ascend together with the internal carotid artery and ophthalmic artery into the orbit, finally reaching and innervating the dilator pupillae, superior and inferior tarsal, and orbitalis muscles (Figs. 4.27 and 4.28). Other sympathetic fibers supply the sweat glands and blood vessels of the ipsilateral half of the face.

Afferent supply of the ciliospinal center: Afferent fibers from the retina travel to the hypothalamus (suprachiasmatic nucleus), in which the central sympathetic pathway arises. The pathway crosses the midline at the level of the midbrain and descends through the brainstem and cervical spinal cord to the ciliospinal center.

Horner syndrome (Fig. 4.28). A lesion affecting the central sympathetic pathway, the ciliospinal center, the superior cervical ganglion, or the postganglionic sympathetic fibers on their way to the eye produces a characteristic constella-

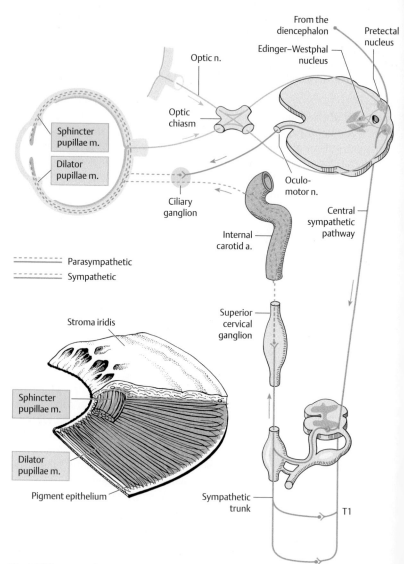

Fig. 4.27 **The sympathetic and parasympathetic innervation of the intraocular muscles.**

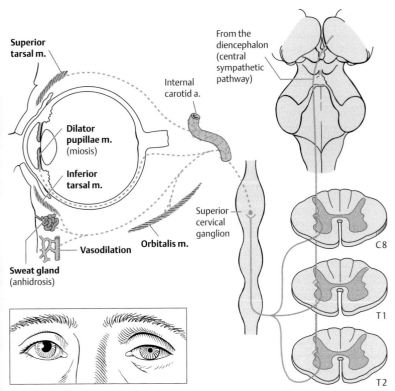

Fig. 4.**28 The sympathetic innervation of the eye and Horner syndrome.** In the region of the eye, sympathetic efferents innervate not only the dilator pupillae muscle (see Fig. 4.**27**), but also the tarsal muscles and the orbitalis muscle. The sympathetic innervation of the sweat glands of the face and of its vasculature (vasoconstrictor fibers) is also shown.

tion of abnormalities, called Horner syndrome. The triad of ocular findings consists of: *narrowing of the palpebral fissure* (due to loss of function of the superior tarsal muscle), *miosis* (due to loss of function of the dilator pupillae muscle, resulting in a preponderance of the constricting effect of the sphincter pupillae muscle), and *enophthalmos* (due to loss of function of the orbitalis muscle). *Anhidrosis* and *vasodilatation* in the ipsilateral half of the face are seen when the sympathetic innervation of the face is also involved, either at the ciliospinal center or in the efferent fibers that emerge from it.

Blink Reflex

If an object suddenly appears before the eyes, reflex eye closure occurs (**blink reflex**). The afferent impulses of this reflex travel from the retina directly to the midbrain tectum and then run, by way of the tectonuclear tract, to the facial nerve nuclei of both sides, whose efferent fibers then innervate the orbicularis oculi muscles. Further impulses may descend in tectospinal fibers to the anterior horn cells of the spinal cord, which innervate the cervical musculature to produce aversion of the head.

Trigeminal Nerve (CN V)

The trigeminal nerve is a mixed nerve. It possesses a larger component (*portio major*) consisting of **sensory fibers** for the face, and a smaller component (*portio minor*) consisting of **motor fibers** for the muscles of mastication.

Trigeminal ganglion and brainstem nuclei. The **trigeminal (gasserian) ganglion** is the counterpart of the spinal dorsal root ganglia for the sensory innervation of the face. Like the dorsal root ganglia, it contains pseudounipolar ganglion cells, whose peripheral processes terminate in receptors for touch, pressure, tactile discrimination, pain, and temperature, and whose central processes project to the **principal sensory nucleus of the trigeminal nerve** (for touch and discrimination) and to the **spinal nucleus of the trigeminal nerve** (for pain and temperature). The **mesencephalic nucleus of the trigeminal nerve** is a special case, in that its cells correspond to spinal dorsal root ganglion cells even though it is located within the brainstem; it is, in a sense, a peripheral nucleus that has been displaced into the central nervous system. The peripheral processes of neurons in this nucleus receive impulses from peripheral receptors in the muscle spindles in the muscles of mastication, and from other receptors that respond to pressure.

The three nuclei just mentioned extend from the cervical spinal cord all the way to the midbrain, as shown in Figure 4.**30**. The trigeminal ganglion is located at the base of the skull over the apex of the petrous bone, just lateral to the posterolateral portion of the cavernous sinus. It gives off the three branches of the trigeminal nerve to the different areas of the face, i.e., the **ophthalmic nerve** (V_1), which exits from the skull through the superior orbital fissure; the **maxillary nerve** (V_2), which exits through the foramen rotundum; and the **mandibular nerve** (V_3), which exits through the foramen ovale.

Somatosensory trigeminal fibers. The peripheral trajectory of the trigeminal nerve is shown in Figure 4.**29**. Its **somatosensory portion** supplies the skin of the face up to the vertex of the head. Figure 4.**30** shows the cutaneous territo-

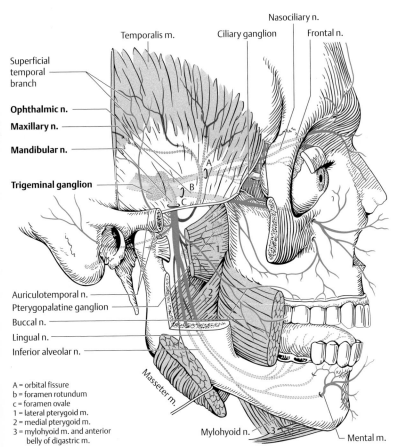

Nasociliary n.

Temporalis m.   Ciliary ganglion   Frontal n.

Superficial
temporal
branch

Ophthalmic n.

Maxillary n.

Mandibular n.

Trigeminal ganglion

Auriculotemporal n.
Pterygopalatine ganglion
Buccal n.
Lingual n.
Inferior alveolar n.

A = orbital fissure
b = foramen rotundum
c = foramen ovale
1 = lateral pterygoid m.
2 = medial pterygoid m.
3 = mylohyoid m. and anterior
    belly of digastric m.

Masseter m.

Mylohyoid n.

Mental m.

Fig. 4.**29 Peripheral course of the somatosensory and motor fibers of the trigeminal nerve**

ries supplied by each of the three trigeminal branches. The cutaneous distribution of the trigeminal nerve borders the dermatomes of the second and third
cervical nerve roots. (The first cervical nerve root, C1, is purely motor and innervates the nuchal muscles that are attached to the skull and the upper cervical vertebrae.)

Furthermore, the mucous membranes of the mouth, nose, and paranasal
sinuses derive their somatosensory innervation from the trigeminal nerve, as
do the mandibular and maxillary teeth and most of the dura mater (in the

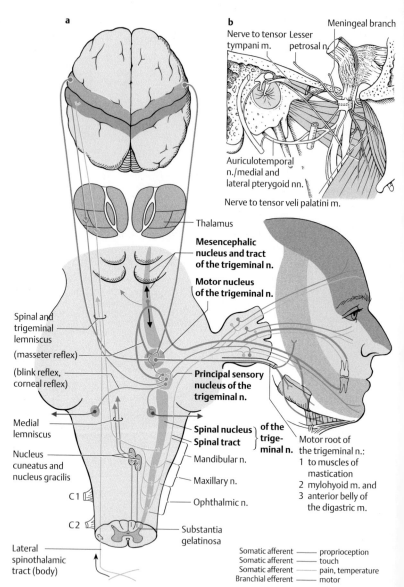

a

b

Nerve to tensor tympani m.   Lesser petrosal n.   Meningeal branch

Auriculotemporal n./medial and lateral pterygoid nn.

Nerve to tensor veli palatini m.

Thalamus

Mesencephalic nucleus and tract of the trigeminal n.

Motor nucleus of the trigeminal n.

Spinal and trigeminal lemniscus

(masseter reflex)

(blink reflex, corneal reflex)

Principal sensory nucleus of the trigeminal n.

Medial lemniscus

Nucleus cuneatus and nucleus gracilis

Spinal nucleus of the **trige-**
Spinal tract minal n.

Motor root of the trigeminal n.:
1 to muscles of mastication
2 mylohyoid m. and
3 anterior belly of the digastric m.

Mandibular n.

Maxillary n.

Ophthalmic n.

C 1

C 2

Substantia gelatinosa

Lateral spinothalamic tract (body)

Somatic afferent	—— proprioception
Somatic afferent	—— touch
Somatic afferent	—— pain, temperature
Branchial efferent	—— motor

Fig. 4.**30 a Central connections of the various trigeminal fibers and their corresponding nuclei** (schematic drawing). **b** Motor root of the trigeminal nerve.

anterior and middle cranial fossae). Around the external ear, however, only the anterior portion of the pinna and the external auditory canal and a part of the tympanic membrane are supplied by the trigeminal nerve. The rest of the external auditory canal derives its somatosensory innervation from the nervus intermedius and the glossopharyngeal and vagus nerves.

Proprioceptive impulses from the muscles of mastication and the hard palate are transmitted by the mandibular nerve. These impulses are part of a feedback mechanism for the control of bite strength.

All trigeminal somatosensory fibers terminate in the **principal sensory nucleus of the trigeminal nerve,** which is located in the dorsolateral portion of the pons (in a position analogous to that of the posterior column nuclei in the medulla). The axons of the second neurons cross the midline and ascend in the contralateral medial lemniscus to the ventral posteromedial nucleus of the thalamus (VPL, Fig. 4.**30**).

The somatosensory fibers of the trigeminal nerve are a component of several important reflex arcs.

Corneal reflex. Somatosensory impulses from the mucous membranes of the eye travel in the ophthalmic nerve to the principal sensory nucleus of the trigeminal nerve (**afferent** arm). After a synapse at this site, impulses travel onward to the facial nerve nuclei and then through the facial nerves to the orbicularis oculi muscles on either side (**efferent** arm). Interruption of this reflex arc in either its afferent component (trigeminal nerve) or its efferent component (facial nerve) abolishes the corneal reflex, in which touching the cornea induces reflex closure of both eyes.

Sneeze and suck reflexes. Other somatosensory fibers travel from the nasal mucosa to the trigeminal nuclear area to form the **afferent** arm of the sneeze reflex. A number of different nerves make up its **efferent** arm: cranial nerves V, VII, IX, and X, as well as several nerves that are involved in expiration. The suck reflex of infants, in which touching of the lips induces sucking, is another reflex with a trigeminal afferent arm and an efferent arm that involves several different nerves.

Pain and temperature fibers of the trigeminal nerve. Fibers subserving pain and temperature sensation travel caudally in the **spinal tract of the trigeminal nerve** and terminate in the **spinal nucleus of the trigeminal nerve,** whose lowest portion extends into the cervical spinal cord. This nucleus is the upper extension of the Lissauer zone and the substantia gelatinosa of the posterior horn, which receive the pain and temperature fibers of the upper cervical segments.

The *caudal portion* (*pars caudalis*) of the spinal nucleus of the trigeminal nerve contains an upside-down somatotopic representation of the face and head: the nociceptive fibers of the ophthalmic nerve terminate most caudally, followed from caudal to rostral by those of the maxillary and mandibular nerves The spinal tract of the trigeminal nerve also contains nociceptive fibers from cranial nerves VII (nervus intermedius), IX, and X, which subserve pain and temperature sensation on the external ear, the posterior third of the tongue, and the larynx and pharynx (see Figs. 4.**48** and 4.**49**).

The *midportion* (*pars interpolaris*) and *rostral portion* (*pars rostralis*) of the spinal nucleus of the trigeminal nerve probably receive afferent fibers subserving touch and pressure sensation (the functional anatomy in this area is incompletely understood at present). The pars interpolaris has also been reported to receive nociceptive fibers from the pulp of the teeth.

The second neurons that emerge from the spinal nucleus of the trigeminal nerve project their axons across the midline in a broad, fanlike tract. These fibers traverse the pons and midbrain, ascending in close association with the lateral spinothalamic tract toward the thalamus, where they terminate in the ventral posteromedial nucleus (Fig. 4.**30**). The axons of the thalamic (third) neurons in the trigeminal pathway then ascend in the posterior limb of the internal capsule to the caudal portion of the postcentral gyrus (Fig. 2.**19**, p. 46).

Motor trigeminal fibers. The motor nucleus from which the motor fibers (portio minor) of the trigeminal nerve arise is located in the lateral portion of the pontine tegmentum, just medial to the principal sensory nucleus of the trigeminal nerve. The portio minor exits the skull through the foramen ovale together with the mandibular nerve and innervates the masseter, temporalis, and medial and lateral pterygoid muscles, as well as the tensor veli palatini, the tensor tympani, the mylohyoid muscle, and the anterior belly of the digastric muscle (Figs. 4.**29** and 4.**30**).

The motor nuclei (and, through them, the muscles of mastication) are under the influence of cortical centers that project to them by way of the corticonuclear tract. This supranuclear pathway is mostly crossed, but there is also a substantial ipsilateral projection. This accounts for the fact that a unilateral interruption of the supranuclear trigeminal pathway does not produce any noticeable weakness of the muscles of mastication.

The supranuclear pathway originates in neurons of the caudal portion of the precentral gyrus (Fig. 3.**2**, p. 58; Fig. 4.**30**).

Lesions of the motor trigeminal fibers. A nuclear or peripheral lesion of the motor trigeminal pathway produces **flaccid weakness of the muscles of mastication.**

This type of weakness, if unilateral, can be detected by palpation of the masseter and temporalis muscles while the patient clamps his or her jaw: the normally palpable muscle contraction is absent on the side of the lesion. When the patient then opens his or her mouth and protrudes the lower jaw, the jaw deviates to the side of the lesion, because the force of the contralateral pterygoid muscle predominates. In such cases, the masseteric or jaw-jerk reflex is absent (it is normally elicitable by tapping the chin with a reflex hammer to stretch the fibers of the masseter muscle).

Disorders Affecting the Trigeminal Nerve

Trigeminal neuralgia. The classic variety of trigeminal neuralgia is characterized by paroxysms of intense, lightninglike (shooting or "lancinating") pain in the distribution of one or more branches of the trigeminal nerve. The pain can be evoked by touching the face in one or more particularly sensitive areas ("trigger zones"). Typical types of stimuli that trigger pain include washing, shaving, and tooth-brushing. This condition is also known by the traditional French designation, *tic douloureux* (which is somewhat misleading, because any twitching movements of the face that may be present are a reflex response to the pain, rather than a true tic). The neurological examination is unremarkable; in particular, there is no sensory deficit on the face.

The pathophysiology of this condition remains imperfectly understood; both central and peripheral mechanisms have been proposed. (The older term **"idiopathic** trigeminal neuralgia" for the classic condition is no longer widely used, because this issue is still unsettled.) Gardner (1959) and, later, Jannetta (1982) attributed trigeminal neuralgia to compression of the trigeminal root by a blood vessel, usually the superior cerebellar artery, looping around the proximal, unmyelinated portion of the root immediately after its exit from the pons (Fig. **4.31**). This hypothesis is supported by the observation that a pain-free state can be achieved in up to 80% of patients with a neurosurgical procedure known as microvascular decompression, in which the vascular loop is exposed and dissected free of the nerve, and a small sponge made of synthetic material is inserted between these two structures to keep them apart.

The pain can be significantly diminished, or even eliminated, in 80-90% of cases by medical treatment alone, either with carbamazepine or with gabapentin, which has recently come into use for this purpose. Neurosurgical intervention is indicated only if the pain becomes refractory to medication. The options for neurosurgical treatment include, among others, microvascular decompression (mentioned above) and selective percutaneous thermocoagulation of the nociceptive fibers of the trigeminal nerve.

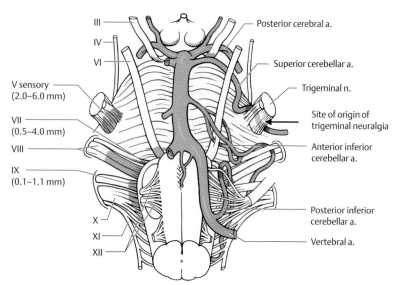

III
IV
VI
Posterior cerebral a.
Superior cerebellar a.
V sensory
(2.0–6.0 mm)
Trigeminal n.
Site of origin of
trigeminal neuralgia
VII
(0.5–4.0 mm)
Anterior inferior
cerebellar a.
VIII
IX
(0.1–1.1 mm)
Posterior inferior
cerebellar a.
X
XI
XII
Vertebral a.

Fig. 4.**31 Unmyelinated portions of the cranial nerve roots** (orange, left) and **nearby vascular loops** (dark red, right) that may irritate the nerve roots at these sites. In particular, the diagram shows **a loop of the superior cerebellar artery that may cause trigeminal neuralgia**.

The most common cause of *symptomatic trigeminal neuralgia* is multiple sclerosis: 2.4% of all MS patients develop trigeminal neuralgia; among these patients, 14% have it bilaterally.

Other, rarer causes of symptomatic pain in the distribution of the trigeminal nerve include dental lesions, sinusitis, bony fractures, and tumors of the cerebellopontine angle, the nose, or the mouth. Pain in the eye or forehead should also arouse suspicion of glaucoma or iritis. The pain of acute glaucoma can mimic that of classic trigeminal neuralgia.

Gradenigo syndrome consists of pain in the distribution of the ophthalmic nerve accompanied by ipsilateral abducens palsy. It is caused by infection in the air cells of the petrous apex.

Differential Diagnosis: Disorders with Facial Pain in the Absence of a Trigeminal Lesion

Charlin neuralgia consists of pain at the inner canthus of the eye and root of the nose accompanied by increased lacrimation. It is thought to be due to irritation of the ciliary ganglion.

Cluster headache is also known as Bing-Horton syndrome, erythroprosopalgia, and histamine headache. It is characterized by brief attacks of pain occurring mainly at night, including during sleep (in distinction to trigeminal neuralgia). These attacks are accompanied by facial erythema, lacrimation, watery nasal secretion, and often Horner syndrome as well. Typical provocative factors include high altitude, alcohol consumption, and the taking of nitroglycerin (glyceryl trinitrate). The attacks occur repeatedly in periods (clusters) characteristically lasting a week or more, separated by headache-free intervals of at least two weeks' duration. There is as yet no consensus on the pathophysiology of this disorder. Its treatment is empirical, with oxygen, triptanes, or other medications.

Facial Nerve (CN VII) and Nervus Intermedius

The facial nerve has two components. The larger component is purely motor and innervates the muscles of facial expression (Fig. 4.**32**). This component is the facial nerve proper. It is accompanied by a thinner nerve, the nervus intermedius, which contains visceral and somatic afferent fibers, as well as visceral efferent fibers (Table 4.**1**, p. 124).

Motor Component of Facial Nerve

The **nucleus** of the motor component of the facial nerve is located in the ventrolateral portion of the pontine tegmentum (Figs. 4.**2** and 4.**3**, and Fig. 4.**33**). The neurons of this motor nucleus are analogous to the anterior horn cells of the spinal cord, but are embryologically derived from the second branchial arch. The **root fibers** of this nucleus take a complicated course. Within the brainstem, they wind around the abducens nucleus (forming the so-called *internal genu of the facial nerve*, Fig. 4.**2**), thereby creating a small bump on the floor of the fourth ventricle (*facial colliculus*) (Fig. 4.**1**). They then form a compact bundle, which travels ventrolaterally to the caudal end of the pons and then exits the brainstem, crosses the subarachnoid space in the cerebellopontine angle, and enters the internal acoustic meatus together with the nervus intermedius and the eighth cranial nerve (the vestibulocochlear nerve). Within the meatus, the **facial nerve** and **nervus intermedius** separate from the eighth nerve and travel laterally in the facial canal toward the geniculate ganglion. At the level of the ganglion, the facial canal takes a sharp downward turn (*external genu of the facial nerve*). At the lower end of the canal, the facial nerve exits the skull through the stylomastoid foramen. Its individual motor fibers are then distributed to all regions of the face (some of them first traveling through the parotid gland). They innervate all of the muscles of facial expression that are derived from the second branchial arch, i.e.,

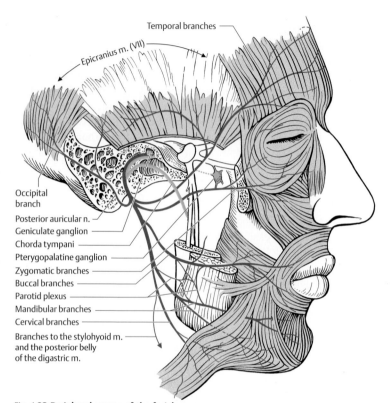

Temporal branches

Epicranius m. (VII)

Occipital
branch
Posterior auricular n.
Geniculate ganglion
Chorda tympani
Pterygopalatine ganglion
Zygomatic branches
Buccal branches
Parotid plexus
Mandibular branches
Cervical branches
Branches to the stylohyoid m.
and the posterior belly
of the digastric m.

Fig. 4.**32 Peripheral course of the facial nerve**

the orbicularis oris and oculi, buccinator, occipitalis, and frontalis muscles and
the smaller muscles in these areas, as well as the stapedius, platysma, stylohyoid
muscle, and posterior belly of the digastric muscle (Fig. 4.**32**).

Reflexes involving the facial nerve. The motor nucleus of the facial nerve participates in a number of reflex arcs. The **corneal reflex** is discussed above (p. 163). In
the **blink reflex**, a strong visual stimulus induces the superior colliculi to send
visual impulses to the facial nucleus in the pons by way of the tectobulbar tract,
with the result that the eyes are immediately closed. Similarly, in the **stapedius
reflex**, auditory impulses are transmitted from the dorsal nucleus of the trapezoid body to the facial nucleus and cause either contraction or relaxation of the
stapedius muscle, depending on the strength of the auditory stimulus.

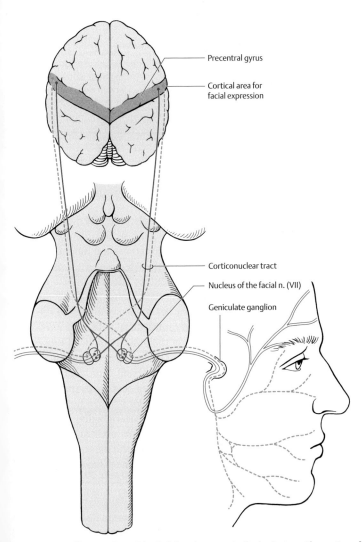

Precentral gyrus

Cortical area for facial expression

Corticonuclear tract

Nucleus of the facial n. (VII)

Geniculate ganglion

Fig. 4.**33 Central innervation of the facial nuclear area in the brainstem.** The portion of the nuclear area controlling the muscles of the forehead is innervated by both cerebral hemispheres. Thus, a lesion affecting the corticonuclear pathway on one side does not cause weakness of the forehead muscles. The remainder of the nuclear area, however, is innervated only by the contralateral hemisphere. A unilateral lesion along the corticonuclear pathway therefore causes contralateral facial weakness with sparing of the forehead muscles.

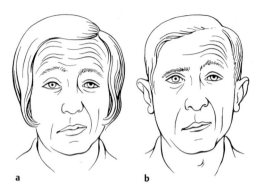

Fig. 4.**34 Facial palsy**
a Central facial palsy: the forehead muscles are not affected.
b Peripheral facial palsy: the forehead muscles are involved along with the rest of the face on the affected side.

Motor lesions involving the distribution of the facial nerve. The muscles of the forehead derive their supranuclear innervation from both cerebral hemispheres, but the remaining muscles of facial expression are innervated only unilaterally, i.e., by the contralateral precentral cortex (Fig. 4.**33**). If the descending supranuclear pathways are interrupted on one side only, e. g., by a cerebral infarct, the resulting facial palsy spares the forehead muscles (Fig. 4.**34a**): the patient can still raise his or her eyebrows and close the eyes forcefully. This type of facial palsy is called **central** facial palsy. In a **nuclear** or **peripheral lesion** (see below), however, all of the muscles of facial expression on the side of the lesion are weak (Fig **4.34b**). One can thus distinguish central from nuclear or peripheral facial palsy by their different clinical appearances.

The motor nuclei of the facial nerve are innervated not only by the facial cortex but also by the diencephalon, which plays a major role in emotion-related facial expressions. Further input is derived from the basal ganglia; in basal ganglia disorders (e. g., Parkinson disease), hypomimia or amimia can be seen. There are also various dyskinetic syndromes affecting the muscles of facial expression with different types of abnormal movement: hemifacial spasm, facial dyskinesias, and blepharospasm, among others. The site of the causative lesion in these syndromes remains unknown.

Idiopathic facial nerve palsy (Bell palsy). This most common disorder affecting the facial nerve arises in about 25 per 100 000 individuals per year. Its cause is still unknown. It is characterized by *flaccid paresis of all muscles of facial expression* (including the forehead muscles), as well as other manifestations depending on the site of the lesion. The various syndromes resulting from nerve damage within the facial canal are depicted in Figure 4.**35**, and a typical MRI correlate of idiopathic facial nerve palsy is shown in Figure 4.**36**. Differential diagno-

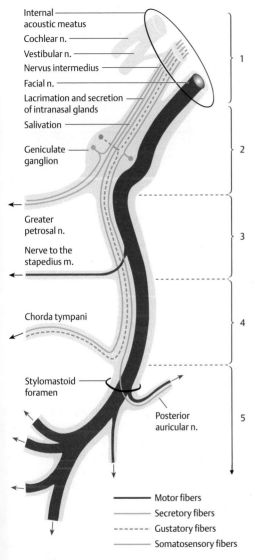

Internal acoustic meatus

Cochlear n.

Vestibular n.

Nervus intermedius

Facial n.

Lacrimation and secretion of intranasal glands

Salivation

Geniculate ganglion

Greater petrosal n.

Nerve to the stapedius m.

Chorda tympani

Stylomastoid foramen

Posterior auricular n.

Motor fibers
Secretory fibers
Gustatory fibers
Somatosensory fibers

Fig. 4.**35 The components of the facial nerve and typical deficits caused by lesions at various sites along its course**

1 Peripheral weakness of the muscles innervated by the facial nerve (muscles of facial expression), hearing loss or deafness, and diminished vestibular excitability.

2 Peripheral weakness and impairment of taste, lacrimation, and salivation.

3 Peripheral weakness of the muscles of facial expression, impairment of taste and salivation, and hearing loss.

4 Peripheral weakness of the muscles of facial expression and impairment of taste and salivation.

5 Peripheral weakness of the muscles of facial expression.

sis is important in cases of acutely arising facial palsy, as not all cases are idiopathic: 10% are due to herpes zoster oticus, 4% to otitis media, and 2% to tumors of various types (parotid tumors, neurinoma, and others).

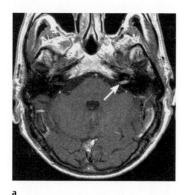
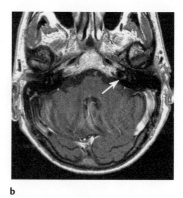

a   b

Fig. 4.**36 MRI in a 73-year-old woman with the acute onset of painless, total left facial nerve palsy** (idiopathic facial nerve palsy, Bell palsy). **a** The contrast-enhanced axial T1-weighted image shows marked contrast uptake along the course of the left facial nerve, as compared to the normal right side. **b** Pathological contrast enhancement is also seen along the further course of the nerve in the petrous bone. Cortisone was given acutely, and the weakness resolved completely within three weeks.

A complete recovery occurs without treatment in 60-80% of all patients. The administration of steroids (prednisolone, 1 mg/kg body weight daily for 5 days), if it is begun within 10 days of the onset of facial palsy, speeds recovery and leads to complete recovery in over 90% of cases, according to a number of published studies.

Partial or misdirected reinnervation of the affected musculature after an episode of idiopathic facial nerve palsy sometimes causes a facial contracture or abnormal accessory movements (*synkinesias*) of the muscles of facial expression. Misdirected reinnervation also explains the phenomenon of "crocodile tears," in which involuntary lacrimation occurs when the patient eats. The reason is presumably that regenerating secretory fibers destined for the salivary glands have taken an incorrect path along the Schwann cell sheaths of degenerated fibers innervating the lacrimal gland, so that some of the impulses for salivation induce lacrimation instead.

Nervus Intermedius

The nervus intermedius contains a number of afferent and efferent components (Table 4.**1**, p. 124).

Gustatory afferent fibers. The cell bodies of the afferent fibers for taste are located in the geniculate ganglion, which contains pseudounipolar cells resembling those of the spinal ganglia. Some of these afferent fibers arise in the taste buds of the anterior two-thirds of the tongue (Fig. 4.**37**). These fibers first accompany the *lingual nerve* (a branch of the mandibular nerve, the lowest division of the trigeminal nerve), and travel by way of the *chorda tympani* to the *geniculate ganglion*, and then in the *nervus intermedius* to the *nucleus of the tractus solitarius*. This nucleus also receives gustatory fibers from the glossopharyngeal nerve, representing taste on the posterior third of the tongue and the vallate papillae, and from the vagus nerve, representing taste on the epiglottis. Thus, taste is supplied by three different nerves (CN VII, IX, and X) on both sides. It follows that complete ageusia on the basis of a nerve lesion is extremely unlikely.

Central propagation of gustatory impulses. The *nucleus of the tractus solitarius* is the common relay nucleus of all gustatory fibers. It sends gustatory impulses to the contralateral *thalamus* (their exact course is unknown) and onward to the most medial component of the *ventral posteromedial nucleus* of the thalamus (VPM, p. 265). From the thalamus, the gustatory pathway continues to the *caudal precentral region* overlying the insula (Fig. 4.**37**).

Afferent somatic fibers. A few somatic afferent fibers representing a small area of the external ear (pinna), the external auditory canal, and the external surface of the tympanum (eardrum) travel in the *facial nerve* to the *geniculate ganglion* and thence to the *sensory nuclei of the trigeminal nerve*. The cutaneous lesion in herpes zoster oticus is due to involvement of these somatic afferent fibers.

Efferent secretory fibers (Fig. 4.**38**). The nervus intermedius also contains efferent parasympathetic fibers originating from the *superior salivatory nucleus* (Fig. 4.**38**), which lies medial and caudal to the motor nucleus of the facial nerve. Some of the root fibers of this nucleus leave the main trunk of the facial nerve at the level of the geniculate ganglion and proceed to the *pterygopalatine ganglion* and onward to the *lacrimal gland* and to the *glands of the nasal mucosa*. Other root fibers take a more caudal route, by way of the chorda tympani and the lingual nerve, to the *submandibular ganglion*, in which a synaptic relay is found. The postganglionic fibers innervate the *sublingual and submandibular glands* (Fig. 4.**38**), inducing salivation. As mentioned above, the superior salivatory nucleus receives input from the olfactory system through the dorsal longitudinal fasciculus. This connection provides the anatomical basis for reflex salivation in response to an appetizing smell. The lacrimal glands receive their central input from the hypothalamus (emotion) by way of the brainstem reticular formation, as well as from the spinal nucleus of the trigeminal nerve (irritation of the conjunctiva).

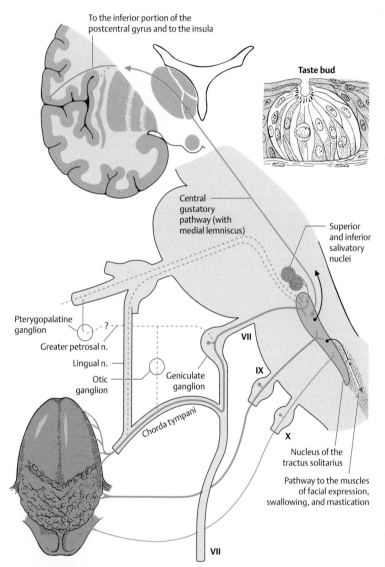

To the inferior portion of the
postcentral gyrus and to the insula

Taste bud

Central
gustatory
pathway (with
medial lemniscus)

Superior
and inferior
salivatory
nuclei

Pterygopalatine
ganglion

?

Greater petrosal n.

Lingual n.

Otic
ganglion

Geniculate
ganglion

VII

IX

Chorda tympani

X

Nucleus of the
tractus solitarius

Pathway to the muscles
of facial expression,
swallowing, and mastication

VII

Fig. 4.**37 Afferent gustatory fibers and the gustatory pathway.** The drawing shows the peripheral receptors (taste buds), the peripheral course of the gustatory fibers (along the nervus intermedius and the glosspharyngeal and vagus nerves), and their central connections with the corresponding brainstem nuclei.

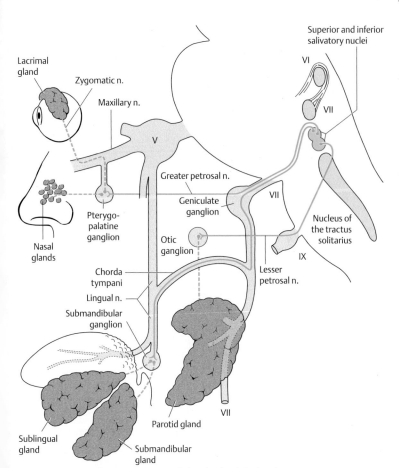

Fig. 4.**38 Parasympathetic innervation of the glands of the head**

Vestibulocochlear Nerve (CN VIII)—Cochlear Component and the Organ of Hearing

The organs of balance and hearing are derived from a single embryological precursor in the petrous portion of the temporal bone: the utriculus gives rise to the vestibular system with its three semicircular canals, while the sacculus gives rise to the inner ear with its snaillike cochlea (Fig. 4.**39**).

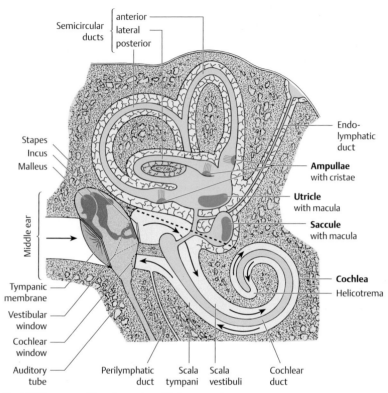

Fig. 4.**39 The organ of hearing and equilibrium**: overview

Auditory perception. Sound waves are vibrations in the air produced by a wide variety of mechanisms (tones, speech, song, instrumental music, natural sounds, environmental noise, etc.). These vibrations are transmitted along the external auditory canal to the eardrum (tympanum or tympanic membrane), which separates the external from middle ear (Fig. 4.**39**).

The *middle ear* (Fig. 4.**39**) contains air and is connected to the nasopharyngeal space (and thus to the outside world) through the auditory tube, also called the eustachian tube. The middle ear consists of a bony cavity (the *vestibulum*) whose walls are covered with a mucous membrane. Its medial wall contains two orifices closed up with collagenous tissue, which are called the oval window or foramen ovale (alternatively, *fenestra vestibuli*) and the round window or foramen rotundum (*fenestra cochleae*). These two windows separate the tympanic cavity from the inner ear, which is filled with perilymph. Incoming sound waves set the tympanic membrane in vibration. The three *ossicles* (malleus, incus, and stapes) then transmit the oscillations of the tympanic membrane to the oval window, setting it in vibration as well and producing oscillation of the perilymph. The tympanic cavity also contains two small muscles, the *tensor tympani muscle* (CN V) and the *stapedius muscle* (CN VII). By contracting and relaxing, these muscles alter the motility of the auditory ossicles in response to the intensity of incoming sound, so that the organ of Corti is protected against damage from very loud stimuli.

Inner ear. The auditory portion of the inner ear has a bony component and a membranous component (Figs. 4.**39**, 4.**40**). The bony cochlea forms a spiral with two-and-a-half revolutions, resembling a common garden snail. (Fig. 4.**39** shows a truncated cochlea for didactic purposes only.) The cochlea contains an antechamber (*vestibule*) and a *bony tube*, lined with epithelium that winds around the modiolus, a tapering bony structure containing the spiral ganglion. A cross section of the cochlear duct reveals **three membranous compartments**: the **scala vestibuli**, the **scala tympani**, and the **scala media** (or cochlear duct), which contains the organ of Corti (Fig. 4.**40**). The **scala vestibuli** and **scala tympani** are filled with perilymph, while the **cochlear duct** is filled with *endolymph*, a fluid produced by the stria vascularis. The cochlear duct terminates blindly at each end (in the cecum vestibulare at its base and in the cecum cupulare at its apex). The upper wall of the cochlear duct is formed by the very thin *Reissner's membrane*, which divides the endolymph from the perilymph of the scala vestibuli, freely transmitting the pressure waves of the scala vestibuli to the cochlear duct so that the *basilar membrane* is set in vibration. The pressure waves of the perilymph begin at the oval window and travel through the scala vestibuli along the entire length of the cochlea up to its apex, where they enter the scala tympani through a small opening called the helicotrema; the waves then travel the length of the cochlea in the scala tympani, finally arriving at the round window, where a thin membrane seals off the inner ear from the middle ear.

The **organ of Corti** (spiral organ) rests on the basilar membrane along its entire length, from the vestibulum to the apex (Fig. 4.**41**). It is composed of hair cells and supporting cells (Fig. 4.**40c** and **d**). The **hair cells** are the *receptors of the organ of hearing*, in which the mechanical energy of sound waves is transduced into electrochemical potentials. There are about 3500 *inner hair cells*, arranged in a single row, and 12 000-19 000 *outer hair cells*, arranged in three or more rows. Each hair cell has about 100 stereocilia, some of which extend into the tectorial membrane. When the basilar membrane oscillates, the stereocilia

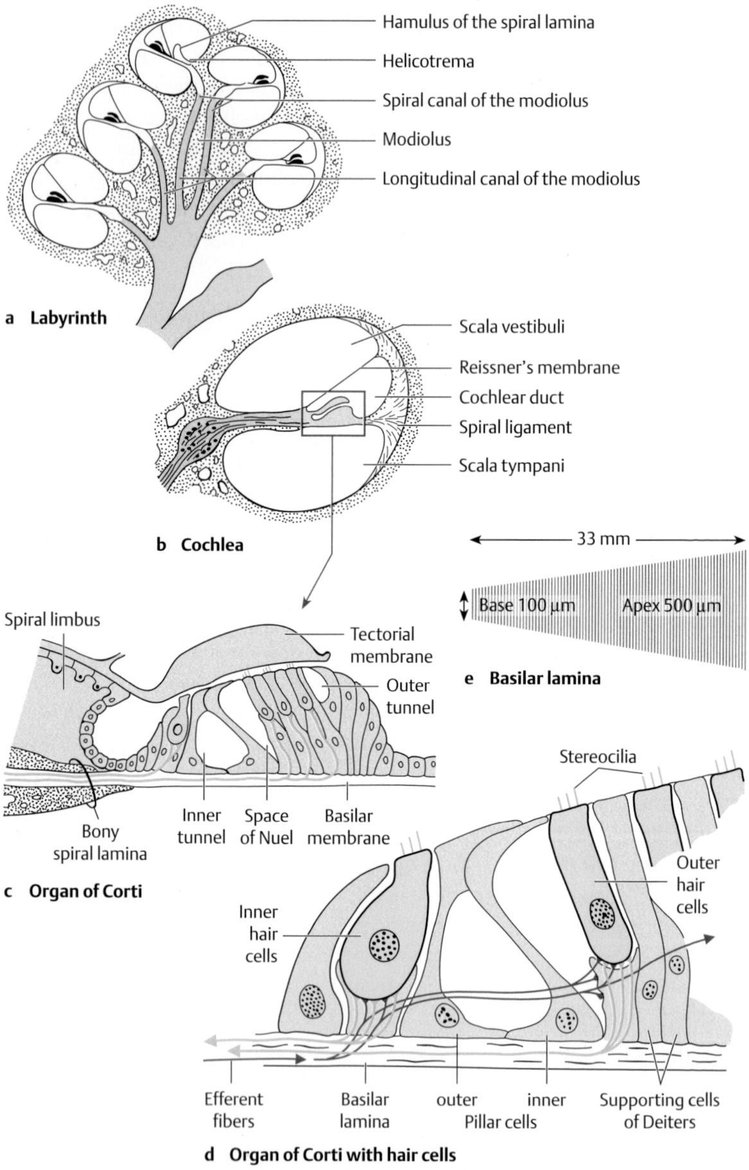

Fig. 4.**40 The microscopic architecture of the organ of hearing. a** Labyrinth. **b** Cochlea. **c** and **d** Organ of Corti. **e** Basilar membrane (lamina).

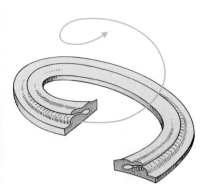

Fig. 4.**41 The course of the basilar lamina**

are bent where they come into contact with the nonoscillating tectorial membrane; this is presumed to be the mechanical stimulus that excites the auditory receptor cells. In addition to the sensory cells (hair cells), the organ of Corti also contains several kinds of *supporting cells*, such as the Deiters cells, as well as empty spaces (tunnels), whose function will not be further discussed here (but see Fig. 4.**40d**). Movement of the footplate of the stapes into the foramen ovale creates a traveling wave along the strands of the basilar membrane, which are oriented transversely to the direction of movement of the wave. An applied pure tone of a given frequency is associated with a particular site on the basilar membrane at which it produces the maximal membrane deviation (i.e., an amplitude maximum). The basilar membrane thus possesses a *tonotopic* organization, in which higher frequencies are registered in the more basal portions of the membrane, and lower frequencies in more apical portions. This may be compared to a piano keyboard, on which the frequency becomes higher from left to right. The basilar membrane is wider at the basilar end than at the apical end (Fig. 4.**40e**).

The **spiral ganglion** (Fig. 4.**42**) contains about 25 000 bipolar and 5 000 unipolar neurons, which have central and peripheral processes. The peripheral processes receive input from the inner hair cells, and the central processes come together to form the cochlear nerve.

Cochlear nerve and auditory pathway. The **cochlear nerve,** formed by the central processes of the spiral ganglion cells, passes along the internal auditory canal together with the vestibular nerve, traverses the subarachnoid space in the cerebellopontine angle, and then enters the brainstem just behind the inferior cerebellar peduncle. In the ventral cochlear nucleus, the fibers of the cochlear nerve split into two branches (like a "T"); each branch then proceeds

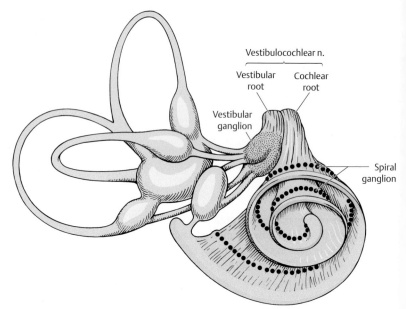

Fig. 4.**42 The spiral ganglion and the vestibular ganglion**

to the site of the next relay (second neuron of the auditory pathway) in the ventral or dorsal cochlear nucleus. The second neuron projects impulses centrally along a number of different pathways, some of which contain further synaptic relays (Fig. 4.**43**).

Neurites (axons) derived from the **ventral cochlear nucleus** cross the midline within the **trapezoid body**. Some of these neurites form a synapse with a further neuron in the trapezoid body itself, while the rest proceed to other relay stations—the superior olivary nucleus, the nucleus of the lateral lemniscus, or the reticular formation. Ascending auditory impulses then travel by way of the lateral lemniscus to the inferior colliculi (though some fibers probably bypass the colliculi and go directly to the medial geniculate bodies).

Neurites arising in the **dorsal cochlear nucleus** cross the midline behind the inferior cerebellar peduncle, some of them in the striae medullares and others through the reticular formation, and then ascend in the lateral lemniscus to the inferior colliculi, together with the neurites from the ventral cochlear nucleus.

The **inferior colliculi** contain a further synaptic relay onto the next neurons in the pathway, which, in turn, project to the **medial geniculate bodies** of the thalamus. From here, auditory impulses travel in the **auditory radiation**, which

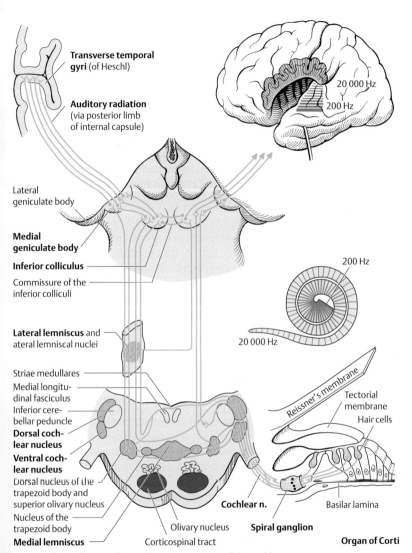

Transverse temporal gyri (of Heschl)

Auditory radiation (via posterior limb of internal capsule)

20 000 Hz

200 Hz

Lateral geniculate body

Medial geniculate body

Inferior colliculus

Commissure of the inferior colliculi

200 Hz

Lateral lemniscus and lateral lemniscal nuclei

20 000 Hz

Reissner's membrane

Striae medullares

Medial longitudinal fasciculus

Inferior cerebellar peduncle

Dorsal cochlear nucleus

Ventral cochlear nucleus

Dorsal nucleus of the trapezoid body and superior olivary nucleus

Nucleus of the trapezoid body

Medial lemniscus

Olivary nucleus

Corticospinal tract

Cochlear n.

Spiral ganglion

Tectorial membrane

Hair cells

Basilar lamina

Organ of Corti

Fig. 4.**43 The auditory pathway.** Central connections of the cochlear nerve.

is located in the posterior limb of the internal capsule (Fig. 3.**2**, p. 58), to the primary auditory cortex in the transverse temporal gyri (area 41 of Brodmann), which are also called the transverse gyri of Heschl (Fig. 9.**10**, p. 358). A tonotopic representation of auditory frequencies is preserved throughout the auditory pathway from the organ of Corti all the way to the auditory cortex (Fig. 4.**43a** and **c**), in an analogous fashion to the somatotopic (retinotopic) organization of the visual pathway.

Bilateral projection of auditory impulses. Not all auditory fibers cross the midline within the brainstem: part of the pathway remains ipsilateral, with the result that injury to a single lateral lemniscus does not cause total unilateral deafness, but rather only partial deafness on the opposite side, as well as an impaired perception of the direction of sound.

Auditory association areas. Adjacent to the primary auditory areas of the cerebral cortex, there are secondary auditory areas on the external surface of the temporal lobe (**areas 42** and **22**; Fig: 9.**26**, p. 385), in which the auditory stimuli are analyzed, identified, and compared with auditory memories laid down earlier, and also classified as to whether they represent noise, tones, melodies, or words and sentences, i.e., speech. If these cortical areas are damaged, the patient may lose the ability to identify sounds or to understand speech (*sensory aphasia*, p. 392).

Integration of auditory processing in various reflex arcs. The pathway from the organ of Corti to the primary auditory cortex is 4-6 neurons long; at each of the relay stations in this pathway (superior olivary nucleus, reticular formation, nucleus of the lateral lemniscus, and inferior colliculi), collateral fibers arise that participate in a number of reflex arcs.

- Some impulses travel to the *cerebellum*, while others pass in the medial longitudinal fasciculus to the *nuclei innervating the extraocular muscles* and bring about conjugate eye movements in the direction of a sound.
- Some impulses pass through the inferior and superior colliculi to the pretectal area and then, by way of the tectobulbar tract, to various brainstem nuclei, including the *nucleus of the facial nerve* (stapedius muscle), or by way of the tectospinal tract to *motor anterior horn cells in the cervical spinal cord.* The impulses that descend to the cervical spinal cord bring about a repositioning of the head toward or away from the origin of a sound.
- Other impulses travel in the ascending reticular activating system to the *reticular formation* (arousal reaction, p. 270).
- Yet others descend in the lateral lemniscus and, via interneurons, exert a regulating influence on the *tension of the basilar lamina.* Some of these de-

scending impulses are thought to have an inhibitory effect; their function is presumably to improve the perception of certain frequencies by suppressing other, neighboring frequencies.

Hearing Disorders

Conductive and Sensorineural Hearing Loss

Two types of hearing loss can be clinically distinguished: middle ear (conductive) hearing loss and inner ear (sensorineural) hearing loss.

Conductive hearing loss is caused by *processes affecting the external auditory canal* or, more commonly, the *middle ear*. Vibrations in the air (sound waves) are poorly transmitted to the inner ear, or not at all. Vibrations in bone can still be conducted to the organ of Corti and be heard (see Rinne test, below).

The **causes** of conductive hearing loss include defects of the tympanic membrane, a serotympanum, mucotympanum, or hemotympanum; interruption of the ossicular chain by trauma or inflammation; calcification of the ossicles (otosclerosis); destructive processes such as cholesteatoma; and tumors (glomus tumor, less commonly carcinoma of the auditory canal).

Inner ear or sensorineural hearing loss is caused by lesions affecting the organ of Corti, the cochlear nerve, or the central auditory pathway.

Inner ear function can be impaired by congenital malformations, medications (antibiotics), industrial poisons (e. g., benzene, aniline, and organic solvents), infection (mumps, measles, zoster), metabolic disturbances, or trauma (fracture, acoustic trauma).

Diagnostic evaluation of hearing loss. In the **Rinne test**, the examiner determines whether auditory stimuli are perceived better if conducted through the air or through bone. The handle of a vibrating tuning fork is placed on the mastoid process. As soon as the patient can no longer hear the tone, the examiner tests whether he or she can hear it with the end of the tuning fork held next to the ear, which a normal subject should be able to do (positive Rinne test = normal finding). In middle ear hearing loss, the patient can hear the tone longer by bone conduction than by air conduction (negative Rinne test = pathological finding).

In the **Weber test**, the handle of a vibrating tuning fork is placed on the vertex of the patient's head, i.e., in the midline. A normal subject hears the tone in the midline; a patient with unilateral conductive hearing loss localizes the tone to the damaged side, while one with unilateral sensorineural hearing loss localizes it to the normal side.

Further diagnostic testing. Middle ear lesions lie in the domain of the otorhinolaryngologist, but lesions of the cochlear nerve and the central auditory pathway are the neurologist's concern.

The bedside tests described above for the differentiation of conductive and sensorineural hearing loss are insufficient for precise diagnostic assessment, which requires **audiometry**, a quantitative and reproducible measurement of hearing ability. The auditory thresholds for air and bone conduction are measured at different frequencies. In conductive hearing loss, the threshold for air conduction is worse than that for bone conduction. In sensorineural hearing loss, the finding depends on the underlying lesion: high-frequency hearing loss is found in old age (presbycusis) and in other forms of acute or chronic hearing loss, but a low-frequency trough of auditory perception is found in Ménière's disease.

Neurological disorders causing hearing loss. **Ménière's disease**, mentioned briefly above, is a disorder of the inner ear causing hearing loss and other neurological manifestations. It is characterized by the clinical triad of rotatory vertigo with nausea and vomiting, fluctuating unilateral partial or total hearing loss, and tinnitus. It is caused by a disturbance of the osmotic equilibrium of the endolymph, resulting in hydrops of the endolymphatic space and rupture of the barrier between the endolymph and the perilymph. The symptoms are treated with antivertiginous medications and intratympanic perfusion with various agents. Beta-histidine is given prophylactically.

Sudden hearing loss, usually accompanied by tinnitus, is presumed to be caused in most cases either by a viral infection or by ischemia in the territory of the labyrinthine artery (an end artery).

The central auditory connections in the brainstem can be affected by vascular processes, inflammation, infection, and tumors. The result is hearing loss. Only bilateral interruption of the auditory pathways in the brainstem can cause total bilateral deafness.

"Acoustic neuroma" is a common, though inaccurate, designation for a tumor that actually arises from the vestibular nerve and is, histologically, a schwannoma. Such tumors will be described in the next section, which deals with the vestibular nerve.

Vestibulocochlear Nerve (CN VIII)—Vestibular Component and Vestibular System

Three different systems participate in the regulation of balance (equilibrium): the vestibular system, the proprioceptive system (i.e., perception of the position of muscles and joints), and the visual system.

The **vestibular system** is composed of the *labyrinth*, the vestibular portion of the eighth cranial nerve (i.e., the *vestibular nerve*, a portion of the vestibulo-cochlear nerve), and the *vestibular nuclei* of the brainstem, with their central connections.

The labyrinth lies within the petrous portion of the temporal bone and consists of the **utricle**, the saccule, and the **three semicircular canals** (Fig. 4.39). The membranous labyrinth is separated from the bony labyrinth by a small space filled with perilymph; the membranous organ itself is filled with endolymph.

The utricle, the saccule, and the widened portions (ampullae) of the semicircular canals contain receptor organs whose function is to maintain balance.

The *three semicircular canals* lie in different planes. The lateral semicircular canal lies in the horizontal plane, and the two other semicircular canals are perpendicular to it and to each other. The posterior semicircular canal is aligned with the axis of the petrous bone, while the anterior semicircular canal is oriented transversely to it. Since the axis of the petrous bone lies at a 45° angle to the midline, it follows that the anterior semicircular canal of one ear is parallel to the posterior semicircular canal of the opposite ear, and vice versa. The two lateral semicircular canals lie in the same plane (the horizontal plane).

Each of the three semicircular canals communicates with the utricle. Each semicircular canal is widened at one end to form an **ampulla**, in which the receptor organ of the vestibular system, the *crista ampullaris*, is located (Fig. 4.**44**). The sensory hairs of the crista are embedded in one end of an elongated gelatinous mass called the *cupula*, which contains no otoliths (see below). Movement of endolymph in the semicircular canals stimulates the sensory hairs of the cristae, which are thus kinetic receptors (movement receptors).

The *utricle* and *saccule* contain further receptor organs, the *utricular* and *saccular macules* (Fig. 4.**45**). The utricular macule lies in the floor of the utricle parallel to the base of the skull, and the saccular macule lies vertically in the medial wall of the saccule. The hair cells of the macule are embedded in a gelatinous membrane containing calcium carbonate crystals, called statoliths. They are flanked by supporting cells.

These receptors transmit static impulses, indicating the position of the head in space, to the brainstem. They also exert an influence on muscle tone.

Impulses arising in the receptors of the labyrinth form the afferent limb of reflex arcs that serve to coordinate the extraocular, nuchal, and body muscles so that balance is maintained with every position and every type of movement of the head.

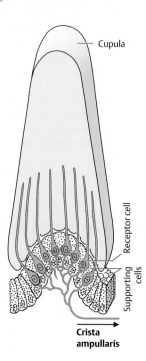

Fig. 4.**44 The crista ampullaris**

Cupula

Receptor cell

Supporting cells

Crista ampullaris

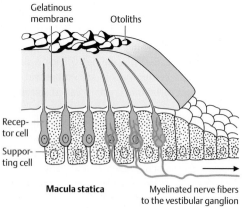

Fig. 4.**45 The macula statica**

Gelatinous membrane

Otoliths

Receptor cell

Supporting cell

Macula statica

Myelinated nerve fibers to the vestibular ganglion

Vestibulocochlear nerve. The next station for impulse transmission in the vestibular system is the vestibulocochlear nerve. The **vestibular ganglion** is located in the internal auditory canal; it contains bipolar cells whose peripheral processes receive input from the receptor cells in the vestibular organ, and whose central processes form the **vestibular nerve**. This nerve joins the cochlear nerve, with which it traverses the internal auditory canal, crosses the subarachnoid space at the cerebellopontine angle, and enters the brainstem at the pontomedullary junction. Its fibers then proceed to the vestibular nuclei, which lie in the floor of the fourth ventricle.

The **vestibular nuclear complex** (Fig. 4.**46a**) is made up of:
- The superior vestibular nucleus (of Bekhterev)
- The lateral vestibular nucleus (of Deiters)
- The medial vestibular nucleus (of Schwalbe)
- The inferior vestibular nucleus (of Roller)

The fibers of the vestibular nerve split into branches before entering the individual cell groups of the vestibular nucleus complex, in which they form a synaptic relay with a second neuron (Fig. 4.**46b**).

Afferent and efferent connections of the vestibular nuclei. The anatomy of the afferent and efferent connections of the vestibular nuclei is not precisely known at present. The current state of knowledge is as follows (Fig. 4.**47**):
- Some fibers derived from the vestibular nerve convey impulses directly to the **flocculonodular lobe of the cerebellum (archicerebellum)** by way of the juxtarestiform tract, which is adjacent to the inferior cerebellar peduncle. The flocculonodular lobe projects, in turn, to the fastigial nucleus and, by way of the uncinate fasciculus (of Russell), back to the vestibular nuclei; some fibers return via the vestibular nerve to the hair cells of the labyrinth, where they exert a mainly inhibitory regulating effect. Moreover, the archicerebellum contains second-order fibers from the superior, medial, and inferior vestibular nuclei (Figs. 4.**47** and 4.**48**) and sends efferent fibers directly back to the vestibular nuclear complex, as well as to spinal motor neurons, via cerebelloreticular and reticulospinal pathways.
- The important lateral vestibulospinal tract originates in the lateral vestibular nucleus (of Deiters) and descends ipsilaterally in the anterior fasciculus to the γ **and** α **motor neurons of the spinal cord**, down to sacral levels. The impulses conveyed in the lateral vestibulospinal tract serve to facilitate the extensor reflexes and to maintain a level of muscle tone throughout the body that is necessary for balance.
- Fibers of the medial vestibular nucleus enter the medial longitudinal fasciculus bilaterally and descend in it to the **anterior horn cells of the cervi-**

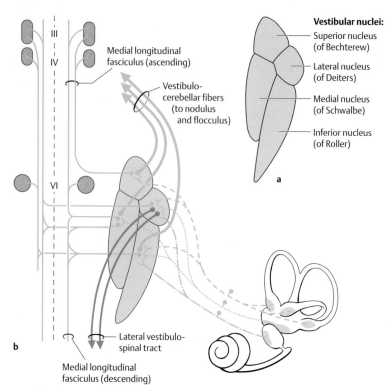

Fig. 4.46 **The vestibular nuclear complex and its central connections. a** Components of the vestibular nuclei. **b** Central connections of the individual components of the vestibular nuclei.

cal spinal cord, or as the medial vestibulospinal tract to the **upper thoracic spinal cord**. These fibers descend in the anterior portion of the cervical spinal cord, adjacent to the anterior median fissure, as the sulcomarginal fasciculus, and distribute themselves to the anterior horn cells at cervical and upper thoracic levels. They affect nuchal muscle tone in response to the position of the head and probably also participate in reflexes that maintain equilibrium with balancing movements of the arms.

- All of the vestibular nuclei project to the nuclei innervating the **extraocular muscles** by way of the medial longitudinal fasciculus. Anatomists have been able to follow some vestibular fibers to the nuclear groups of Cajal (interstitial nucleus) and Darkschewitsch and further on into the thalamus (Fig. 4.**47**).

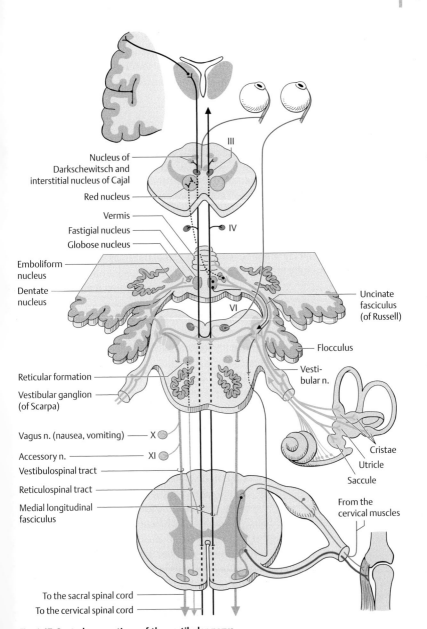

Nucleus of
Darkschewitsch and
interstitial nucleus of Cajal

III

Red nucleus

Vermis

Fastigial nucleus

Globose nucleus

Emboliform
nucleus

Dentate
nucleus

IV

VI

Uncinate
fasciculus
(of Russell)

Flocculus

Vesti-
bular n.

Reticular formation

Vestibular ganglion
(of Scarpa)

Vagus n. (nausea, vomiting) — X

Accessory n. — XI

Vestibulospinal tract

Reticulospinal tract

Medial longitudinal
fasciculus

Cristae

Utricle

Saccule

From the
cervical muscles

To the sacral spinal cord

To the cervical spinal cord

Fig. 4.**47 Central connections of the vestibular nerve**

The complex of structures consisting of the vestibular nuclei and the flocculonodular lobe of the cerebellum plays an important role in the maintenance of equilibrium and muscle tone. Equilibrium is also served by spinocerebellar and cerebellocerebellar projections, which will be discussed later in Chapter 5.

Disturbances of Equilibrium

Dizziness and dysequilibrium are, after headache, the symptoms that most commonly lead patients to seek medical attention. In colloquial speech, "dizziness" refers to a wide variety of abnormal feelings. "Dizziness" sometimes means true vertigo, i.e., a sensation of movement or rotation in some direction: patients may describe feeling as if they were on a carousel, a shifting boat, or an elevator starting to move or coming to a halt. Many patients, however, use the word loosely for other conditions, such as being dazed, feeling one is about to faint, being unsteady on one's feet (a common complaint of the elderly), or mild anxiety, as in claustrophobia. Patients complaining of "dizziness" should, therefore, be carefully interviewed to determine the precise nature of the complaint. **Vertigo** is, by definition, the abnormal and disturbing feeling that one is moving with respect to the environment (subjective vertigo), or that the environment is moving when it is actually stationary (objective vertigo; note that the words "subjective" and "objective" do not have their common meanings in these two expressions). Patients with vertigo may also have **oscillopsia**, a visual illusion in which objects seem to move back and forth. Only when "dizziness" is truly vertigo, according to the strict definition of the term, is it likely to be due to a disturbance in the vestibular or visual systems, or both, and to require evaluation by a neurologist. Nondirected feelings of unsteadiness or presyncope, on the other hand, are more likely to be nonspecific manifestations of a cardiovascular disorder, intoxication, or depression.

The cause of most cases of vertigo is presumed to be an imbalance of the sensory impulses relating to motion that reach the brain through three different perceptual systems—visual, vestibular, and somatosensory (proprioceptive). This is known as the hypothesis of **sensory conflict** or *polysensory mismatch*.

Even in normal individuals, "unusual" movement of various kinds can induce vertigo. The most bothersome manifestations of motion sickness are autonomic (nausea, pallor, hypotension, fatigue, yawning, diaphoresis, and vomiting), while the vertigo itself usually causes less suffering for the patient and may be barely noticed. Normal persons can suffer from severe motion sickness when there is a blatant sensory conflict, e. g., when the individual is below deck on a large ship. In this situation, the visual system reports that the environment is stationary, in contradiction to the continual movement signaled by the vestibular system. Once the inciting stimulus is removed, motion sickness subsides slowly within the following 24 hours.

Vestibular disorders cause vertigo rather than nonspecific dizziness. The responsible lesion may be anywhere in the **vestibular system** (a collective term for the vestibular organ, the vestibulocochlear nerve, and the vestibular nuclei, as well as their central connections). Vestibular vertigo is felt as either rotatory or translational (corresponding to the roles of the semicircular canals and the otoliths, respectively), and is associated with **nystagmus**. A lesion of the vestibular organ or the vestibulocochlear nerve on one side produces a difference in the level of activity of the vestibular nuclei on the two sides, which is interpreted by the central vestibular apparatus as indicating movement to the side of the higher activity (i.e., the normal side). This, in turn, induces the vestibulo-ocular reflex (VOR), i.e., nystagmus, with a rapid component toward the normal ear and a slow component toward the side of the lesion (but see also vestibular neuritis, p. 193). Vestibular nystagmus often has a rotatory (torsional) component, which is easiest to see when the fixation of gaze is eliminated with Frenzel goggles, and which increases further when the patient gazes in the direction of the rapid phase (*Alexander's law*).

Vestibular vertigo causes **nausea and vomiting**, at least initially, as well as a **tendency to fall to the side of the lesion**. The accompanying nystagmus induces illusory motion of the environment (oscillopsia). The patient, therefore, prefers to keep his or her eyes closed, and to avoid further irritation of the vestibular system by keeping the head in a fixed position, with the abnormal ear upper-

Autoinduction of Vestibular Vertigo (an Experiment)

Instructions: Put a coin or other small object on the floor, stand directly over it, bend the head about 30° forward to keep the coin in view, and then rotate rapidly 5 or 6 times to the right around the axis of your own body. Stop suddenly, stand up, and extend both arms forward.

What happens? The subject suddenly feels as if he or she is rotating to the left and tends to fall to the right, while the arms deviate to the right. This experiment might cause the subject to fall, so at least one other person should be present to lend support, if necessary. It might also induce nausea or even vomiting. Nystagmus is observed, in the opposite direction to the rotation. *Explanation*: Keeping the head bent 30° forward during the rotation puts the horizontal

semicircular canals exactly into the plane of rotation. Rapid turning sets the fluid (endolymph) in the canals in motion. The inertia of the fluid keeps it moving in the same direction for a little while after the individual suddenly stops turning. The fluid moves past the now stationary cristae, producing the illusion of continued movement.

When this experiment is performed, excitatory impulses from the semicircular canals also travel to the nuclei controlling eye movement (producing nystagmus), to the spinal cord (causing unsteadiness of stance and gait, with a tendency to fall), and to the autonomic centers in the reticular formation.

most. Lesions affecting the vestibular nuclei in the floor of the fourth ventricle can produce similar symptoms.

One can gain some idea of what it feels like to have a vestibular lesion by performing the experiment described on p. 191 on oneself.

Proprioceptive vertigo (or, more accurately, proprioceptive unsteadiness) is usually motion-dependent and non-directional and is due to an abnormality of the proprioceptive impulses arising in the cervical spinal cord. It can also be caused by peripheral neuropathy or by lesions of the posterior columns, either of which can impair central transmission of proprioceptive impulses from the lower limbs. Proprioceptive unsteadiness of the latter type is characterized by prominent unsteadiness of gait, without nystagmus. The gait disturbance characteristically worsens when the eyes are closed, or in the dark, because the individual can no longer use visual input to compensate for the missing proprioceptive information.

Peripheral Vestibular Lesions

Positioning Vertigo

Benign paroxysmal positioning vertigo (BPPV) is the most common cause of directional vertigo, accounting for 20% of all cases.

Patients with BPPV typically report **brief attacks of intense rotatory vertigo** arising a short time after **rapid movements of the head**, usually when the head is leaned backward or turned to one side, with the affected ear upward (e. g., when the patient turns in bed). The vertigo subsides in 10-60 seconds. This type of vertigo is caused by detachment of statoliths from the statolith membrane. Under the influence of gravity, the statoliths migrate to the lowest part of the labyrinth, where they can easily be swept into the entrance to the posterior semicircular canal when the patient lies supine. The detached statoliths can also (rarely) enter the lateral semicircular canal.

Movement in the plane of the affected semicircular canal sets the crystals within it in motion, producing relative motion of the endolymph (**canalolithiasis**; piston effect), which is transmitted to the cupula. The impulses that originate in the affected semicircular canal produce a sensation of movement and nystagmus in the plane of the stimulated semicircular canal, which begins after a short latency interval and subsides within 60 seconds. Repetition of the precipitating head movement leads to a transient diminution of the symptomatic response (habituation).

The treatment consists of rapid repositioning maneuvers in the plane of the affected semicircular canal, by means of which the statoliths can be drawn out of the canal.

In the differential diagnosis of BPPV, one must consider **central positional vertigo** due to lesions in the region of the floor of the fourth ventricle involving the vestibular nuclei or their connections. A lesion of the cerebellar nodulus, for example, produces downbeat positional nystagmus when the head is bowed. Central positional vertigo is sometimes accompanied by severe vomiting, but more commonly by relatively mild nausea. In central positional vertigo, unlike BPPV, nystagmus and vertigo are often dissociated: the nystagmus is largely independent of the speed at which the patient is repositioned, it tends to persist for a longer time, it may change direction depending on the position of the head, and it is usually accompanied by further abnormalities of gaze fixation and pursuit.

Vestibular Neuropathy

An acute, unilateral vestibular deficit (vestibular neuropathy or neuritis = acute loss of function of, usually, a single vestibular organ or vestibular nerve) is the second most common cause of rotatory vertigo. Although, in most cases, no cause can be definitively identified, much evidence suggests that such episodes are of *viral origin*, in similar fashion to idiopathic facial palsy (Bell palsy) and acute hearing loss.

The main symptom of vestibular neuropathy is **severe rotatory vertigo of acute onset and several days' duration**, which is exacerbated by movements of the head. This is accompanied by horizontal torsional nystagmus that beats away from the side of the lesion, as well as a tendency to fall to the affected side, nausea, vomiting, and intense malaise. A mild prodrome in the form of brief, transient sensations of vertigo occasionally precedes the acute attack by a few days. Hearing is most often unaffected, but if hearing loss is found, the differential diagnosis must include infectious illnesses such as mumps, measles, mononucleosis, borreliosis, neurosyphilis, and herpes zoster oticus; an acoustic neuroma; ischemia in the territory of the labyrinthine artery; and Ménière's disease. Vestibular neuropathy tends to affect persons between the ages of 30 and 60 years and does not become more common in old age, which implies that it is probably not due to ischemia. The diagnosis is established by a finding of impaired excitability of the affected labyrinth on caloric testing in the absence of other neurological manifestations (such as other cranial nerve, cerebellar, or brainstem deficits). The vertigo and unsteadiness improve slowly over 1-2 weeks, and all symptoms generally resolve completely by three weeks after their onset. Treatment with bed rest and antivertiginous agents is indicated only in the first two or three days. Patients should start a specific, directed gymnastics program as soon as possible, including balance exercises that are easy to learn and to perform at home, to help speed their recovery.

Acoustic Neuroma

As already stated, the common (indeed almost universal) designation "acoustic neuroma" is actually a misnomer for a schwannoma arising from the vestibular fibers of the vestibulocochlear nerve. The tumor destroys these fibers first, slowly and progressively impairing the excitability of the vestibular organ on the affected side; patients rarely suffer from vertigo, because this deficit can be compensated for at higher levels of vestibular processing, but the asymmetric excitability can be demonstrated by caloric testing. Depending on whether the tumor grows rapidly or slowly, irritation and/or compression of the fibers of the cochlear nerve leads sooner or later to clinically evident **high-frequency hearing loss**. The diagnosis of acoustic neuroma is supported by the finding of high-frequency hearing loss by audiometry, and of a prolonged conduction time by measurement of brainstem auditory evoked potentials (BAEP); it can be confirmed by MRI. There is, however, no direct and reliable relationship between the size of the tumor and the severity of the hearing loss that it causes.

Further growth of the tumor can compress neighboring structures (brainstem, facial nerve, trigeminal nerve), leading to further cranial nerve deficits (e. g., impaired lacrimation and taste due to dysfunction of the chorda tympani) and, finally, to symptomatic compression of the brainstem and cerebellum.

Patients with bilateral acoustic neuroma most likely suffer from neurofibromatosis type II (also called bilateral acoustic neuromatosis).

The treatment of acoustic neuroma is currently the subject of intense discussion among neurosurgeons. Many lesions that previously could only have been treated by open surgery can now be treated with as good or better results by stereotactic radiosurgery (i.e., with the Gamma Knife or a stereotactic linear accelerator).

Vagal System (CN IX, X, and the Cranial Portion of XI)

Glossopharyngeal Nerve (CN XI)

The glossopharyngeal nerve shares so many of its functions with the nervus intermedius, the vagus nerve, and the cranial portion of the accessory nerve that these nerves can be considered together as a single "vagal system" to avoid making the presentation unnecessarily repetitive. These nerves are all mixed (sensory and motor) nerves, and some of their components arise from common brainstem nuclei (the nucleus ambiguus and nucleus solitarius) (cf. Table 4.**1** and Figs. 4.**2** and 4.**3**).

Anatomical course and distribution (Fig. 4.**48**). The glossopharyngeal, vagal, and accessory nerves exit the skull together through the jugular foramen,

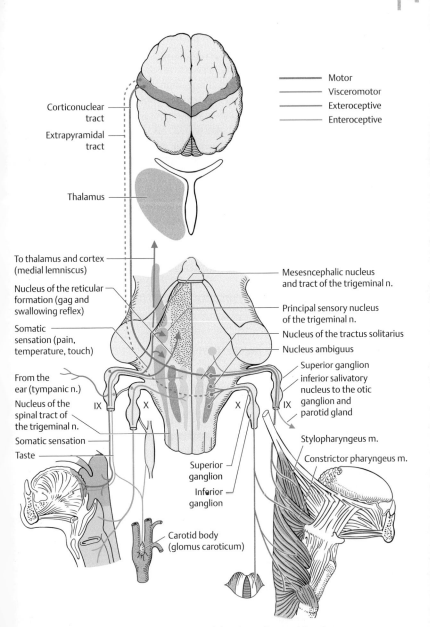

Corticonuclear tract

Extrapyramidal tract

Thalamus

To thalamus and cortex (medial lemniscus)

Nucleus of the reticular formation (gag and swallowing reflex)

Somatic sensation (pain, temperature, touch)

From the ear (tympanic n.)

Nucleus of the spinal tract of the trigeminal n.

Somatic sensation

Taste

Motor
Visceromotor
Exteroceptive
Enteroceptive

Mesesncephalic nucleus and tract of the trigeminal n.

Principal sensory nucleus of the trigeminal n.

Nucleus of the tractus solitarius

Nucleus ambiguus

Superior ganglion inferior salivatory nucleus to the otic ganglion and parotid gland

Stylopharyngeus m.

Constrictor pharyngeus m.

Superior ganglion

Inferior ganglion

Carotid body (glomus caroticum)

IX   X   X   IX

Fig. 4.**48 Distribution and central connections of the glossopharyngeal and vagus nerves**

which is also the site of both ganglia of the glossopharyngeal nerve, the *superior* (*intracranial*) ganglion and the *inferior* (*extracranial*) ganglion. After leaving the foramen, the glossopharyngeal nerve travels between the internal carotid artery and the jugular vein toward the stylopharyngeus muscle. It continues between the stylopharyngeus and styloglossus muscles and onward to innervate the root of the tongue, the pharyngeal mucosa, the tonsils, and the posterior third of the tongue. Along its course, it gives off the following branches:

- The *tympanic nerve* runs from the inferior ganglion to the tympanic cavity and tympanic plexus (of Jacobson), and then onward in the lesser petrosal nerve, by way of the otic ganglion, to the parotid gland (Fig. 4.**38**). It supplies sensation to the mucosa of the tympanic cavity and eustachian tube.
- *Stylopharyngeal branches* to the stylopharyngeus muscle.
- *Pharyngeal branches,* which, together with branches of the vagus nerve, form the pharyngeal plexus. This plexus supplies the striated muscles of the pharynx.
- *Branches to the carotid sinus,* which run with the carotid artery to the carotid sinus and carotid body.
- *Lingual branches* conveying gustatory impulses from the posterior third of the tongue.

Lesions of the Glossopharyngeal Nerve

Isolated lesions of the glossopharyngeal nerve are rare; the vagus and accessory nerves are usually involved as well.

The **causes** of glossopharyngeal nerve lesions include basilar skull fracture, sigmoid sinus thrombosis, tumors of the caudal portion of the posterior fossa, aneurysms of the vertebral or basilar arteries, iatrogenic lesions (caused, e. g., by surgical procedures), meningitis, and neuritis.

The clinical syndrome of a glossopharyngeal nerve lesion is characterized by:
- Impairment or loss of taste (ageusia) on the posterior third of the tongue
- Diminution or absence of the gag and palatal reflexes
- Anesthesia and analgesia in the upper portion of the pharynx and in the area of the tonsils and the base of the tongue
- A mild disturbance of swallowing (dysphagia)
- Impaired salivation from the parotid gland

Glossopharyngeal neuralgia is approximately 1% as common as trigeminal neuralgia; like trigeminal neuralgia, it is characterized by **intense, paroxysmal pain**. The painful attacks generally begin suddenly in the **pharynx, neck, tonsils, or tongue**, and last a few seconds or minutes. They can be provoked by swallowing, chewing, coughing, or speaking. The patient is afraid to eat because of the pain and rapidly loses weight. This syndrome usually resolves spontaneously within six months of onset. Persistence suggests a possible anatomical cause, such as a tumor in the pharynx, which must be ruled out by radiological study. In analogous fashion to trigeminal neuralgia, it is generally treated medically with carbamazepine or gabapentin at first. In refractory cases, a neurosurgical procedure called microvascular decompression can be considered (Jannetta 1977); this involves opening the posterior fossa and moving a loop of the vertebral or posterior inferior cerebellar artery away from the ninth cranial nerve.

Vagus Nerve (CN X)

Like the glossopharyngeal nerve, the vagus nerve also possesses two ganglia, the *superior (jugular) ganglion* and the *inferior (nodose) ganglion*, both of which are found in the region of the jugular foramen.

Anatomical course. The vagus nerve is derived from the fourth and lower branchial arches. Below the inferior (nodose) ganglion, it follows the internal carotid and common carotid arteries downward, and then passes through the superior thoracic aperture into the mediastinum. Here, the right vagal trunk crosses over the subclavian artery, while the left trunk runs behind the hilum and past the aortic arch. Both then become applied to the esophagus, with the fibers of the right vagal trunk running on its posterior side, and those of the left vagal trunk on its anterior side. The terminal vagal branches then accompany the esophagus through the esophageal hiatus of the diaphragm into the abdominal cavity.

Branches of the vagus nerve. Along its way to the abdominal cavity, the vagus nerve gives off the following branches (Figs. 4.**48**, 4.**49**; and Fig. 6.**14**, p. 290):

- *Dural branch:* running from the superior ganglion back through the jugular foramen to the dura mater of the posterior fossa.
- *Auricular branch:* from the superior ganglion of the vagus nerve to the skin on the posterior surface of the external ear and the inferoposterior portion of the external auditory canal. This is the only cutaneous branch of the vagus nerve.
- *Pharyngeal branches:* these accompany the fibers of the glossopharyngeal nerve and the sympathetic chain into the pharyngeal plexus to supply the muscles of the pharynx and soft palate.
- *Superior laryngeal nerve:* from the inferior ganglion to the larynx. This nerve splits into two branches of its own. The external branch gives off branches to the pharyngeal constrictor muscle and then goes on to innervate the cri-

cothyroid muscle. The internal branch is a sensory nerve supplying the laryngeal mucosa as far downward as the vocal folds, as well as the mucosa of the epiglottis. It also contains gustatory fibers for the epiglottis and parasympathetic fibers innervating the mucosal glands.

- *Recurrent laryngeal nerve:* This branch runs around the subclavian artery on the right side and the aortic arch on the left (Fig. 4.**49**), then proceeds upward between the trachea and the esophagus toward the larynx. It supplies motor innervation to the internal laryngeal musculature, with the exception of the cricothyroid muscle, as well as sensory innervation to the laryngeal mucosa below the vocal folds.
- *Superior cervical cardiac branches and thoracic cardiac branches:* these accompany sympathetic fibers to the heart, by way of the cardiac plexus.
- *Bronchial branches:* these form the pulmonary plexus in the wall of the bronchi.
- *Anterior and posterior gastric branches, and hepatic, celiac, and renal branches:* these travel, by way of the celiac and superior mesenteric plexuses, and together with sympathetic fibers, to the abdominal viscera (stomach, liver, pancreas, spleen, kidneys, adrenal glands, small intestine, and proximal portion of large intestine). In the abdominal cavity, the fibers of the right and left vagus nerves become closely associated with those of the sympathetic nervous system and can no longer be clearly distinguished from them.

Syndrome of a Unilateral Lesion of the Vagus Nerve

- The soft palate hangs down on the side of the lesion, the gag reflex is diminished, and the patient's speech is nasal because the nasal cavity can no longer be closed off from the oral cavity. Paresis of the pharyngeal constrictor muscle causes the palatal veil to be pulled over to the normal side when the patient phonates.
- Hoarseness results from paresis of the vocal folds (lesion of the recurrent laryngeal nerve with paresis of the internal muscles of the larynx, with the exception of the cricothyroid muscle).
- Further components of the syndrome are dysphagia and occasionally tachycardia, and cardiac arrhythmia.

Causes. Many diseases can cause a central vagal lesion, including malformations (Chiari malformation, Dandy-Walker syndrome, etc.), tumors, hemorrhage, thrombosis, infection/inflammation, amyotrophic lateral sclerosis, and aneurysms. Peripheral vagal lesions can be caused by neuritis, tumors, glandular disturbances, trauma, and aortic aneurysms.

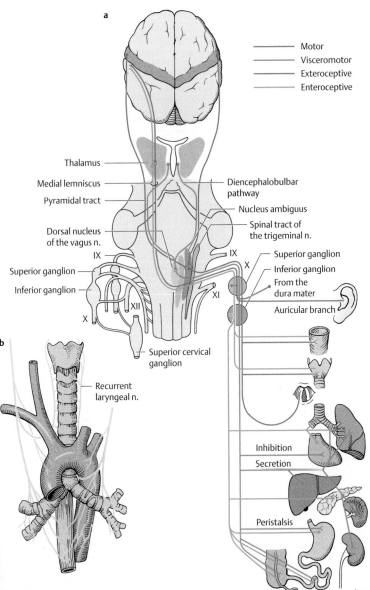

a

Motor
Visceromotor
Exteroceptive
Enteroceptive

Thalamus
Medial lemniscus
Pyramidal tract

Diencephalobulbar pathway
Nucleus ambiguus
Spinal tract of the trigeminal n.

Dorsal nucleus of the vagus n.

IX

IX

Superior ganglion
Inferior ganglion

Superior ganglion
Inferior ganglion
From the dura mater
Auricular branch

X

XI

XII

X

Superior cervical ganglion

b

Recurrent laryngeal n.

Inhibition

Secretion

Peristalsis

Fig. 4.**49 Distribution and central connections of the vagus nerve. a** Overview. **b** Topographic relations of the recurrent laryngeal nerve.

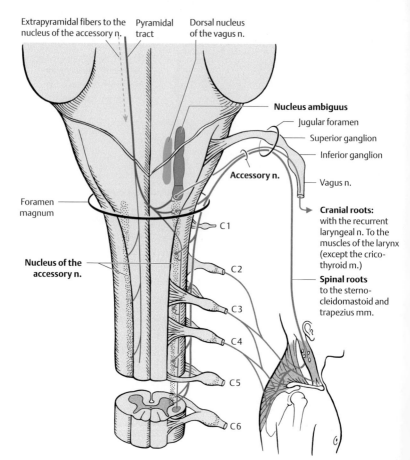

Extrapyramidal fibers to the nucleus of the accessory n.

Pyramidal tract

Dorsal nucleus of the vagus n.

Nucleus ambiguus

Jugular foramen

Superior ganglion

Inferior ganglion

Accessory n.

Vagus n.

Foramen magnum

Cranial roots:
with the recurrent laryngeal n. To the muscles of the larynx (except the crico-thyroid m.)

C1

Nucleus of the accessory n.

C2

Spinal roots
to the sterno-cleidomastoid and trapezius mm.

C3

C4

C5

C6

Fig. 4.**50** **Distribution and central connections of the accessory nerve**

Cranial Roots of the Accessory Nerve (CN XI)

The accessory nerve has two sets of roots, cranial and spinal (Fig. 4.**50**). The neurons giving rise to the cranial roots lie in the nucleus ambiguus next to the neurons whose processes run in the vagus nerve. This portion of the eleventh cranial nerve is best considered a functional component of the vagus nerve, as its functions are essentially the same as those of the portion of the vagus nerve that arises in the nucleus ambiguus. (The spinal roots of the accessory nerve, on the other hand, have an entirely different function.) The cranial roots separate off from the spinal roots within the jugular foramen to join the vagus nerve. This portion of the accessory nerve thus belongs to the "vagal system." The spinal roots and their function will be discussed below.

Common Nuclear Areas and Distribution of CN IX and X

Nucleus Ambiguus

The nucleus ambiguus is the common motor nucleus of the glossopharyngeal and vagus nerves and of the cranial portion of the accessory nerve (Figs. 4.**48**, 4.**49**, and 4.**50**). It receives descending impulses from the cerebral cortex of both hemispheres by way of the corticonuclear tract. Because of this bilateral innervation, unilateral interruption of these central descending fibers does not produce any major deficit in the motor distribution of the nucleus ambiguus.

The axons that originate in the nucleus ambiguus travel in the glossopharyngeal and vagus nerves and the cranial portion of the accessory nerve to the muscles of the soft palate, pharynx, and larynx, and to the striated muscle of the upper portion of the esophagus. The nucleus ambiguus also receives afferent input from the spinal nucleus of the trigeminal nerve and from the nucleus of the tractus solitarius. These impulses are the afferent limb of the important reflex arcs by which mucosal irritation in the respiratory and digestive tracts produces coughing, gagging, and vomiting.

Parasympathetic Nuclei of CN IX and X

The dorsal nucleus of the vagus nerve and the inferior salivatory nucleus are the two parasympathetic nuclei that send fibers into the glossopharyngeal and vagus nerves. The superior salivatory nucleus is the parasympathetic nucleus for the nervus intermedius, as discussed above (Figs. 4.**48** and 4.**49**).

Dorsal nucleus of the vagus nerve. The **efferent** axons of the dorsal nucleus of the vagus nerve travel as preganglionic fibers with the vagus nerve to the parasympathetic ganglia of the head, thorax, and abdomen. After a synaptic relay, the short postganglionic fibers convey visceromotor impulses to the smooth musculature of the respiratory tract and of the gastrointestinal tract as far down as the left colic flexure, as well as to the cardiac muscle. Stimulation of the vagal parasympathetic fibers causes slowing of the heartbeat, constriction of the bronchial smooth muscle, and secretion from the bronchial glands. Peristalsis in the gastrointestinal tract is promoted, as is secretion from the glands of the stomach and pancreas.

The dorsal nucleus of the vagus nerve receives **afferent** input from the hypothalamus, the olfactory system, autonomic centers in the reticular formation, and the nucleus of the tractus solitarius. These connections are important components of the reflex arcs for the control of cardiovascular, respiratory, and alimentary function. Impulses from the baroreceptors in the wall of the carotid sinus, which reach the dorsal nucleus of the vagus nerve through the glossopharyngeal nerve, serve to regulate arterial blood pressure. Chemoreceptors in the glomus caroticum participate in the regulation of the partial pressure of oxygen in the blood. Other receptors in the aortic arch and para-aortic bodies send afferent impulses to the dorsal nucleus of the vagus nerve by way of the vagus nerve, and have similar functions.

Inferior salivatory nucleus. The parasympathetic fibers arising in the inferior salivatory nucleus and traveling by way of the glossopharyngeal nerve to the parotid gland have already been discussed (pp. 175 and 196).

Visceral Afferent Fibers of CN IX and X

Special visceral afferent fibers. The perikarya (cell bodies) of the afferent gustatory fibers of the glossopharyngeal nerve (pseudounipolar neurons) are found in the *inferior (extracranial) ganglion*, while those of the vagus nerve are found in the *inferior (nodose) ganglion*. Both groups of fibers convey gustatory impulses from the epiglottis and the posterior third of the tongue. The glossopharyngeal nerve is the main nerve of taste. Its central processes travel in the tractus solitarius to the nucleus of the tractus solitarius, which also receives gustatory impulses from the anterior two-thirds of the tongue, conveyed by the nervus intermedius (Fig. 4.**37**). From the nucleus of the tractus solitarius, gustatory impulses ascend to the ventral posteromedial nucleus of the thalamus (VPM) and then onward to the gustatory cortex at the lower end of the postcentral gyrus (Fig. 4.**37**).

Visceral afferent fibers of the glossopharyngeal nerve belong to the pseudounipolar cells of the superior (intracranial) ganglion, while those of the vagus nerve are derived from its inferior ganglion. These fibers conduct sensory impulses from the mucosa of the posterior third of the tongue, the pharynx (CN IX), and the thoracic and abdominal viscera (CN X) (Figs. 4.**48** and 4.**49**).

Somatic Afferent Fibers of CN IX and X

Pain and temperature fibers. Nociceptive and probably also temperature-related impulses from the posterior third of the tongue, the upper portion of the pharynx, the eustachian tube, and the middle ear travel by way of the glossopharyngeal nerve and the superior (intracranial) ganglion to the nucleus of the spinal tract of the trigeminal nerve. Impulses of this type from the lower portion of the pharynx, the skin behind the ear and in part of the external auditory canal, the tympanic membrane, and the dura mater of the posterior fossa arrive at the same brainstem nucleus by way of the vagus nerve and its superior ganglion (the jugular ganglion).

Fibers for touch perception (somatosensory fibers) from the areas just named probably terminate in the principal sensory nucleus of the trigeminal nerve. Somatosensory impulses ascend from this nucleus in the medial lemniscus to the thalamus, and thence to the postcentral cortex.

Spinal Roots of the Accessory Nerves (CN XI)

The spinal portion of the accessory nerve is *purely motor* and arises in a cell column in the ventrolateral portion of the anterior horn, extending from C2 down to C5 or C6 (Fig. 4.**50**). The root fibers climb one or two segments in the lateral funiculus and then exit the spinal cord between the anterior and posterior roots, just dorsal to the denticulate ligament. They then ascend in the subarachnoid space and join with root fibers from higher levels to form a common trunk, which enters the skull through the foramen magnum and unites, over a short stretch, with the cranial roots of the accessory nerve. As the accessory nerve passes through the jugular foramen, the spinal portion splits off again as the **external branch** (ramus externus), while the cranial portion joins the vagus nerve. The external branch then descends into the nuchal region to innervate the **sternocleidomastoid** and **trapezius muscles**. It is joined along its course by spinal somatic efferent fibers from C2 through C4.

The literature offers conflicting views regarding the relative importance of the accessory nerve and spinal nerves C2 through C4 in the innervation of the trapezius muscle. Some authors assert that the accessory nerve mainly supplies the lower portion of the muscle, others that it mainly supplies the upper portion. Lesions of the accessory nerve are followed by atrophy mainly affecting the upper portion of the trapezius muscle.

The external branch also contains a few afferent fibers that conduct proprioceptive impulses toward the brainstem.

Lesions Affecting the Spinal Roots of the Accessory Nerve

Causes. The most common cause of a peripheral extracranial accessory nerve palsy is iatrogenic injury as a complication of surgical procedures in the lateral triangle of the neck (e. g., lymph node biopsy), followed by pressure- and radiation-induced lesions. Other causes include trauma with or without basilar skull fracture, skull base tumors (particularly in the region of the foramen magnum), and anomalies of the craniocervical junction.

Intramedullary lesions of the spinal cord are rarely extensive enough to destroy the gray matter of the anterior horn on one side from C1 to C4, producing a central extracranial accessory nerve palsy (syringomyelia, amyotrophic lateral sclerosis, poliomyelitis, other causes).

Typical deficits. Unilateral *interruption of the external branch after its exit from the jugular foramen* has different effects on the sternocleidomastoid and trapezius muscles: the sternocleidomastoid muscle is paralyzed (flaccid) in its entirety, while the trapezius muscle is affected only in its upper half, because it also receives innervation from the spinal nerves of segments C2 through C4. *Injury to the accessory nerve distal to the sternocleidomastoid muscle* causes weakness of the trapezius muscle exclusively; such injuries sometimes occur during lymph node biopsies at the posterior edge of the sternocleidomastoid muscle. No sensory deficit arises, because the spinal portion of the accessory nerve is purely motor.

In unilateral weakness of the sternocleidomastoid muscle, the patient has difficulty turning the head to the opposite side. Bilateral weakness makes it difficult to hold the head erect, or to raise the head when lying supine. Weakness of the trapezius muscle causes a shoulder drop with downward and outward displacement of the scapula. Lateral raising of the arm beyond 90° is impaired, because the trapezius muscle normally assists the serratus anterior muscle with this movement. Simple visual inspection of a patient with an accessory nerve palsy reveals atrophy of the sternocleidomastoid muscle as well as a drooping shoulder.

Paresis of central origin. The spinal portion of the accessory nerve receives central descending impulses by way of the corticonuclear and corticospinal tracts. These impulses are derived mainly, but not exclusively, from the contralateral cerebral hemisphere. Thus, a central lesion of the descending pathways sometimes causes contralateral weakness of the sternocleidomastoid and trapezius muscles, but the weakness is only partial because of the preserved ipsilateral innervation and is, therefore, easily overlooked.

Hypoglossal Nerve (CN XII)

The nucleus of the hypoglossal nerve (Figs. 4.**2** and 4.**3**, and Fig. 4.**51**) is located in the lower third of the medulla, abutting the midline and just below the floor of the fourth ventricle (in the so-called hypoglossal triangle or trigone). It con-

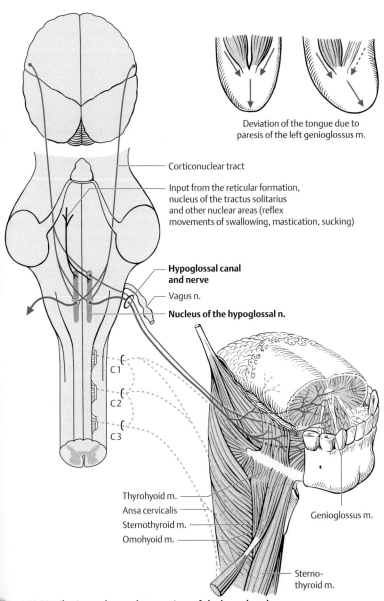

Deviation of the tongue due to
paresis of the left genioglossus m.

Corticonuclear tract

Input from the reticular formation,
nucleus of the tractus solitarius
and other nuclear areas (reflex
movements of swallowing, mastication, sucking)

**Hypoglossal canal
and nerve**

Vagus n.

Nucleus of the hypoglossal n.

C1

C2

C3

Thyrohyoid m.
Ansa cervicalis
Sternothyroid m.
Omohyoid m.

Genioglossus m.

Sterno-
thyroid m.

Fig. 4.**51 Distribution and central connections of the hypoglossal nerve**

sists of a number of cell groups supplying the individual muscles of the tongue. The cells are analogous to the motor anterior horn cells of the spinal cord.

Supranuclear innervation of the nucleus of the hypoglossal nerve. Voluntary movements of the tongue are subserved by the *corticonuclear tract*, which descends through the internal capsule in association with the corticospinal tract and terminates in the nucleus of the hypoglossal nerve.

The nucleus of the hypoglossal nerve derives its afferent input mainly from the *contralateral cerebral hemisphere*, though there is some ipsilateral input as well. It derives further input from the reticular formation, the nucleus of the tractus solitarius (taste), the midbrain (tectospinal tract), and the trigeminal nuclei. These connections participate in reflexes concerned with swallowing, chewing, sucking, and licking.

Because the muscles of the two sides of the tongue constitute a functional unit and are innervated by both cerebral hemispheres (albeit mainly contralaterally), a unilateral supranuclear lesion produces no significant deficit of tongue motility.

Course and distribution of the hypoglossal nerve. The hypoglossal nerve is a *somatic efferent* (motor) nerve. Its axons descend in the medulla and emerge from the brainstem as root fibers in the anterolateral sulcus between the inferior olive and the pyramid (Fig. 4.1). The hypoglossal nerve exits the skull through the hypoglossal canal (Figs. 4.6 and 4.51) and runs in the lower cervical region between the jugular vein and carotid artery together with the fibers of the first three cervical segments (ansa hypoglossi). These fibers, which make no connection with the hypoglossal nerve, separate from it again a short distance later to supply the muscles of the hyoid bone, i.e., the thyrohyoid, sternohyoid, and omohyoid muscles.

The hypoglossal nerve proper innervates the *muscles of the tongue*, the *styloglossus muscle*, the *hyoglossus muscle*, and the *genioglossus muscle*.

Hypoglossal nerve palsy. In unilateral hypoglossal nerve palsy, the tongue usually deviates a little toward the paretic side when it is protruded. The genioglossus muscle is responsible for protrusion (Fig. 4.51). If the genioglossus muscle of one side is weak, the force of the opposite muscle prevails and pushes the tongue to the side of the lesion. In hemiplegia, the patient's speech is dysarthric at first, but swallowing is not impaired. Bilateral supranuclear palsy produces severe dysarthria and dysphagia (pseudobulbar palsy).

Nuclear lesions affecting the hypoglossal nerve are usually manifested by bilateral flaccid paralysis of the tongue with atrophy and fasciculations, because the nuclei of the two sides lie so close to each other that they are usually affected together. In advanced cases, the tongue lies limply in the floor of the mouth and fasciculates intensely. Speech and swallowing are profoundly impaired. Causes include progressive bulbar palsy, amyotrophic lateral sclerosis, syringobulbia, poliomyelitis, and vascular processes.

Peripheral lesions of the hypoglossal nerve have the same consequences as nuclear lesions, but the paralysis is usually only unilateral. Causes include tumors, infection/inflammation, and vascular disease.

Topographical Anatomy of the Brainstem

Up to this point, we have discussed the ascending and descending pathways of the spinal cord and the positions of the cranial nerve nuclei in the brainstem, along with their emerging root fibers and their central connections. This section deals with the topography of the *pathways* that traverse the brainstem, as well as the *site and function of other nuclei* besides those that have already been described. Knowledge of the topographical anatomy of the brainstem is essential for a proper understanding of the clinical syndromes produced by lesions affecting the medulla, pons, and midbrain.

Internal Structure of the Brainstem

The brainstem contains important nuclei, including the *reticular formation*, the *olives*, the *red nucleus*, the *substantia nigra*, and others, each of which will be described in the subsection dealing with the part of the brainstem in which it is located. The *connections* that these nuclei make with each other and with the cerebrum, cerebellum, and spinal cord will also be discussed.

Figures 4.**52** and 4.**53** contain longitudinal and cross-sectional diagrams of the brainstem, showing the individual nuclei, the ascending and descending pathways, and their spatial relationships.

Figures 4.**54** and 4.**55** depict the spatial relationships of the individual fiber pathways in lateral and dorsal views of the brainstem.

Medulla

The spatial arrangement of the gray and white matter in the medulla already differs from that in the spinal cord at the lowest medullary level, i.e., at the level of the pyramidal decussation (Fig. 4.**52**). The anterior horns can still be seen: they contain the motor nuclei for the first cervical nerve and for the roots of the accessory nerve. The descending fibers of the corticospinal tracts are lo-

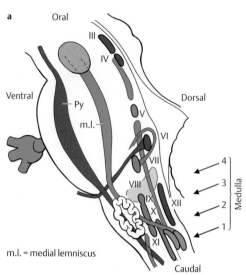

a

Oral

III

IV

Ventral — Py

m.l.

Dorsal

V

VI

VII

VIII

IX

X

XII

4

3

2

1

Medulla

XI

m.l. = medial lemniscus

Caudal

Fig. 4.**52 Cross sections of the medulla at four different levels. a** The four planes of section.

cated in the pyramids; most of these fibers cross the midline at this level, then descend in the contralateral lateral funiculus of the spinal cord. In the region of the posterior columns, two nuclei are found, i.e., the **nucleus cuneatus** and the **nucleus gracilis**. These are the relay nuclei for the ascending posterior column fibers of the spinal cord. They, in turn, project impulses by way of the medial lemniscus to the contralateral thalamus. These two nuclei possess a somatotopic arrangement (point-to-point projection), in which the nucleus cuneatus contains fibers for the upper limbs, while the nucleus gracilis contains fibers for the lower limbs. This somatotopy is preserved in the medial lemniscus, in the thalamus, and all the way up to the primary sensory cortex. Figure 4.**55c** shows the twisting course of the medial lemniscus: the fibers carrying impulses for the lower limb are more lateral, and those carrying impulses for the upper limb are more medial.

The **lateral spinothalamic tract** (pain, temperature), **anterior spinothalamic tract** (touch, pressure), and **spinotectal tract** (to the quadrigeminal region) have essentially the same position in the caudal medulla as in the cervical spinal cord.

An extensive network of cells, the **lateral reticular nucleus**, receives incoming fibers from the reticular formation of the spinal cord. This nucleus lies dorsal to the inferior olivary nucleus. The spinoreticular fibers carry sensory im-

b

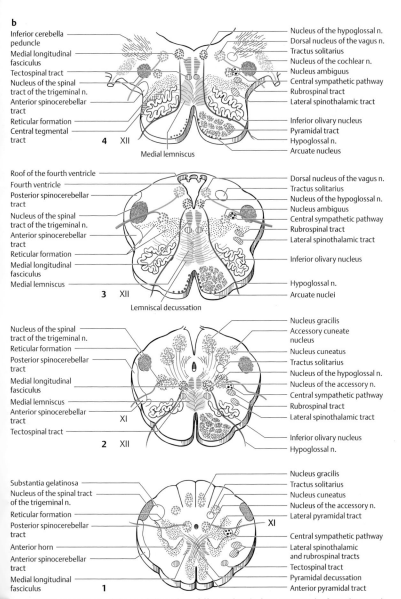

Inferior cerebella peduncle
Medial longitudinal fasciculus
Tectospinal tract
Nucleus of the spinal tract of the trigeminal n.
Anterior spinocerebellar tract
Reticular formation
Central tegmental tract

Nucleus of the hypoglossal n.
Dorsal nucleus of the vagus n.
Tractus solitarius
Nucleus of the cochlear n.
Nucleus ambiguus
Central sympathetic pathway
Rubrospinal tract
Lateral spinothalamic tract
Inferior olivary nucleus
Pyramidal tract
Hypoglossal n.
Arcuate nucleus

4   XII
Medial lemniscus

Roof of the fourth ventricle
Fourth ventricle
Posterior spinocerebellar tract
Nucleus of the spinal tract of the trigeminal n.
Anterior spinocerebellar tract
Reticular formation
Medial longitudinal fasciculus
Medial lemniscus

Dorsal nucleus of the vagus n.
Tractus solitarius
Nucleus of the hypoglossal n.
Nucleus ambiguus
Central sympathetic pathway
Rubrospinal tract
Lateral spinothalamic tract
Inferior olivary nucleus
Hypoglossal n.
Arcuate nuclei

3   XII
Lemniscal decussation

Nucleus of the spinal tract of the trigeminal n.
Reticular formation
Posterior spinocerebellar tract
Medial longitudinal fasciculus
Medial lemniscus
Anterior spinocerebellar tract
Tectospinal tract

Nucleus gracilis
Accessory cuneate nucleus
Nucleus cuneatus
Tractus solitarius
Nucleus of the hypoglossal n.
Nucleus of the accessory n.
Central sympathetic pathway
Rubrospinal tract
Lateral spinothalamic tract
Inferior olivary nucleus
Hypoglossal n.

XI
2   XII

Substantia gelatinosa
Nucleus of the spinal tract of the trigeminal n.
Reticular formation
Posterior spinocerebellar tract
Anterior horn
Anterior spinocerebellar tract
Medial longitudinal fasciculus

Nucleus gracilis
Tractus solitarius
Nucleus cuneatus
Nucleus of the accessory n.
Lateral pyramidal tract
Central sympathetic pathway
Lateral spinothalamic and rubrospinal tracts
Tectospinal tract
Pyramidal decussation
Anterior pyramidal tract

XI
1

Fig. 4.52 Cross-sections of the medulla at four different levels. b Sections in the four planes indicated in **a**, showing the important nuclei and fiber pathways.

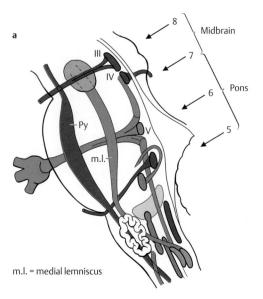

Fig. 4.**53 Cross sections of the pons and midbrain at four different levels. a** The four planes of section.

m.l. = medial lemniscus

pulses from the skin and internal organs. These fibers run more diffusely in the spinal cord, some of them in association with the spinothalamic tract.

The **posterior spinocerebellar tract**, which originates in Clarke's column (the thoracic nucleus) and ascends ipsilaterally in the spinal cord, at first keeps its position in the caudal medulla, then takes a progressively more dorsal position and finally accompanies the olivocerebellar tract as it travels, via the inferior cerebellar peduncle, to the cerebellum (Figs. 4.**54b** and **4.55b**). The **anterior spinocerebellar tract**, part of which is crossed, traverses the medulla and pons and finally enters the cerebellum by way of the superior cerebellar peduncle and the superior medullary velum (Figs. 4.**54b** and **4.55b**).

The **olivary nuclear complex** is located in the rostral portion of the medulla. The inferior olive (Figs. 4.**54** and 4.**55**), which resembles a sheet of gray matter that has been folded up to form a bag, receives most of its afferent input from the red nucleus of the midbrain, by way of the central tegmental tract. It receives further afferent input from the striatum, the periaqueductal gray matter, the reticular formation, and the cerebral cortex, by way of the cortico-olivary tract, which runs together with the corticospinal tract. Efferent fibers from the inferior olive cross the midline and form the olivocerebellar tract, which enters the cerebellum through the inferior cerebellar peduncle (Figs. 4.**54b** and **4.55b**) and conveys impulses to the entire neocerebellar cortex. This olivocerebellar

b

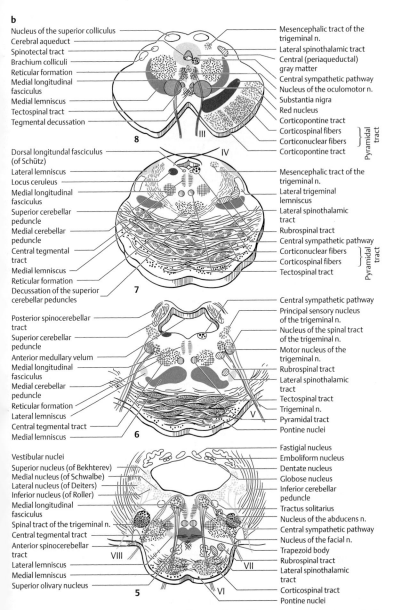

Nucleus of the superior colliculus
Cerebral aqueduct
Spinotectal tract
Brachium colliculi
Reticular formation
Medial longitudinal fasciculus
Medial lemniscus
Tectospinal tract
Tegmental decussation

Mesencephalic tract of the trigeminal n.
Lateral spinothalamic tract
Central (periaqueductal) gray matter
Central sympathetic pathway
Nucleus of the oculomotor n.
Substantia nigra
Red nucleus
Corticopontine tract
Corticospinal fibers
Corticonuclear fibers
Corticopontine tract

Pyramidal tract

8

III

IV

Dorsal longitundal fasciculus (of Schütz)
Lateral lemniscus
Locus ceruleus
Medial longitudinal fasciculus
Superior cerebellar peduncle
Medial cerebellar peduncle
Central tegmental tract
Medial lemniscus
Reticular formation
Decussation of the superior cerebellar peduncles

Mesencephalic tract of the trigeminal n.
Lateral trigeminal lemniscus
Lateral spinothalamic tract
Rubrospinal tract
Central sympathetic pathway
Corticonuclear fibers
Corticospinal fibers
Tectospinal tract

Pyramidal tract

7

Posterior spinocerebellar tract
Superior cerebellar peduncle
Anterior medullary velum
Medial longitudinal fasciculus
Medial cerebellar peduncle
Reticular formation
Lateral lemniscus
Central tegmental tract
Medial lemniscus

Central sympathetic pathway
Principal sensory nucleus of the trigeminal n.
Nucleus of the spinal tract of the trigeminal n.
Motor nucleus of the trigeminal n.
Rubrospinal tract
Lateral spinothalamic tract
Tectospinal tract
Trigeminal n.
Pyramidal tract
Pontine nuclei

6

V

Vestibular nuclei
Superior nucleus (of Bekhterev)
Medial nucleus (of Schwalbe)
Lateral nucleus (of Deiters)
Inferior nucleus (of Roller)
Medial longitudinal fasciculus
Spinal tract of the trigeminal n.
Central tegmental tract
Anterior spinocerebellar tract
Lateral lemniscus
Medial lemniscus
Superior olivary nucleus

Fastigial nucleus
Emboliform nucleus
Dentate nucleus
Globose nucleus
Inferior cerebellar peduncle
Tractus solitarius
Nucleus of the abducens n.
Central sympathetic pathway
Nucleus of the facial n.
Trapezoid body
Rubrospinal tract
Lateral spinothalamic tract
Corticospinal tract
Pontine nuclei

VIII

5

VI

VII

Fig. 4.53 Cross-sections of the pons and midbrain at four different levels. b Sections in the four planes indicated in **a**, showing the important nuclei and fiber pathways.

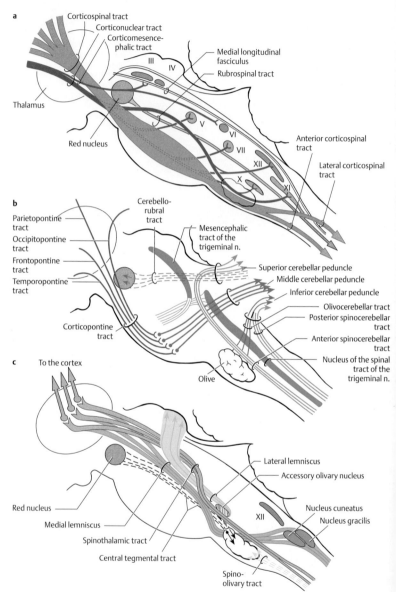

a

Corticospinal tract
Corticonuclear tract
Corticomesence-
phalic tract
Thalamus
Red nucleus

Medial longitudinal
fasciculus
Rubrospinal tract

III   IV

V
VI
VII
XII
X
XI

Anterior corticospinal
tract

Lateral corticospinal
tract

b

Cerebello-
rubral
tract

Parietopontine
tract
Occipitopontine
tract
Frontopontine
tract
Temporopontine
tract

Corticopontine
tract

Mesencephalic
tract of the
trigeminal n.

Superior cerebellar peduncle
Middle cerebellar peduncle
Inferior cerebellar peduncle
Olivocerebellar tract
Posterior spinocerebellar
tract
Anterior spinocerebellar
tract
Nucleus of the spinal
tract of the
trigeminal n.

Olive

c

To the cortex

Red nucleus
Medial lemniscus
Spinothalamic tract
Central tegmental tract

Lateral lemniscus
Accessory olivary nucleus

XII

Nucleus cuneatus
Nucleus gracilis

Spino-
olivary tract

Fig. 4.**54 Fiber connections in the brainstem, lateral view. a** Efferent pathways. **b** Cerebellar
pathways. **c** Afferent pathways.

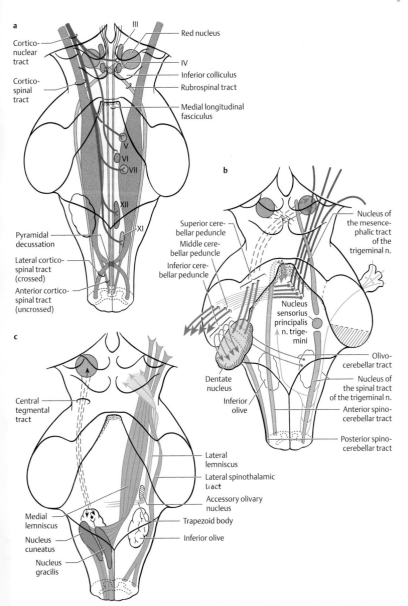

Fig. 4.55 Fiber connections in the brainstem, dorsal view. a Efferent pathways. **b** Cerebellar pathways. **c** Afferent pathways.

projection belongs to the system for coordination of voluntary movement; it will be discussed further in the chapters concerning the cerebellum (Chapter 5) and basal ganglia (Chapter 8).

The **accessory olive** is phylogenetically older than the inferior olive. It is connected to the archicerebellum and plays a role in the maintenance of balance.

Lesions of the inferior olive or of the central tegmental tract produce rhythmic twitching of the soft palate, the pharynx, and sometimes the diaphragm (myorhythmia, myoclonus, singultus). Ischemia is the usual cause.

The courses of the **corticospinal and corticonuclear tracts** are depicted in the cross-sectional diagrams of the brainstem and in Figures 4.**54a** and **4.55a**.

The **rubrospinal tract** also passes through the medulla. This tract originates in the red nucleus of the midbrain and crosses the midline a short distance below it in the ventral tegmental decussation (of Forel). It accompanies the lateral corticospinal tract as it descends in the lateral funiculus of the spinal cord (Fig. 4.**55**).

The **tectospinal tract** originates in the midbrain tectum and immediately crosses the midline, swinging around the periaqueductal gray in the so-called dorsal tegmental decussation (of Meynert). The tectospinal tract at first descends near the midline and then gradually takes a more ventral and lateral position, coming to lie in the ventrolateral portion of the medulla, near the rubrospinal tract. Along its way into the medulla, the tectospinal tract gives off collaterals to the nuclei innervating the extraocular muscles, as well as to the nucleus of the facial nerve and the cerebellum. It ends in the cervical spinal cord. **Function:** The superior colliculi receive visual input from the retina and auditory input from the inferior colliculi. Intense visual and auditory stimuli evoke reflex closure of the eyes, turning of the head away from the stimulus, and sometimes also raising of the arms (defense position); these reflexes are mediated by the tectonuclear and tectospinal pathways. The functional interaction of the occipital lobe and the superior collicular plate was mentioned in an earlier section. These two structures work together with the tectospinal pathways to enable *automatic pursuit movements of the eyes and head when the individual looks at a moving object.*

On the various cross-sectional images of the medulla, pons, and midbrain, one can see, in the spaces between the larger nuclei and the ascending and descending pathways, a number of diffusely distributed nuclei of varying size that occasionally cluster into nuclear groups, with an extensive network of fibers connecting them. These interconnected groups of neurons are known collectively as the **reticular formation**, a structure whose great importance was first recognized by Moruzzi and Magoun (1949). The reticular formation extends from the spinal cord (where it lies between the lateral and posterior funiculi) upward, through the medulla and pons, to the oral part of the midbrain (Figs. 4.**52** and 4.**53**). We will discuss its function later (p. 219).

One of the important nuclei in the medulla is the **dorsal nucleus of the vagus nerve**, which lies beneath the floor of the fourth ventricle (Fig. 4.**1b**). It contains autonomic motor (i.e., parasympathetic) neurons, which are analogous to the (sympathetic) neurons of the lateral horns of the spinal cord from T1 to L2. The more laterally lying **nucleus of the tractus solitarius** is a somatosensory and special sensory nucleus. Its rostral portion receives gustatory input from cranial nerves VII, IX, and X. Its caudal portion, which receives afferent fibers from the thoracic and abdominal viscera, is interconnected with the dorsal nucleus of the vagus nerve, with visceral centers in the reticular formation, and with neurons projecting to the autonomic nuclei in the lateral horns of the spinal cord. All of these nuclei can thus participate in reflex arcs that regulate and control cardiovascular, respiratory, and alimentary function, and other vegetative processes (see Fig. 4.**56**).

The **nucleus of the hypoglossal nerve** and the **nucleus ambiguus** have already been discussed in the section dealing with the cranial nerves, as have the **vestibular nuclei** and the **nucleus of the spinal tract of the trigeminal nerve**. The medial longitudinal fasciculus is found in a dorsal position near the midline; ventral to it lie the tectospinal tract and the medial lemniscus (Fig. 4.**52**).

Pons

The **pons** has two components: the *pontine tegmentum* is dorsal, and the *ventral portion of the pons* (*basis pontis*) is ventral.

Ventral portion of the pons. Many fiber bundles traverse the pons from one side to the other in the basis pontis, thereby fragmenting the descending corticospinal tracts into many little fascicles (Fig. 4.**53**). These horizontally running tracts give the pons its name ("bridge"), though they do not, in fact, constitute a bridge. They are pontocerebellar fibers, arising in nuclei of the basis pontis that contain the second neurons of the **corticopontocerebellar** pathway. These nuclei receive input via descending corticopontine fibers from the ipsilateral frontal, parietal, and temporal cerebral cortex (which are found in the lateral portion of the cerebral peduncle on either side, accompanying the corticospinal and corticonuclear fibers), and they receive further input from collateral fibers of the pyramidal tracts. The pontocerebellar fibers project across the midline and then enter the cerebellum through the middle cerebellar peduncle.

All cortically derived impulses related to voluntary movement are relayed by the pontine nuclei to the cerebellar cortex, which then projects back to the cerebral cortex by way of the dentate nucleus, superior cerebellar peduncle, and thalamus (feedback mechanism, cf. Fig. 5.**6**, p. 250). This regulatory circuit enables smooth and precise coordination of voluntary movement.

The structure of the pontine tegmentum is similar to that of the medullary tegmentum. The most ventral portion of the tegmentum contains the **medial lemniscus** (Figs. 4.**53b** and 4.**55c**), a transversely oriented band that has twisted itself around so that the fibers derived from the nucleus cuneatus are now more medial, and those from the nucleus gracilis more lateral. Thus, from lateral to medial, the parts of the body represented in the medial lemniscus are the lower limb, trunk, upper limb, and neck. The **spinothalamic tract** abuts the medial lemniscus laterally (Fig. 4.**55c**), as does the lateral lemniscus (auditory pathway). The last-named structure is the continuation of a fiber bundle that decussates in the caudal pons, the so-called **trapezoid body** (Figs. 4.**53b** and 4.**55**). The trapezoid body contains fibers derived from the cochlear nuclei and transmits auditory impulses to the inferior colliculi, both directly and indirectly. The **vestibular nuclear complex** lies at the far lateral end of the floor of the fourth ventricle (Fig. 4.**53b**). The lateral vestibular nucleus gives off the vestibulospinal tract to neurons of the spinal cord. The vestibular nuclei are also connected, through the medial longitudinal fasciculus, to the somatomotor and visceromotor nuclei of the brainstem (Fig. 4.**46**).

The spinal nucleus of the trigeminal nerve ends at a mid-pontine level, above which the **principal sensory nucleus of the trigeminal nerve** is found. The **motor trigeminal nucleus**, which innervates the muscles of mastication, is ventrolateral to the principal sensory nucleus. The second neurons of the spinal nucleus of the trigeminal nerve (pain and temperature) and the principal sensory nucleus of the trigeminal nerve (epicritic sensation) project to the contralateral thalamus through the **ventral trigeminothalamic tract**. The principal sensory nucleus also sends uncrossed fibers to the thalamus through the **dorsal trigeminothalamic tract**. The **nucleus of the mesencephalic tract of the trigeminal nerve** continues rostrally into the midbrain (Fig. 4.**55b**). This trigeminal nucleus differs from the rest—as already mentioned—in that it contains first sensory neurons, and can thus be thought of as a sensory ganglion that is exceptionally located within the brainstem. The remainder of the first sensory neurons of the trigeminal system are located in the **trigeminal (gasserian) ganglion**. The afferent fibers of the nucleus of the mesencephalic tract of the trigeminal nerve convey proprioceptive input mainly derived from the sensory receptors of the muscles of mastication and the jaw joint.

Midbrain

The midbrain lies rostral to the pons. Its internal structure is shown in Figure 4.**53b** (section 8). The midbrain has four parts: (1) the **tectum** ("roof"), delimited by an imaginary horizontal line through the aqueduct, which contains the superior and inferior colliculi (quadrigeminal plate); (2) the **tegmentum**, lying between the tectum and the substantia nigra; (3) the **substantia nigra**; and (4) the **cerebral peduncles** (crura cerebri).

Tectum. The **quadrigeminal plate** consists of the *superior and inferior colliculi*. These, particularly the superior colliculi, are highly specialized organs with seven cellular layers and numerous afferent and efferent connections that can only be discussed here in broad outline.

The nuclear area of the *inferior colliculi* receives numerous afferent fibers of the auditory pathway (lateral lemniscus) and projects onward, by way of the brachia of the inferior colliculi, to the medial geniculate bodies on either side. These, in turn, project to the primary auditory cortex in the temporal lobe (transverse gyri of Heschl).

The nuclear area of the *superior colliculi* receives afferent fibers from the visual pathway as well as from the cerebral cortex (occipital lobe), spinal cord (spinotectal tract), and inferior colliculi. It projects efferent fibers to the spinal cord (tectospinal tract) and to the cranial nerve nuclei (tectonuclear tract), as well as to the red nucleus and reticular formation.

Reflexes mediated by the superior and inferior colliculi. Fibers projecting from the inferior colliculus to the superior colliculus form part of a reflex arc that turns the head and eyes toward the source of an incoming sound. Retinal impulses that reach the superior colliculi by way of the lateral geniculate body participate in a further reflex arc that makes the eyes close in response to a sudden visual stimulus, and may also cause the head to turn away from the stimulus. The tectonuclear and tectospinal tracts form the efferent arms of these reflex arcs.

The small **pretectal nuclei** are found immediately anterolateral to the superior colliculi on both sides. These nuclei receive afferent fibers from the retina and project efferent fibers, after a synaptic relay, around the periaqueductal gray matter to the parasympathetic Edinger-Westphal nuclei (= accessory [autonomic] nuclei). They participate in the reflex arc that regulates the size of the pupil in response to the intensity of the incident light (p. 155).

In the middle of the **tegmentum**, between the substantia nigra and the periaqueductal gray matter, one finds a large, ellipsoidally shaped nucleus that is red in fresh anatomical sections, partly because it is well vascularized, and partly because it contains iron. This is the red nucleus (nucleus ruber).

The *red nucleus* has two parts, a caudal *magnocellular part* and a rostral *parvocellular part*. It receives **afferent** input from the *emboliform* and *dentate nuclei* of the cerebellum by way of the brachia conjunctiva (superior cerebellar peduncles). The fibers that originate in the phylogenetically older emboliform nucleus participate in reflex arcs controlling body posture and various types of movement. The fibers that originate in the dentate nucleus are especially numerous in humans and participate in other reflex arcs. One regulatory circuit for the smooth and precise execution of voluntary movement consists of connections from the cortex to the cerebellum and then back to the cortex by way of the dentate nucleus, red nucleus, and thalamus (cf. p. 249). Another group of dentatorubral fibers terminates primarily in the parvocellular part of the red nucleus. All cerebellorubral fibers cross the midline in the midbrain, in the decussation of the superior cerebellar peduncles. The red nucleus receives further afferent input from the *cerebral cortex* (*corticorubral tract*) and from the *tectum*.

The main **efferent** projections of the red nucleus (the *rubrospinal* and *rubroreticular tracts*) exert an influence on the spinal motor neurons; both of these tracts cross the midline, just after they emerge from the red nucleus, in the ventral tegmental decussation (of Forel). Further efferent fibers travel by way of the central tegmental tract to the olive (rubro-olivary fibers), from which a recurrent projection returns to the cerebellum.

Other tegmental nuclei and fiber tracts. The lateral portion of the tegmentum contains the *mesencephalic tract of the trigeminal nerve*, the *trigeminal lemniscus*, the *medial lemniscus*, and the *spinothalamic tract*, all of which project to the thalamus. The *trochlear nerve* emerges from the brainstem dorsally (it is the only cranial nerve to do so); its *root fibers* cross the midline just caudal to the inferior colliculi, then circle around the cerebral peduncle to the base of the brain, and continue, below the tentorial edge, to the cavernous sinus. The *nuclear complex of the oculomotor nerve*, as well as the parasympathetic *Edinger-Westphal nucleus* (accessory [autonomic] nucleus) and *nucleus of Perlia*, lie in the midbrain tegmentum at the level of the superior colliculi, anterior to the aqueduct and periaqueductal gray matter and medial to the medial longitudinal fasciculus. Some of the root fibers of the third cranial nerve traverse the red nucleus before they emerge from the brainstem into the interpeduncular fossa. Impulses from the vestibular nuclei are carried downward toward the spinal cord in the *medial longitudinal fasciculus*—a bundle that incorporates a number of different fiber systems and is present along the entire extent of the brainstem, as well as in the cervical spinal cord. Its fibers lie near the midline below the floor of the fourth ventricle (at medullary and pontine levels), and ventral to the aqueduct and periaqueductal gray matter (at midbrain levels); some of them terminate on the nuclei innervating the extraocular muscles (the nuclei of the oculomotor, trochlear, and abducens nerves) and connect these nuclei with one another. Other fibers of the medial longitudinal fasciculus terminate in nuclei of the reticular formation, including the interstitial nucleus (of Cajal) and the nucleus of Darkschewitsch.

The *central sympathetic pathway* is thought to originate in multiple nuclei of the hypothalamus and reticular formation. It passes through the midbrain and pons just anterior to the aqueduct and below the floor of the fourth ventricle. In the medulla, it occupies a more lateral position, from which it then passes into the lateral horns of the spinal gray matter. Interruption of the central sympathetic pathway produces Horner syndrome (p. 157).

The **substantia nigra** is a large motor nucleus that lies between the tegmentum and the crus cerebri on either side. Its dark coloration is due to a melanin pigment contained in the neuronal cell bodies. The substantia nigra is an important component of the extrapyramidal motor system and thus has an intimate functional relationship with the basal ganglia. It will be discussed further, together with the basal ganglia, in Chapter 9.

The **cerebral peduncles** (crura cerebri is the plural form; singular, crus cerebri) are large fiber bundles, one on either side, made up of corticospinal, corticonuclear, and corticopontine fibers (Fig. 3.**7**, p. 65, and Fig. 4.**53b**). Each cerebral peduncle is formed by fibers from these three tracts, which twist toward the midline as they descend in the internal capsule. The corticospinal and corticonuclear fibers occupy the midportion of the cerebral peduncle and are flanked, both medially and laterally, by corticopontine fibers (Fig. 4.**53b**).

Reticular Formation

The cell groups and fibers of the netlike reticular formation are found throughout the entire length of the brainstem, where they fill up the interstices between the cranial nerve nuclei, olives, and ascending and descending nerve pathways (Figs. 4.**52b**, 4.**53b**, and 4.**56a**). The reticular formation receives afferent fibers from the spinal cord, the cranial nerve nuclei, the cerebellum, and the cerebral hemispheres, and projects efferent fibers back to these same structures. Some of the nuclei of the reticular formation have descending projections to the spinal cord that influence both motor and autonomic function.

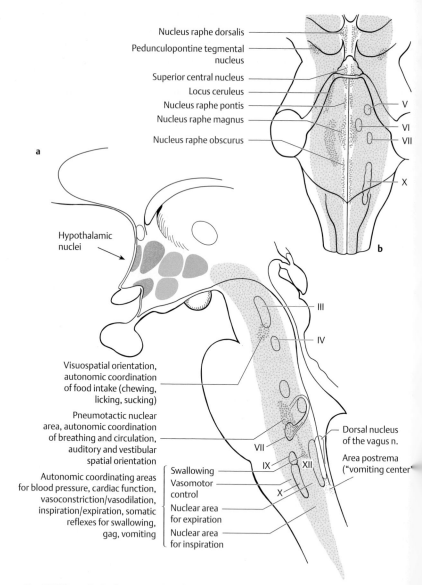

Nucleus raphe dorsalis
Pedunculopontine tegmental nucleus
Superior central nucleus
Locus ceruleus
Nucleus raphe pontis
Nucleus raphe magnus
Nucleus raphe obscurus

V
VI
VII
X

a

b

Hypothalamic nuclei

III

IV

Visuospatial orientation, autonomic coordination of food intake (chewing, licking, sucking)

Pneumotactic nuclear area, autonomic coordination of breathing and circulation, auditory and vestibular spatial orientation

VII

Dorsal nucleus of the vagus n.

IX   XII

Area postrema ("vomiting center"

Autonomic coordinating areas for blood pressure, cardiac function, vasoconstriction/vasodilation, inspiration/expiration, somatic reflexes for swallowing, gag, vomiting

Swallowing
Vasomotor control
Nuclear area for expiration
Nuclear area for inspiration

X

Fig. 4.**56 The reticular formation: dorsal (a) and lateral (b) views. a** Diagram of the major regulatory centers in the medulla, pons, and midbrain. **b** Additional depiction of the raphe nuclei.

Ascending reticular activating system. Other nuclei of the reticular formation, particularly in the midbrain, project to higher centers, mainly by way of the intralaminar nuclei of the thalamus, and by way of the subthalamus. These nuclei receive collateral input from many different ascending fiber tracts (among them the spinothalamic tract, the spinal tract of the trigeminal nerve, the tractus solitarius, and fibers from the vestibular and cochlear nuclei, as well as from the visual and olfactory systems); they relay these impulses upward, over a polysynaptic pathway, to extensive areas of the cerebral cortex, where they exert an activating function. Experimental stimulation of these nuclei in animals produces an "arousal reaction," in which the sleeping animal is awakened. The pioneering study of Moruzzi and Magoun (1949), and the subsequent work of numerous others, have provided overwhelming evidence that this system plays an important role in setting the **level of consciousness** in humans, as well as in maintaining the **sleep-wake cycle**. It has, therefore, been named the "ascending reticular activating system" (ARAS, cf. p. 270). Lesions affecting this system can impair or abolish consciousness. Even today, not much is known about the neuron groups that influence ARAS activity; the maintenance of wakefulness is presumed to depend, at least in part, on neurons of the reticular formation that can synthesize monoamine neurotransmitters such as norepinephrine (noradrenaline), dopamine, and serotonin. Neurons synthesizing norepinephrine are found in the lateral portion of the reticular formation, which includes the locus ceruleus. Serotonin is produced by the neurons of the raphe nuclei (Fig. 4.**56b**).

Neurons of the nucleus basalis (of Meynert) and of the substantia innominata send cholinergic fibers to extensive areas of the cerebral cortex (Fig. 6.**7**, p. 274).

The precise roles played by the ARAS and the cholinergic system just mentioned in consciousness and the sleep-wake cycle are not yet well enough understood to be presented in detail in this book. One thing that is certain is that unconsciousness can be produced by lesions of multiple brain structures.

The **descending reticular pathways** (ventral and lateral reticulospinal tracts) originate in the reticular formation and exert both excitatory and inhibitory effects on the motor neurons of the spinal cord. The cells of origin of these pathways receive afferent input from the cerebral cortex, particularly the frontal lobes, as well as from the cerebellum and the basal ganglia. Excitatory impulses from the brainstem (lateral portion of the reticular formation, mainly in the pons but also in the midbrain) are carried by both the reticulospinal and the vestibulospinal tracts in the anterolateral funiculus of the spinal cord, while inhibitory impulses, derived mainly from the ventromedial portion of the medulla, reach the spinal motor neurons over multiple synaptic relays, mainly by way of the lateral reticulospinal tract (adjacent to the corticospinal tract). Both the excitatory and the inhibitory systems impinge, through interneurons, on the γ motor neurons of the spinal cord. Thus, by regulating the function of the spinal reflex arcs, the reticular formation plays an important role in the maintenance of adequate muscle tone for standing and walking, as well as in the maintenance of balance.

Autonomic nuclei and pathways. Many neurons in the reticular formation have autonomic functions. Nuclei containing such cells are scattered throughout the pons and medulla and receive input from the somatic cranial nerve nuclei (Fig. 4.**56**, p. 220). These autonomic nuclei receive input from the hypothalamus and send projections to the cranial nerve nuclei and the spinal cord.

Regulation of salivation. Salivation is controlled by the *superior and inferior salivatory nuclei.* It can be evoked in reflex fashion by an appetizing smell or taste. The individual's mental state can also inhibit salivation under some circumstances, causing a dry mouth.

Regulation of blood pressure. Other nuclei regulate blood pressure. Afferent impulses arising in the carotid sinus travel over the glossopharyngeal and vagal nerves to the corresponding reticular nuclear areas in the medulla (autonomic centers for the regulation of blood pressure, cardiac activity, and vasoconstriction/vasodilation), which are located near the nuclei of cranial nerves IX and X. Efferent impulses mediated by the vagus nerve inhibit cardiac activity, resulting in slowing of the heart rate and a fall in blood pressure.

Regulation of other autonomic bodily functions. Some descending impulses from the reticular formation inhibit the sympathetic nuclei of the spinal cord, causing vasodilation. Reticular nuclei dorsal to the inferior olive control *respiration*; there are distinct expiratory and aspiratory centers. Yet other reticular nuclei control and coordinate *gastrointestinal motility*. Reflex *swallowing* is a complicated process involving many different muscles, which must be activated in the proper sequence and at the proper intensity to propel a bolus of food smoothly from the mouth into the stomach; coordinating the multiple nerves involved in this process is the function of the so-called medullary swallowing center, which lies in the vicinity of the motor cranial nerve nuclei that it activates. Nearby, there is also a nucleus responsible for gagging (the *gag reflex*). The area postrema contains an important area for the regulation of *vomiting*. There is presumed to be a higher center for *cardiorespiratory* function (a pneumotactic nucleus) in the vicinity of the locus ceruleus, as well as a higher center for *food intake* (chewing, licking, sucking) in the midbrain (Fig. 4.**56a**).

Brainstem Disorders

Ischemic Brainstem Syndromes

The anatomy of the arterial blood supply of the brainstem is depicted in Figure 4.**57**, and the territories of individual arteries supplying the medulla, pons, and midbrain are shown in Figure 4.**58**. A thorough discussion of the arterial blood supply and venous drainage of the brainstem is found in Chapter 11, on pages 418 ff. Knowledge of the pattern of blood supply is essential for an understanding of the vascular syndromes to be described in this section.

Inadequate perfusion of discrete regions of the brainstem can be either **transient** (e. g., the transient ischemia of subclavian steal syndrome, see below) or **permanent** (causing tissue necrosis, i.e., **brainstem infarction**). Infarction is usually due to arterial occlusion. It produces different patterns of clinical deficits, depending on the particular vessel that has been occluded (**vascular syndromes**). Because the nuclei and fiber pathways of the brainstem are numerous, compactly arranged, and highly diverse in function, a correspondingly wide variety of vascular syndromes can be observed. To understand each vascular syndrome, one must first understand the complex topographical anatomy of the brainstem in the region that it affects. This is why the brainstem vascular syndromes are presented here in the chapter on the brainstem, rather than in Chapter 11 together with the vascular disorders of the rest of the brain.

Subclavian steal syndrome will be discussed first, as an example of a syndrome with transient brainstem ischemia. The major arterial occlusion syndromes of the brainstem will be presented thereafter.

Subclavian Steal Syndrome

This syndrome occurs as the result of **occlusion of the right or left subclavian artery** proximal to the origin of the vertebral artery Despite the occlusion, the cardiovascular system maintains adequate perfusion of the ipsilateral arm by "tapping" the ipsilateral vertebral artery in retrograde fashion: blood flows up the contralateral vertebral artery to its junction with the ipsilateral vertebral artery (where the two arteries join to form the basilar artery), and then back down the ipsilateral vertebral artery into the axillary artery and onward into the brachial artery. In rare cases, a situation may arise in which exercise of the arm diverts so much blood from the vertebrobasilar system that clinically evident brainstem ischemia ensues. The diagnosis of subclavian steal syndrome requires *both* the characteristic clinical manifestations *and* a clinically corre-

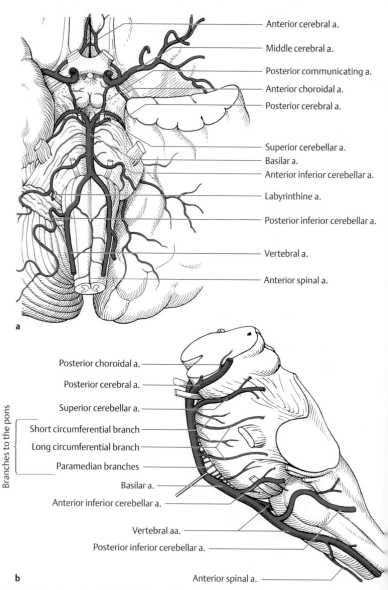

Anterior cerebral a.
Middle cerebral a.
Posterior communicating a.
Anterior choroidal a.
Posterior cerebral a.

Superior cerebellar a.
Basilar a.
Anterior inferior cerebellar a.
Labyrinthine a.
Posterior inferior cerebellar a.
Vertebral a.
Anterior spinal a.

a

Posterior choroidal a.
Posterior cerebral a.
Superior cerebellar a.
Branches to the pons
Short circumferential branch
Long circumferential branch
Paramedian branches
Basilar a.
Anterior inferior cerebellar a.
Vertebral aa.
Posterior inferior cerebellar a.
b
Anterior spinal a.

Fig. 4.**57 Blood supply of the brainstem. a** Basal view. **b** Lateral view.

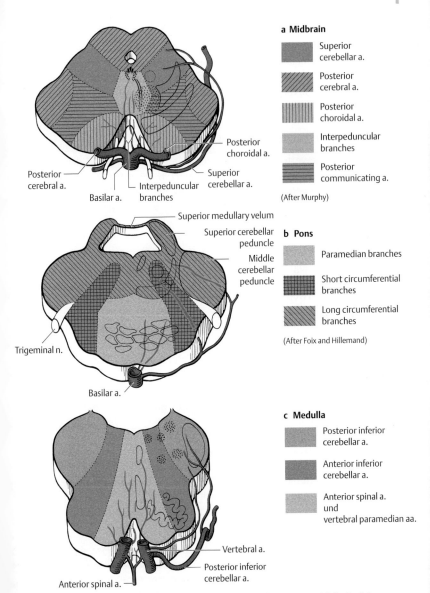

a **Midbrain**

- Superior cerebellar a.
- Posterior cerebral a.
- Posterior choroidal a.
- Interpeduncular branches
- Posterior communicating a.

(After Murphy)

Posterior choroidal a.

Posterior cerebral a.

Superior cerebellar a.

Basilar a.

Interpeduncular branches

Superior medullary velum

Superior cerebellar peduncle

Middle cerebellar peduncle

b **Pons**

- Paramedian branches
- Short circumferential branches
- Long circumferential branches

(After Foix and Hillemand)

Trigeminal n.

Basilar a.

c **Medulla**

- Posterior inferior cerebellar a.
- Anterior inferior cerebellar a.
- Anterior spinal a. und vertebral paramedian aa.

Vertebral a.

Posterior inferior cerebellar a.

Anterior spinal a.

Fig. 4.**58 Distribution of the individual arteries supplying the brainstem. a** Midbrain. **b** Pons. **c** Medulla.

lated angiographic finding of **retrograde flow in the vertebral artery**. Subclavian artery occlusion needs to be treated only if it causes ischemia in the hand or frank subclavian steal syndrome, with manifestations of ischemia in the vertebrobasilar territory, such as loss of consciousness or vertigo.

The traditional term "vertebrobasilar insufficiency" is now obsolete and should no longer be used.

Individual Brainstem Vascular Syndromes

Infarction in the vertebrobasilar distribution, as in the carotid distribution, is usually due to **embolism** (for a discussion, cf. p. 466). The responsible emboli may arise from the heart, from atheromatous plaques in the vertebral arteries, or from an arterial dissection with secondary thrombosis. The once-current notion that kinking of the vertebral arteries during sleep might cause ischemia is no longer tenable today.

A number of different brainstem vascular syndromes can be identified on clinical and radiological grounds. Very recently, high-resolution magnetic resonance imaging with T2-weighted and diffusion-weighted sequences has enabled the direct visualization of brainstem infarcts in their acute phase. Although there is a degree of variation among individuals, the vascular architecture of the brainstem is sufficiently uniform that the syndromes described here are well-defined clinical entities.

Brainstem infarction in a number of different locations often becomes manifest clinically as **alternating hemiplegia** (crossed weakness), which is defined as a combination of cranial nerve deficits on the side of the lesion with weakness of the opposite hemibody. In Figure 4.**59**, three different alternating hemiplegia syndromes are shown, each the result of ischemia in a particular region of the brainstem, with corresponding clinical deficits.

We now list the individual vascular syndromes that can be considered, in simplified terms, to be "variations" of the alternating hemiplegia syndrome, albeit with extraordinarily diverse manifestations. To make the presentation as clear as possible, the discussion of each syndrome is accompanied by a drawing of the affected structures in the brainstem, and by a schematic diagram of the resulting clinical deficits.

Dorsolateral medullary syndrome (Wallenberg syndrome, Figs. 4.**60** and 4.**61**). *Cause:* occlusion or embolism in the territory of the posterior inferior cerebellar artery or vertebral artery. *Clinical features:* sudden onset with vertigo, nystagmus (inferior vestibular nucleus and inferior cerebellar peduncle), nausea and vomiting (area postrema), dysarthria and dysphonia (nucleus ambiguus), singultus (respiratory center of the reticular formation). For further details, see Figure 4.**60**.

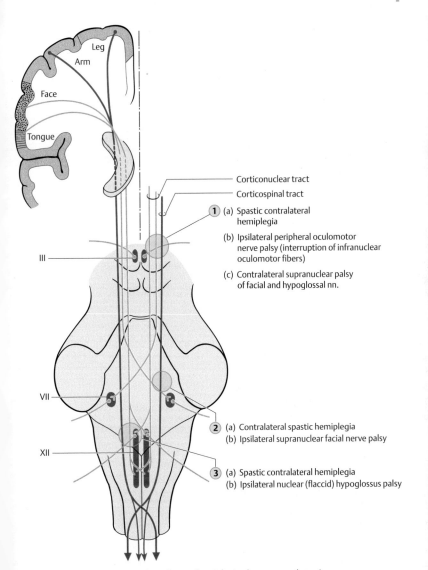

Corticonuclear tract
Corticospinal tract

1 (a) Spastic contralateral hemiplegia

(b) Ipsilateral peripheral oculomotor nerve palsy (interruption of infranuclear oculomotor fibers)

(c) Contralateral supranuclear palsy of facial and hypoglossal nn.

2 (a) Contralateral spastic hemiplegia
(b) Ipsilateral supranuclear facial nerve palsy

3 (a) Spastic contralateral hemiplegia
(b) Ipsilateral nuclear (flaccid) hypoglossus palsy

Leg
Arm
Face
Tongue
III
VII
XII

Fig. 4.**59 Lesions causing crossed weakness** (hemiplegia alternans syndrome)

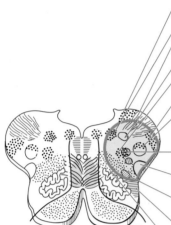

Inferior vestibular nucleus: nystagmus and tendency to fall to ipsilateral side

Dorsal nucleus of the vagus n.: tachycardia and dyspnea

Inferior cerebellar peduncle: ipsilateral ataxia and asynergia

Nucleus of the tractus solitarius: ageusia

Nucleus ambiguus: ipsilateral paresis of palate, larynx, and pharynx; hoarseness

Nucleus of the cochlear n.: hearing loss

Nucleus of the spinal tract of the trigeminal n.: ipsilateral analgesia and thermanesthesia of the face; absent corneal reflex

Central sympathetic pathway: Horner's syndrome, hypohidrosis, ipsilateral facial vasodilatation

Anterior spinocerebellar tract: ataxia, ipsilateral hypotonia

Lateral spinothalamic tract: analgesia and thermanesthesia of contralateral hemibody

Central tegmental tract: palatal and pharyngeal myorhythmia

Reticular formation (respiratory center): singultus (hiccups)

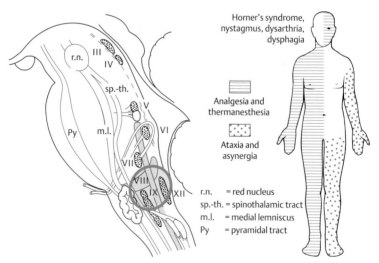

Horner's syndrome, nystagmus, dysarthria, dysphagia

Analgesia and thermanesthesia

Ataxia and asynergia

r.n. = red nucleus
sp.-th. = spinothalamic tract
m.l. = medial lemniscus
Py = pyramidal tract

Fig. 4.**60 Dorsolateral medullary syndrome** (Wallenberg syndrome)

Case Presentation 4: *Wallenberg Syndrome*

The MRI findings in this case are typical of Wallenberg syndrome. Some 20 hours before the scan was obtained, this 56-year-old man suddenly became dizzy and unsteady, with a tendency to fall to the left. Examination revealed left-sided ataxia and asynergia as well as a deficit of protopathic sensation on the right side of the body. A CT scan of the head was normal.

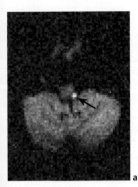 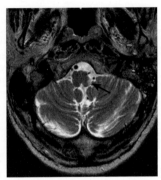

a   b

Fig. 4.**61 Wallenberg syndrome. a** The diffusion-weighted MR image shows a lesion in the left dorsolateral portion of the medulla. **b** Hyperintensity is seen at this site on the T2-weighted image. The finding was found to be an infarct in the territory of the left PICA territory due to occlusion of the left vertebral artery.

Medial medullary syndrome (Dejerine syndrome) (Fig. 4.**62**). *Cause:* occlusion of paramedian branches of the vertebral or basilar artery (Fig. 4.**58**), often bilaterally. *Clinical features:* ipsilateral flaccid hypoglossal nerve palsy, contralateral hemiplegia (not spastic) with Babinski's sign, contralateral posterior column hypesthesia (i.e., hypesthesia to touch and pressure, with impaired position sense), and nystagmus (in case the medial longitudinal fasciculus is involved by the lesion).

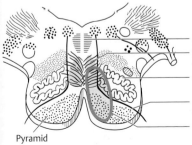

Medial longitudinal fasciculus: nystagmus
Medial lemniscus: contralateral impairment of touch, vibration, and position sense
Olive: ipsilateral palatal and pharyngeal myorhythmia
Hypoglossal n.: ipsilateral hypoglossal palsy with hemiatrophy of the tongue
Pyramidal tract: contralateral hemiplegia without spasticity but with present Babinski reflex

Pyramid

Fig. 4.**62 Medial medullary syndrome** (Dejerine syndrome).

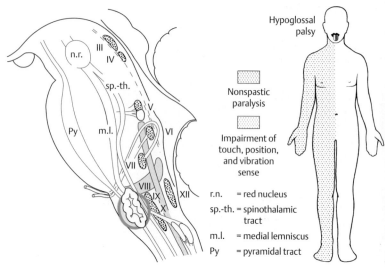

Fig. 4.**62** (continued) **Medial medullary syndrome** (Dejerine syndrome)

Case Presentation 5: *Medial Medullary Syndrome (Dejerine Syndrome)*

The MRI findings in this case are typical of a medial medullary infarct. This 58-year-old woman suddenly developed flaccid right hemiparesis, a deficit of epicritic sensation, and left hypoglossal nerve palsy. No infarct was seen on cranial CT. The MRI scan was obtained 19 hours later.

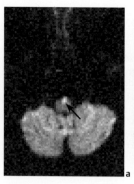
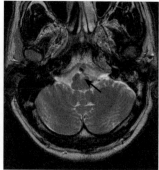

Fig. 4.**63 Medial medullary syndrome. a** The diffusion-weighted image shows an abnormality of diffusion in the oral paramedian portion of the medulla.
b The T2-weighted image reveals hyperintensity at this site.

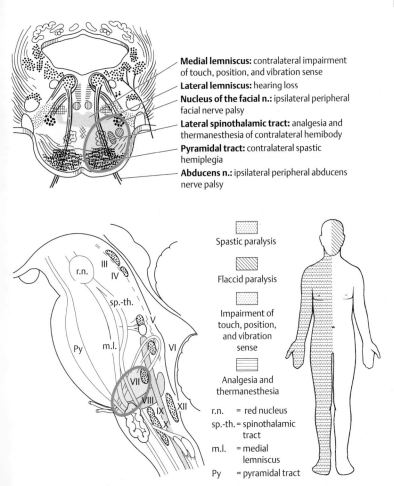

Medial lemniscus: contralateral impairment of touch, position, and vibration sense

Lateral lemniscus: hearing loss

Nucleus of the facial n.: ipsilateral peripheral facial nerve palsy

Lateral spinothalamic tract: analgesia and thermanesthesia of contralateral hemibody

Pyramidal tract: contralateral spastic hemiplegia

Abducens n.: ipsilateral peripheral abducens nerve palsy

Spastic paralysis

Flaccid paralysis

Impairment of touch, position, and vibration sense

Analgesia and thermanesthesia

r.n. = red nucleus

sp.-th. = spinothalamic tract

m.l. = medial lemniscus

Py = pyramidal tract

Fig. 4.**64 Syndrome of the caudal basis pontis** (Millard–Gubler syndrome)

Syndrome of the caudal basis pontis (Millard-Gubler or Foville syndrome). *Cause:* occlusion of the circumferential branches of the basilar artery, tumor, abscess, etc. *Clinical features:* ipsilateral abducens palsy (peripheral) and facial palsy (nuclear); contralateral hemiplegia; contralateral analgesia, thermanesthesia, and impairment of touch, position, and vibration sense (Fig. 4.**64**).

Syndrome of the caudal pontine tegmentum (Fig. 4.**65**). *Cause:* occlusion of branches of the basilar artery (short and long circumferential branches). *Clini-*

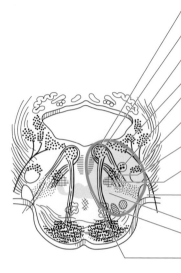

Medial longitudinal fasciculus: nystagmus, gaze paresis to side of lesion

Nucleus of the abducens n.: ipsilateral nuclear abducens palsy

Middle cerebellar peduncle: hemiataxia, intention tremor, adiadochokinesia, cerebellar dysarthria

Vestibular nuclei: nystagmus, rotatory vertigo

Central sympathetic pathway: Horner syndrome, hypohidrosis, ipsilateral vasodilatation

Nucleus of the spinal tract of the trigeminal n.: ipsilateral facial analgesia and thermanesthesia

Nucleus of the facial n.: ipsilateral nuclear facial palsy (atrophy)

Central tegmental tract: ipsilateral palatal and pharyngeal myorhythmia

Anterior spinocerebellar tract: ipsilateral asynergia and hypotonia

Lateral lemniscus: hearing loss

Lateral spinothalamic tract: analgesia and thermanesthesia of contralateral hemibody

Medial lemniscus: impairment of touch, vibration, and position sense of the contralateral hemibody; atax

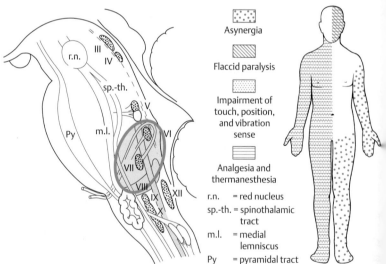

Asynergia

Flaccid paralysis

Impairment of touch, position, and vibration sense

Analgesia and thermanesthesia

r.n. = red nucleus
sp.-th. = spinothalamic tract
m.l. = medial lemniscus
Py = pyramidal tract

Fig. 4.**65** Syndrome of the caudal pontine tegmentum

cal features: ipsilateral nuclear abducens and facial palsy, nystagmus (medial longitudinal fasciculus), gaze paresis toward the side of the lesion; ipsilateral hemiataxia and asynergia (medial cerebellar peduncle); contralateral analge-

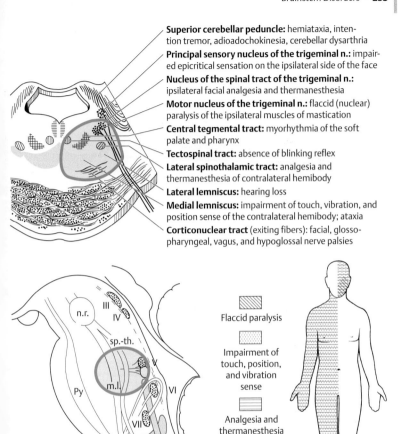

Superior cerebellar peduncle: hemiataxia, intention tremor, adioadochokinesia, cerebellar dysarthria

Principal sensory nucleus of the trigeminal n.: impaired epicritical sensation on the ipsilateral side of the face

Nucleus of the spinal tract of the trigeminal n.: ipsilateral facial analgesia and thermanesthesia

Motor nucleus of the trigeminal n.: flaccid (nuclear) paralysis of the ipsilateral muscles of mastication

Central tegmental tract: myorhythmia of the soft palate and pharynx

Tectospinal tract: absence of blinking reflex

Lateral spinothalamic tract: analgesia and thermanesthesia of contralateral hemibody

Lateral lemniscus: hearing loss

Medial lemniscus: impairment of touch, vibration, and position sense of the contralateral hemibody; ataxia

Corticonuclear tract (exiting fibers): facial, glossopharyngeal, vagus, and hypoglossal nerve palsies

Flaccid paralysis

Impairment of touch, position, and vibration sense

Analgesia and thermanesthesia

r.n. = red nucleus
sp.-th. = spinothalamic tract
m.l. = medial lemniscus
Py = pyramidal tract

Fig. 4.**66 Syndrome of the oral pontine tegmentum**

sia and thermanesthesia (lateral spinothalamic tract); contralateral hypesthesia and impairment of position and vibration sense (medial lemniscus); ipsilateral palatal and pharyngeal myorhythmia (central tegmental tract).

Syndrome of the oral pontine tegmentum (Fig. 4.**66**). *Cause:* occlusion of the long circumferential branches of the basilar artery and superior cerebellar artery. *Clinical features:* ipsilateral loss of facial sensation (interruption of all

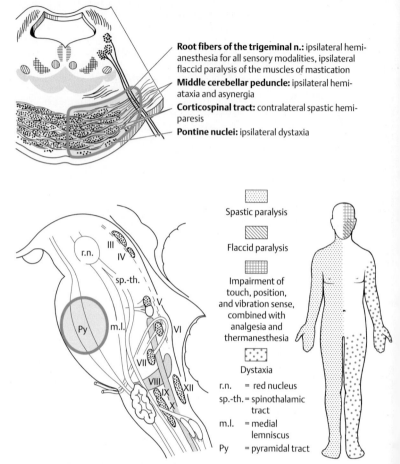

Root fibers of the trigeminal n.: ipsilateral hemi-anesthesia for all sensory modalities, ipsilateral flaccid paralysis of the muscles of mastication
Middle cerebellar peduncle: ipsilateral hemi-ataxia and asynergia
Corticospinal tract: contralateral spastic hemi-paresis
Pontine nuclei: ipsilateral dystaxia

Spastic paralysis

Flaccid paralysis

Impairment of touch, position, and vibration sense, combined with analgesia and thermanesthesia

Dystaxia

r.n. = red nucleus
sp.-th. = spinothalamic tract
m.l. = medial lemniscus
Py = pyramidal tract

Fig. 4.**67 Syndrome of the midportion of the basis pontis**

trigeminal fibers) and paralysis of the muscles of mastication (motor nucleus of the trigeminal nerve), hemiataxia, intention tremor, adiadochokinesia (superior cerebellar peduncle); contralateral impairment of all sensory modalities.

Syndrome of the midportion of the basis pontis (Fig. 4.**67**). *Cause:* occlusion of the paramedian and short circumferential branches of the basilar artery. *Clinical features:* ipsilateral flaccid paresis of the muscles of mastication, as well as facial hypesthesia, analgesia, and thermanesthesia; ipsilateral hemiataxia and asynergia; contralateral spastic hemiparesis.

Case Presentation 6: *Paramedian Pontine Infarct*

The MRI findings in this case are typical of a paramedian pontine infarct. Twelve hours before the scan was obtained, the patient had suddenly developed left hemiparesis accompanied by a deficit of both protopathic and epicritic sensation.

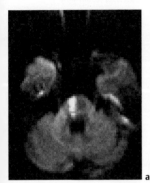 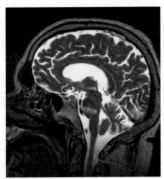

Fig. 4.**68 Paramedian pontine infarct. a** The axial, diffusion-weighted image shows a wedge-shaped region in the right paramedian area of the pons sparing the trigeminal nerve, which exits the brainstem at this level. **b** The sagittal T2-weighted image shows a pontine lesion of typical configuration, corresponding to the territory of one of the pontine arteries.

Syndrome of the red nucleus (Benedikt syndrome) (Fig. 4.**69**). *Cause:* occlusion of the interpeduncular branches of the basilar and posterior cerebral arteries. *Clinical features:* ipsilateral oculomotor nerve palsy with mydriasis (interruption of the root fibers of CN III); contralateral impairment of touch, position, and vibration sense, as well as of two-point discrimination (involvement of the medial lemniscus); contralateral hyperkinesia (tremor, chorea, athetosis) due to involvement of the red nucleus; contralateral rigidity (substantia nigra).

Syndrome of the cerebral peduncle (Weber syndrome) (Fig. 4.**70**). *Cause:* occlusion of the interpeduncular branches of the posterior cerebral and posterior choroidal arteries; rarely also tumor (glioma). *Clinical features:* ipsilateral oculomotor nerve palsy; contralateral spastic hemiparesis; contralateral parkinsonian rigidity (substantia nigra); contralateral dystaxia (corticopontine tract); possible cranial nerve deficits due to interruption of the supranuclear innervation of CN VII, IX, X, and XII.

Small infarcts of the **oral region of the pons**, caused by the occlusion of perforating arteries, can produce a wide variety of circumscribed and often transient deficits. Arteriosclerosis of the basilar artery can cause multiple small in-

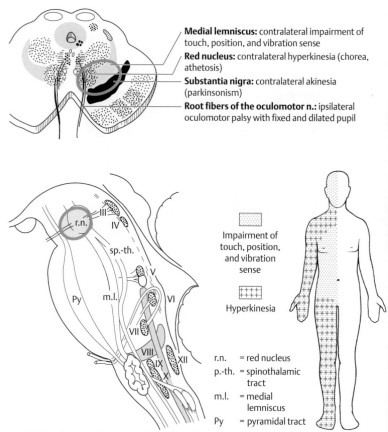

Medial lemniscus: contralateral impairment of touch, position, and vibration sense

Red nucleus: contralateral hyperkinesia (chorea, athetosis)

Substantia nigra: contralateral akinesia (parkinsonism)

Root fibers of the oculomotor n.: ipsilateral oculomotor palsy with fixed and dilated pupil

Impairment of touch, position, and vibration sense

Hyperkinesia

r.n. = red nucleus
p.-th. = spinothalamic tract
m.l. = medial lemniscus
Py = pyramidal tract

Fig. 4.**69 Syndrome of the red nucleus** (Benedikt syndrome)

farcts on one or both sides of the brainstem, occurring stepwise over time and eventually producing the clinical picture of microangiopathic pseudobulbar palsy. In this syndrome, dysarthria and dysphagia result from interruption of the supranuclear innervation of the motor cranial nerve nuclei. Microangiopathic brainstem disease is most often due to generalized arterial hypertension; it is, therefore, usually accompanied by further lesions above the tentorium.

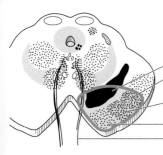

Substantia nigra: akinesia (parkinsonism)
Corticospinal fibers: contralateral spastic hemiplegia
Corticonuclear fibers: contralateral supranuclear facial and hypoglossal nerve palsies
Corticopontine tract: contralateral dystaxia
Root fibers of the oculomotor n.: ipsilateral oculomotor palsy with fixed and dilated pupil

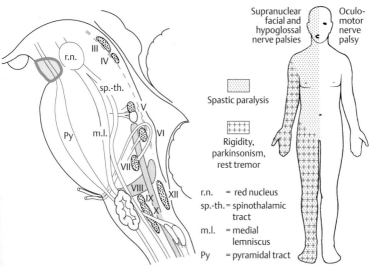

Supranuclear facial and hypoglossal nerve palsies

Oculomotor nerve palsy

Spastic paralysis

Rigidity, parkinsonism, rest tremor

r.n. = red nucleus
sp.-th. = spinothalamic tract
m.l. = medial lemniscus
Py = pyramidal tract

Fig. 4.**70 Syndrome of the cerebral peduncle** (Weber syndrome)

5 Cerebellum

5   Cerebellum

The cerebellum is a central organ for **fine motor control**. It processes information from multiple sensory channels (particularly vestibular and proprioceptive), together with motor impulses, and modulates the activity of motor nuclear areas in the brain and spinal cord.

Anatomically, the cerebellum is made up of **two hemispheres** and the **vermis** that lies between them. It is connected to the brainstem by **the three cerebellar peduncles**. An anatomical section reveals the cerebellar cortex and the underlying white matter, in which the deep cerebellar nuclei are embedded. The **cerebellar cortex** is primarily responsible for the integration and processing of afferent impulses. It projects to the **deep cerebellar nuclei**, which then emit most of the efferent fibers that leave the cerebellum.

Functionally (and phylogenetically), the cerebellum is divided into three components: the vestibulocerebellum, spinocerebellum, and cerebrocerebellum. The **vestibulocerebellum** is phylogenetically oldest. It receives afferent input mainly from the vestibular organ, and its function is to regulate balance. The **spinocerebellum** mainly processes proprioceptive impulses from the spinocerebellar pathways and controls stance and gait. The youngest component of the cerebellum, the **cerebrocerebellum**, has a close functional relationship with the motor cortex of the telencephalon and is responsible for the smooth and precise execution of all finely controlled movements. **Cerebellar lesions** manifest themselves clinically with disturbances of movement and balance.

Surface Anatomy

The cerebellum lies in the *posterior fossa*. Its superior surface is covered by the *tentorium cerebelli*, a tentlike double fold of the dura mater that separates the cerebellum from the cerebrum.

The **surface** of the cerebellum (Fig. 5.**1**), unlike that of the cerebrum, displays numerous small, horizontally running convolutions (*folia*), which are separated from each other by *fissures*. The narrow central portion of the cerebellum connecting the two hemispheres on either side is called the *vermis* because of its fancied resemblance to a worm.

A view of the cerebellum from below (Fig. 5.**2**) reveals the upper portion of the fourth ventricle lying between the cerebellar peduncles. The fourth ventricle communicates with the subarachnoid space through a single *median aperture* (foramen of Magendie) and two *lateral apertures* (foramina of Luschka). Caudal to the inferior and middle cerebral peduncles, there is a structure on either side called the *flocculus*; the two flocculi are connected across the midline through a portion of the vermis called the *nodulus*. Together, these structures constitute the *flocculonodular* lobe.

The subdivisions of the cerebellar vermis and hemispheres were given individual names by the old anatomists (culmen, declive, etc.), which are indicated in Figs. 5.**1** and 5.**2**, although they have little functional significance and are generally not clinically relevant. Today, it is more common to distinguish **three major components of the cerebellum** on phylogenetic and functional grounds:

The archicerebellum (phylogenetically oldest portion of the cerebellum) is intimately related to the vestibular apparatus. It receives most of its afferent input from the vestibular nuclei of the brainstem and is thus also called the **vestibulocerebellum**. Anatomically, it consists mainly of the flocculus and nodulus (*flocculonodular lobe*).

The paleocerebellum (next oldest portion of the cerebellum, after the archicerebellum) receives most of its afferent input from the spinal cord and is, therefore, also called the **spinocerebellum** (the term we will use in the following sections). It consists of the culmen and central lobule of the *anterior lobe* of the vermis, as well as the uvula and pyramid of its *inferior lobe*, and the paraflocculus. One can state, as a mild simplification, that the spinocerebellum is composed of most of the vermis and paravermian zone (pars intermedialis).

The neocerebellum (youngest portion of the cerebellum) is its largest part. Its phylogenetic development occurred together with the expansion of the cerebrum and the transition to an upright stance and gait. It is formed by the two cerebellar hemispheres and has an intimate functional connection to the cerebral cortex, which projects to it by way of the pontine nuclei. Thus, the neocerebellum is also termed the pontocerebellum or **cerebrocerebellum**, as we will call it in the following sections.

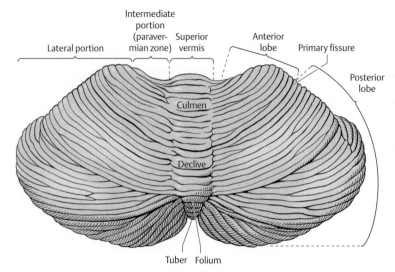

Fig. 5.**1 The cerebellum, viewed from above.** *Left side:* division into vermis, pars intermedialis, and pars lateralis. *Right side:* division into vermis, anterior lobe, and posterior lobe. The anterior and posterior lobes are separated by the primary fissure.

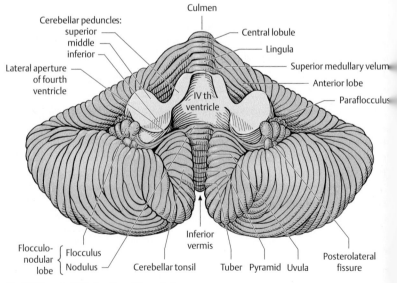

Fig. 5.**2 The cerebellum, viewed from below**

Internal Structure

Although the cerebellum accounts for only about 10% of the brain by weight, it contains more than 50% of all the brain's neurons. The neurons of the cerebellum are located in the gray matter of the highly convoluted cerebellar cortex and in the four deep cerebellar nuclei on either side (see below).

Cerebellar Cortex

The cerebellar cortex is composed of three layers (Fig. 5.**3**). Proceeding from the outermost inward, these layers are:

Molecular layer (stratum moleculare). This layer consists mainly of cellular processes, of which the majority are granule cell axons—*parallel fibers*, see below—and *Purkinje cell dendrites*. A few neurons are found among the fibers (stellate cells, basket cells, Golgi cells), which function as inhibitory interneurons.

Pukinje cell layer (stratum ganglionare). This thin layer contains nothing but the large cell bodies of the Purkinje cells, arranged side by side in rows. The elaborate, highly branched dendritic trees of these cells are directed outward into the molecular layer, where the dendritic tree of each individual Purkinje cell lies in a plane perpendicular to the long axis of the folium. The Purkinje cell axons are the only efferent fibers leaving the cerebellar cortex. They project mainly to the deep cerebellar nuclei and release the inhibitory neurotransmitter GABA (γ-aminobutyric acid). Efferent fibers from the cortex of the vestibulocerebellum bypass the deep cerebellar nuclei and project directly to sites outside the cerebellum.

Granule cell layer (stratum granulosum). This layer consists almost entirely of the densely packed cell bodies of the small granule cells, which account for more than 95% of all cerebellar neurons. The axons of these cells are mainly found in the molecular layer, where they travel along individual folia as parallel fibers and form synapses with the perpendicularly oriented dendritic trees of the Purkinje cells (approximately 200 000 parallel fibers form synapses with a single Purkinje cell). The cerebellar granule cells are glutamatergic and are the only neurons of the cerebellar cortex that exert an excitatory influence on their target cells.

Afferent Input to the Cerebellar Cortex

The afferent input to the cerebellar cortex is mainly derived from the *ipsilateral vestibular nuclei* (a small part, in fact, comes directly from the *vestibular organ*,

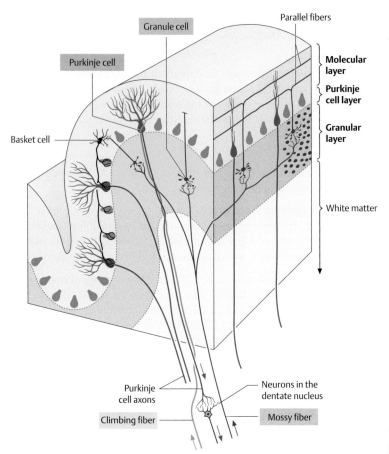

Fig. 5.**3 Structure of the cerebellar cortex** with its afferent and efferent connections (schematic drawing)

without any intervening synaptic relay), the *ipsilateral spinal cord*, the *contralateral pontine nuclei* (and thus, indirectly, from the contralateral cerebral cortex), and the *contralateral olivary nuclear complex* in the medulla (olive, for short). The olivary fibers are the so-called **climbing fibers**, which terminate on the Purkinje cells of the cerebellar cortex, climbing up their dendritic trees like ivy. All other afferent fibers terminate as **mossy fibers** on the granule cells of the cerebellar cortex, which then relay further impulses along their axons (parallel fibers of the molecular layer) to the Purkinje cell dendrites. Both mossy fibers and climbing fibers give off important collaterals to the deep cerebellar nuclei on their way to the cortex.

In view of the fact that both the mossy fibers and the granule cells (and thus the overwhelming majority of synapses in the cerebellum) are glutamatergic, it is not surprising that the **administration of glutamate antagonists** causes a marked worsening of cerebellar function in patients with cerebellar lesions.

Cerebellar Nuclei

A horizontal section of the cerebellum reveals four deep nuclei within each cerebellar hemisphere (see Fig. 5.**5**). The **fastigial nucleus** ("roof nucleus") is found most medially, in the roof of the fourth ventricle. It receives most of its *afferent* fibers from the Purkinje cells of the flocculonodular lobe (vestibulocerebellum). Its *efferent* fibers travel directly to the vestibular nuclei (*fastigiobulbar tract*) (Fig. 5.**5**) or cross to the opposite side of the cerebellum and then continue to the reticular formation and the vestibular nuclei (*uncinate fasciculus*).

Lateral to the fastigial nucleus, one finds two smaller nuclei, the **globose nucleus** (usually divided into two or three subnuclei) and the **emboliform nucleus**. Both of these nuclei receive *afferent* input from the cortex of the paravermian zone and vermis (spinocerebellum) and send *efferent* fibers to the contralateral red nucleus (Fig. 5.**5**).

The largest of the cerebellar nuclei, the **dentate nucleus**, occupies a lateral position in the deep white matter of each cerebellar hemisphere. Its *afferent* input comes mainly from the cortex of the cerebellar hemispheres (cerebrocerebellum), and, to a lesser extent, from the cortex of the paravermian zone. Its *efferent* fibers travel by way of the superior cerebellar peduncle to the contralateral red nucleus and thalamus (ventral lateral nucleus, VL) (Fig. 5.**5**). The thalamus is the site of a synaptic relay, with further projection to the motor areas of the cerebral cortex (Brodmann areas 4 and 6) (Fig. 6.**4**, p. 266).

Afferent and Efferent Projections of the Cerebellar Cortex and Nuclei

Synaptic transmission *within* the cerebellum follows a uniform scheme (Fig. 5.**4**): the cerebellar afferent pathways project to the cerebellar cortex and, through collateral fibers, to the deep cerebellar nuclei. In the cortex, afferent information is processed in a complex polysynaptic pathway that eventually converges onto the Purkinje cells. The Purkinje cells, in turn, transmit the results of this processing to the deep cerebellar nuclei, in the form of inhibitory, GABAergic impulses. In the deep nuclei, integrative processing of both primary

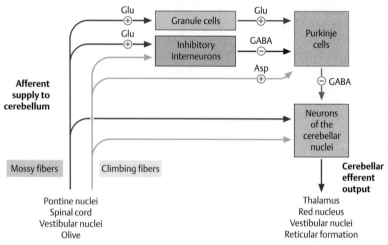

Fig. 5.**4 The basic scheme of neuronal connections within the cerebellum**

information (from the collateral fibers of the cerebellar afferent pathways) and modulated information (from the Purkinje cells/from the cortex) takes place and the result is then transmitted, by way of cerebellar efferent fibers, to the targets of the cerebellar projections.

Connections of the Cerebellum with Other Parts of the Nervous System

All sensory modalities that are important for orientation in space (vestibular sense, touch, proprioception, vision, and hearing) convey information to the cerebellum. The cerebellum receives input from widely diverse sensory areas of the nervous system by way of the three cerebellar peduncles, and sends its output by way of the deep cerebellar nuclei to all motor areas.

This section concerns the many afferent and efferent connections of the cerebellum and their distribution among the three cerebellar peduncles. The more important pathways are shown schematically in Fig. 5.**5**.

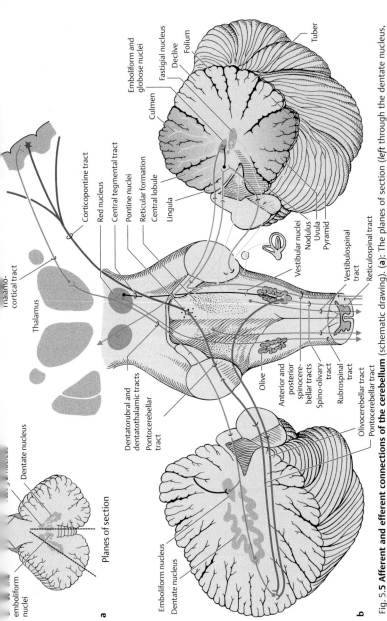

Fig. 5.5 **Afferent and efferent connections of the cerebellum** (schematic drawing). (**a**): The planes of section (*left* through the dentate nucleus, *right* through the vermis).

Inferior Cerebellar Peduncle

The inferior cerebellar peduncle (restiform body) contains the following **afferent** pathways:

- Fibers from the *vestibulocochlear nerve* and the *vestibular nuclei* to the flocculonodular lobe and fastigial nucleus (Fig. 5.**5**).
- Axons from the contralateral olive in the *olivocerebellar tract*, which continue as climbing fibers to the dendrites of the Purkinje cells of all areas of the cerebellar cortex (the inferior olivary nucleus projects mainly to the cerebrocerebellum, while the accessory olivary nuclei project mainly to the vestibulo- and spinocerebellum).
- The *posterior spinocerebellar tract*, whose fibers arise in the neurons of the nucleus dorsalis (thoracic nucleus or Clarke's column) at the base of the posterior horn of the spinal gray matter (Figs. 2.**16** and 2.**17**, pp. 42 f.); this tract mainly conveys impulses from the muscle spindles of the lower limbs and trunk to the paravermian zone of the anterior and posterior lobes.
- A pathway arising in neurons of the cervical spinal cord above the level of the thoracic nucleus, which ascends in the lateral portion of the fasciculus cuneatus and undergoes a synaptic relay in the *accessory cuneate nucleus* of the medulla; this pathway accompanies the posterior spinocerebellar tract on its way into the cerebellum.
- Fibers from the reticular formation (not shown in Fig. 5.**5**).
  The inferior cerebellar peduncle contains the following *efferent* pathways:
- The *fastigiobulbar tract* (largest efferent pathway of the inferior cerebellar peduncle) to the vestibular nuclei; this tract closes a vestibulocerebellar regulatory feedback loop through which the cerebellum influences the motor function of the spinal cord.
- Fibers from the fastigial nucleus to the reticular formation (*cerebelloreticular tract*) and from the dentate nucleus to the olive (*cerebello-olivary tract*).

Middle Cerebellar Peduncle

The middle cerebellar peduncle (brachium pontis) exclusively contains **afferent fibers**, of the following types:

- The *pontocerebellar tract* decussates in the pons and then travels in a thick bundle, by way of the middle cerebellar peduncle, to the cerebellar hemispheres. These fibers originate in the basal pontine nuclei and are thus the continuation, after a synaptic relay, of the corticocerebellar projections, which are derived from all of the lobes of the cerebrum, but in greatest number from the frontal lobe. The fibers cross the midline as soon as they emerge from the relay nuclei in the basis pontis.

- Further afferent fibers from the monoaminergic raphe nuclei travel by way of the middle cerebellar peduncle to the cerebellum.

Superior Cerebellar Peduncle

Efferent pathways. The superior cerebellar peduncle (brachium conjunctivum) contains most of the **cerebellar efferent fibers**. These fibers originate in the deep cerebellar nuclei and project mainly to the following structures:
- The contralateral thalamus (ventral lateral and centromedian nuclei, Figs. 6.**4** and 6.**6**, p. 266 ff.)
- The contralateral red nucleus
- The reticular formation

Efferent fibers to the thalamus. Efferent fibers in the superior cerebellar peduncle traveling to the thalamus arise mainly in the dentate nucleus (cerebrocerebellum). After a synaptic relay in the thalamus, further fibers ascend to the motor and premotor cerebral cortex, which, in turn, projects back to the pontine nuclei by way of the corticopontine tract. A long regulatory loop is thus created, traveling from the cerebral cortex to the pontine nuclei, cerebellar cortex, dentate nucleus, thalamus, and finally back to the cortex (Figs 5.**5** and 5.**6**).

Efferent fibers to the red nucleus and reticular formation. A further regulatory circuit comprises the so-called triangle of Guillain and Mollaret, traveling from the red nucleus by way of the central tegmental tract to the olive, then to the cerebellum and back to the red nucleus (Fig. 5.**7**). The cerebellum influences spinal motor function by way of fibers traveling from the red nucleus and reticular formation down into the spinal cord (cf. Fig. 3.**5**, p. 62).

Afferent pathways. One of the few afferent pathways in the superior cerebellar peduncle is the *anterior spinocerebellar tract*, which terminates in the same area (spinocerebellum) as the posterior spinocerebellar tract. Both convey proprioceptive impulses from the periphery, i.e., from muscle spindles, Golgi tendon organs, and joint receptors.

Fibers from the tectum travel to the cerebellar vermis in the *tectocerebellar tract*, which occupies a medial position in the superior cerebellar peduncle, at its transition to the superior medullary velum. These fibers convey auditory information from the inferior colliculi, and probably also visual information from the superior colliculi.

Topography of Cerebellar Afferent Pathways

Each half of the cerebellum is responsible for motor function on the *ipsilateral* half of the body. Some of the efferent fiber systems are doubly crossed: thus,

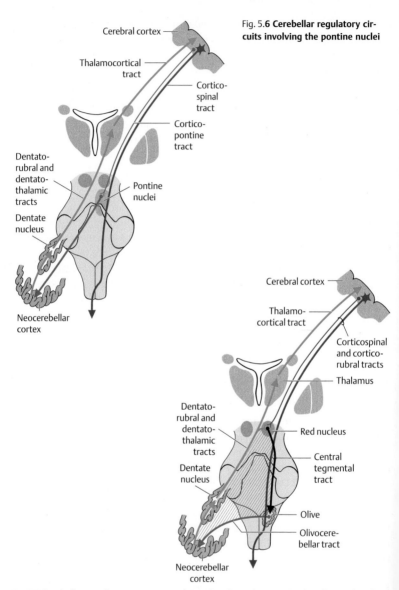

Fig. 5.**6 Cerebellar regulatory circuits involving the pontine nuclei**

Fig. 5.**7 Cerebellar regulatory circuits involving the olive.** The triangle of Guillain and Mollaret passes from the red nucleus by way of the central tegmental tract, the olive, and the cerebellum back to the red nucleus.

the cerebellorubral tract crosses the midline as soon as it enters the brainstem from behind, and the rubrospinal tract crosses the midline again just after its origin from the red nucleus (in the decussation of Forel). Similarly, the cerebellothalamic fibers travel from one side of the cerebellum to the opposite side of the thalamus and then proceed to the ipsilateral cerebral cortex, whose efferent fibers enter the pyramidal tract and decussate once more before they reach the spinal cord on the original side.

Cerebellar Function and Cerebellar Syndromes

Three important points must be grasped for a proper understanding of cerebellar function:
- The cerebellum receives a very large amount of general and special sensory input, but does not participate to any significant extent in conscious perception or discrimination.
- Although the cerebellum influences motor function, cerebellar lesions do not produce paralysis.
- The cerebellum is unimportant for most cognitive processes but nonetheless plays a major role in motor learning and memory.

Essentially, the cerebellum is a coordination center that **maintains balance** and **controls muscle tone** through regulatory circuits and complex feedback mechanisms, and **assures the precise**, **temporally well-coordinated execution of all directed motor processes**. Cerebellar coordination of movement occurs unconsciously.

The individual components of the cerebellum (vestibulocerebellum, spinocerebellum, and cerebrocerebellum) have different functions in the coordination of movement. These particular functions can be determined from experimental studies in animals on the one hand, and from clinical studies of patients with cerebellar lesions on the other. The constellations of signs and symptoms accompanying cerebellar disease that will be described here are seldom observed in pure form, both because it is rare for only one of the functional components of the cerebellum to be affected in isolation, and because slowly expanding processes (such as benign tumors) may induce functional compensation. Other portions of the brain can apparently assume some of the functions of the cerebellum, if necessary. Yet, if the disturbance affects not just the cerebellar cortex but also the deep cerebellar nuclei, only minimal recovery is likely to occur.

This being said, it is still best, from the didactic point of view, to consider the functions and typical clinical syndromes of each of the three parts of the cerebellum separately.

Vestibulocerebellum

Function. The vestibulocerebellum receives impulses from the vestibular apparatus carrying information about the position and movements of the head. Its efferent output influences the motor function of the eyes and body in such a way that equilibrium can be maintained in all positions and with any movement.

Synaptic connections. The following reflex arcs participate in the maintenance of equilibrium (balance). From the vestibular organ, impulses travel both directly and indirectly (by way of the vestibular nuclei) to the vestibulocerebellar cortex, and onward to the fastigial nucleus. The vestibulocerebellar cortex transmits impulses back to the vestibular nuclei, as well as to the reticular formation; from these sites, the *vestibulospinal* and *reticulospinal* tracts and the *medial longitudinal fasciculus* enter the brainstem and spinal cord to control spinal motor and oculomotor function (Fig. 5.**5**). These reflex arcs assure stability of stance, gait, and eye position and enable the fixation of gaze.

Lesions of the Vestibulocerebellum

Functional impairment of the flocculonodular lobe or fastigial nucleus renders the patient less capable of orienting himself or herself in the Earth's gravitational field, or of keeping his or her gaze fixed on a stationary object when the head is moving.

Dysequilibrium. The patient has difficulty standing upright (**astasia**) and walking (**abasia**), and the gait is broad-based and unsteady, resembling the gait of a drunken individual (**truncal ataxia**). Heel-to-toe walking can no longer be performed. The unsteadiness is not due to a deficiency of proprioceptive impulses reaching consciousness, but rather to faulty coordination of the musculature in response to gravity.

Oculomotor disturbances, nystagmus. Cerebellar disturbances of oculomotor function are manifest as an impaired ability to hold one's gaze on a stationary or moving target (lesions of the flocculus and paraflocculus). The result is **saccadic pursuit movements** and **gaze-evoked nystagmus:** if the patient tries to follow a moving object with his or her eyes, *square-wave jerks* can be observed, i.e., the amplitude of the microsaccades that normally occur in ocular pursuit is abnormally increased, so that they become visible to the examiner. Gaze-evoked nystagmus is more prominent when the eyes move toward the side of the cerebellar lesion and diminishes somewhat if the gaze is held to that side; if the eyes are then brought back to the midline, nystagmus in the opposite direction may be seen (*rebound nystagmus*).

Lesions of the vestibulocerebellum may impair the patient's ability to suppress the vestibulo-ocular reflex (VOR, p. 191), in which turning the head produces saccadic jerks of the eyes. A healthy individual can suppress this reflex by fixing the gaze upon an object, but a patient with a vestibulocerebellar lesion cannot (**impaired suppression of the VOR by fixation**). Furthermore, lesions of the nodulus and uvula impair the ability of the VOR (rotatory nystagmus) to habituate and may lead to the appearance of *periodic alternating nystagmus* that changes directions every 2-4 minutes.

Cerebellar lesions can also produce various types of **complex nystagmus**, such as opsoclonus (rapid conjugate movements of the eyes in multiple planes) or *ocular flutter* (opsoclonus in the horizontal plane only), whose precise localization has not yet been determined.

Spinocerebellum

Function. The spinocerebellum controls muscle tone and coordinates the actions of antagonistic muscle groups that participate in stance and gait. Its efferent output affects the activity of the anti-gravity muscles and controls the strength of forces induced by movement (e. g., inertia and centrifugal force).

Connections. The cortex of the spinocerebellum receives its afferent input from the spinal cord by way of the *posterior spinocerebellar tract*, the *anterior spinocerebellar tract*, and the *cuneocerebellar tract* (from the accessory cuneate nucleus). The cortex of the paravermian zone mainly projects to the *emboliform and globose nuclei*, while the vermian cortex mainly projects to the *fastigial nucleus*. The efferent output of these nuclei then proceeds through the *superior cerebellar peduncle* to the *red nucleus* and the *reticular formation*, from which modulating impulses are conveyed over the *rubrospinal, rubroreticular, and reticulospinal tracts* to the spinal motor neurons (Fig. 5.5). Each half of the body is served by the *ipsilateral* cerebellar cortex, but there is no precise somatotopic arrangement. Recent studies suggest that the neural organization of the cerebellar cortex resembles a patchwork rather than an exact somatotopic map.

Some of the efferent output of the emboliform nucleus travels by way of the thalamus to the motor cortex—mainly the portion of it that controls the proximal musculature of the limbs (pelvic and shoulder girdles) and the trunk. By this means, the spinocerebellum also exerts an influence on *voluntary, directed movements* of these muscle groups.

Lesions of the Spinocerebellum

The major manifestations of lesions of the cerebellar vermis and paravermian zone are as follows.

Lesions of the anterior lobe and of the superior portion of the vermis in and near the midline produce ataxia of stance and gait. The gait ataxia (abasia) produced by such lesions is worse than the ataxia of stance (astasia). Affected patients suffer from a **broad-based**, **unsteady gait** that deviates to the side of the lesion, and there is a **tendency to fall to that side**. The ataxia of stance is revealed by the Romberg test: when the patient stands with eyes closed, a gentle push on the sternum causes the patient to sway backwards and forwards at a frequency of 2-3 Hz. If the lesion is strictly confined to the superior portion of the vermis, the finger-nose test and the heel-knee-shin test may still be performed accurately.

Lesions of the inferior portion of the vermis produce an **ataxia of stance** (astasia) that is more severe than the ataxia of gait. The patient has difficulty sitting or standing steadily, and, in the Romberg test, sways slowly back and forth, without directional preference.

Cerebrocerebellum

Connections. The cerebrocerebellum receives most of its neural input indirectly from extensive portions of the cerebral cortex, mainly from *Brodmann areas 4 and 6* (the motor and premotor cortex) via the *corticopontine tract* (Fig. 5.**6**), but also, to a lesser extent, from the *olive* via the *olivocerebellar tract* (Fig. 5.**7**). The cerebellum receives advance notice of any planned voluntary movement initiated in the cerebral cortex, so that it can immediately send modulating and corrective impulses back to the motor cortex through the **dentatothalamocortical pathway** (Fig. 5.**5**, p. 247, and Fig. 5.**6**). The dentate nucleus also projects to the parvocellular portion of the red nucleus. Unlike the rest of the red nucleus, this part does not send fibers to the spinal cord by way of the rubrospinal tract. Rather, it projects through the central tegmental tract to the inferior olive, which then projects back to the cerebrocerebellum. This **dentato-rubro-olivo-cerebellar neural feedback loop** plays an important role in neocerebellar impulse processing.

Function. The complex connections of the cerebrocerebellum enable it to regulate all directed movements smoothly and precisely. By way of the very rapidly conducting afferent spinocerebellar pathways, it continuously receives real-time information about motor activity in the periphery. It can thus take action to correct any errors in the course of voluntary movement to ensure that they are executed smoothly and accurately. The executive patterns of a large number of different types of movement are probably stored in the cerebellum, as in a computer, over the life of the individual, so that they can be recalled from it at any time. Thus, once we have reached a certain stage of development, we can perform difficult learned movements rapidly, relatively effortlessly, and at will by calling upon the precise regulatory function of the cerebellum.

The functions of the cerebellum extend beyond the coordination of movement to the processing of sensory stimuli and of information that is relevant to memory. A further discussion of these aspects is beyond the scope of this book.

Lesions of the Cerebrocerebellum

It follows from the discussion of cerebellar function in the preceding sections that lesions of the cerebrocerebellum do not produce paralysis but nonetheless severely impair the execution of voluntary movements. The clinical manifestations are always ipsilateral to the causative lesion.

Decomposition of voluntary movements. The movements of the limbs are atactic and uncoordinated, with dysmetria, dyssynergia, dysdiadochokinesia, and intention tremor. These abnormalities are more pronounced in the upper than in the lower limbs, and complex movements are more severely affected than simple ones. **Dysmetria**, i.e., the inability to stop a directed movement on time, is manifested (for example) by a moving finger going past the location of its target (past-pointing, overshoot; *hypermetria*). **Dyssynergia** is the loss of the precise cooperation of multiple muscle groups in the execution of a particular movement; each muscle group contracts, but the individual groups fail to work together correctly. **Dysdiadochokinesia** is an impairment of rapid alternating movements caused by a breakdown of the precisely timed coordination of antagonistic muscle groups: movements such as rapid pronation and supination of the hand are slow, halting, and arrhythmic. **Intention tremor**, or more properly—**action tremor**, is seen mainly in directed movements and becomes more intense the nearer the finger comes to its target. There may also be a postural tremor at a frequency of 2-3 Hz, particularly when the patient tries to hold the pronated hands directly in front, with arms extended.

Rebound phenomenon. When the patient presses against the examiner's hand with maximum strength and the examiner suddenly pulls his or her own hand away, the patient's movement fails to be braked as normal, and the arm lurches toward the examiner.

Hypotonia and hyporeflexia. In an acute lesion of the cerebellar hemisphere, the muscular resistance to passive movement is diminished, and abnormal postures (e. g., of the hand) may result. The intrinsic muscle reflexes are also diminished in the hypotonic muscles.

Scanning dysarthria and dysarthrophonia. These manifestations arise mainly as a result of paravermian lesions and reflect impaired synergy of the musculature of speech. The patient speaks slowly and haltingly, with poor articulation, and with an abnormal, unvarying stress on each syllable.

Cerebellar Disorders

Cerebellar Ischemia and Hemorrhage

Arterial blood reaches the cerebellum through the three cerebellar arteries: the superior cerebellar, anterior inferior cerebellar, and posterior inferior cerebellar arteries. The origin and anatomical course of these arteries and the typical clinical manifestations of occlusions of each of them are presented in Chapter 11 on p. 427 ff. The typical manifestations of cerebellar hemorrhage are presented on p. 480 f.

Cerebellar Tumors

Cerebellar tumors are only rarely confined to a single subdivision of the cerebellum.

Benign cerebellar tumors (such as pilocytic astrocytoma) may be problematic in that they often grow quite large before producing symptoms, because of the plasticity of the cerebellum. Papilledema, an indirect sign of an intracranial mass, may be lacking for a long time, particularly in adults; it is present in about 75 % of affected children. In most cases (90 %), cerebellar tumors manifest themselves initially with occipitocervical headache and nausea and vomiting on an empty stomach (dry heaves). A forced head tilt is a clinical sign of impending herniation of the cerebellar tonsils through the foramen magnum.

Medulloblastoma is a malignant tumor that preferentially affects children and adolescents and accounts for one-third of all brain tumors in this age group (8 % of all brain tumors regardless of age). It often arises from the roof of the fourth ventricle and then grows into the vermian portion of the flocculonodular lobe, possibly metastasizing to other regions of the brain and spinal cord

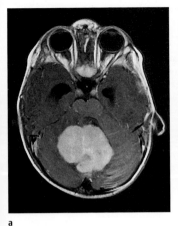 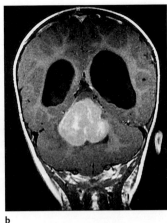

a   b

Fig. 5.**8 Medulloblastoma**, seen in T1-weighted MR images after intravenous administration of contrast material. **a** A large, markedly and homogeneously contrast-enhancing tumor is seen in the superior portion of the vermis. The tumor compresses the fourth ventricle and causes occlusive hydrocephalus, as manifested by the enlarged temporal horns of the lateral ventricles. **b** The coronal image shows the origin of the tumor from the superior vermis and reveals marked dilatation of the lateral ventricles.

through the cerebrospinal fluid (*drop metastases*). Because this type of tumor often begins in the vestibulocerebellum, its typical initial sign is dysequilibrium: the affected child has a broad-based, swaying, and staggering gait. Further cerebellar manifestations including ataxia, dysmetria, asynergia, adiadochokinesia, and intention tremor gradually arise as the tumor grows further and begins to affect the lateral portions of the cerebellum (the hemispheres). In advanced stages of tumor growth, blockage of the fourth ventricle or of the cerebral aqueduct causes occlusive hydrocephalus, with clinical signs of intracranial hypertension (Fig. 5.8).

Astrocytoma and hemangioblastoma. Similar manifestations are produced by **pilocytic astrocytoma**, a further characteristic type of posterior fossa tumor arising near the midline. On the other hand, **hemangioblastoma** in the setting of von Hippel-Lindau disease and **cystic astrocytoma** tend to arise in the cerebellar hemispheres and, therefore, to produce appendicular ataxia and gaze-evoked nystagmus as their typical manifestations.

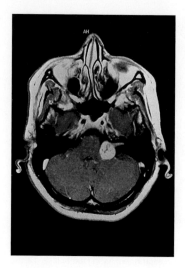

Fig. 5.**9 Acoustic neuroma,** seen in an axial, T1-weighted MR image at the level of the internal acoustic meatus, obtained after intravenous administration of contrast material. Note the typical intrameatal and extrameatal extension of the left-sided tumor, with expanded extrameatal portion ("ice-cream cone" appearance).

Acoustic neuroma (i.e., vestibular schwannoma). This tumor arises from the *Schwann cells of the eighth cranial nerve* (usually its vestibular portion) and is thus found in the cerebellopontine angle. It expands slowly and may reach a considerable size, producing the clinical manifestations described above on p. 194 f.

6 Diencephalon and Autonomic Nervous System

6 Diencephalon and Autonomic Nervous System

The diencephalon lies between the brainstem and the telencephalon. It has four components: the thalamus, epithalamus, subthalamus, and hypothalamus.

The **thalamus** is found on both sides of the third ventricle and consists of numerous nuclei with different functions. It is the relay station for most of the afferent pathways that ascend to the cerebral cortex. Some types of impulses (e. g., nociceptive impulses) may already be perceived, integrated, and given an affective coloring, in an imprecise way, in the thalamus, but actual conscious experiences do not seem to be generated until sensory impulses reach the cerebral cortex. Moreover, the thalamus has extensive connections with the basal ganglia, brainstem, cerebellum, and motor cortical areas of the cerebrum and is thus a major component of the motor regulatory system.

The most important nucleus of the **subthalamus** is the subthalamic nucleus, which is closely functionally related to the basal ganglia.

The **epithalamus** is mainly composed of the epiphysis (pineal gland/pineal body) and the habenular nuclei; it plays a role in the regulation of circadian rhythms.

The most basal portion of the diencephalon is the **hypothalamus**, which coordinates vital bodily functions such as respiration, circulation, water balance, temperature, and nutritional intake and is thus the hierarchically uppermost regulatory organ of the autonomic nervous system. It also influences the activity of the endocrine glands by way of the hypothalamic-pituitary axis.

The **autonomic nervous system** is responsible for the nerve supply of the internal organs, blood vessels, sweat glands, and salivary and lacrimal glands. It is called "autonomic" because it functions largely independently of consciousness; it is alternatively (less commonly) called the vegetative nervous system. Its efferent arm in the periphery is composed of two anatomically and functionally distinct parts, the sympathetic and parasympathetic nervous systems. The afferent arm is not divided in this way.

Because of the multiplicity of functions that the diencephalon performs, **diencephalic lesions** can have very diverse effects, depending on their site and extent. Thalamic lesions produce hemiparesis and hemisensory deficits, movement disorders, disturbances of consciousness, and pain syndromes, while hypothalamic lesions impair various vital functions singly or in combination, and cause endocrine dysfunction.

Location and Components of the Diencephalon

Location. The position of the diencephalon is just oral to that of the midbrain; the diencephalon does not continue along the brainstem axis, but rather takes a rostral bend, so that it comes to lie nearly in the longitudinal axis of the cerebrum (Fig. 6.**1**). It is located in the middle of the brain, ventrally and caudally to the frontal lobe, and encloses the lower portion of the third ventricle from both sides (Fig. 6.**2**).

The *thalamus* forms the **upper** portion of the third ventricular wall, the *hypothalamus* its **lower** portion. **Dorsally**, the diencephalon is enclosed by the corpus callosum, the lateral ventricles, and the cerebral hemispheres (Fig. 6.**2**). The roof of the third ventricle is formed by the thin tela choroidea and the attached choroid plexus. The **rostral** extent of the diencephalon is delimited by the lamina terminalis and anterior commissure, its **caudal** extent by the posterior commissure, habenular commissure, and pineal body (epiphysis). The interventricular foramen of Monro, which connects the lateral ventricle with the third ventricle, is found on either side anterior to the rostral portion of the thalamus, just below the genu of the fornix. The basal portion of the dien-

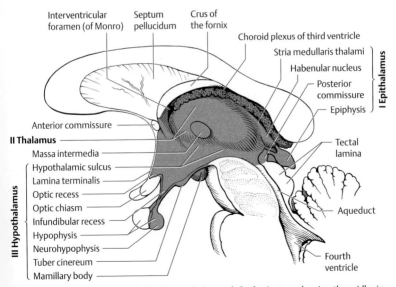

Fig. 6.1 **Sagittal section through the diencephalon and the brainstem** showing the midbrain–diencephalic junction and the structures surrounding the third ventricle

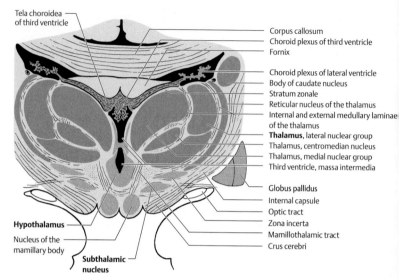

Fig. 6.**2 Coronal section through the diencephalon**

cephalon is its only externally visible part: it can be seen on the undersurface of the brain between the optic chiasm, the optic tract, and the cerebral peduncles. The visible diencephalic structures in this area are the mamillary bodies and the tuber cinereum, together with its infundibulum (pituitary stalk), which leads downward to the pituitary gland (cf. Fig. 4.**8**, p. 129).

The two halves of the thalamus facing each other across the third ventricle are connected in 70-80% of cases by the interthalamic adhesion (*massa intermedia*) (Fig. 6.**1**), which is not a fiber pathway but rather a secondary adhesion of the gray matter coming from either side. **Laterally**, the diencephalon is delimited by the internal capsule.

The globus pallidus is embryologically a part of the diencephalon, though it is separated from it by the internal capsule (Fig. 8.**4**, p. 334) and is thus located in the basal ganglia. It will be discussed along with the rest of the basal ganglia in Chapter 8 (p. 332). Likewise, a discussion of the hypophysis (pituitary gland), which is linked to the hypothalamus by the infundibulum, will be deferred to the section on the autonomic nervous system (p. 289).

Subdivisions. The diencephalon has the following components (Fig. 6.**1**):
- The **epithalamus**, which consists of the habenula and habenular nuclei, the habenular commissure, the epiphysis, and the epithalamic (posterior) commissure.

- The **thalamus**, a large complex of neurons that accounts for four-fifths of the volume of the diencephalon.
- The **hypothalamus**, which is demarcated from the thalamus by the hypothalamic sulcus, and contains various functionally distinct groups of neurons. It is the hierarchically uppermost center ("head ganglion") of the autonomic nervous system; on each side, the column of the fornix descends through the lateral wall of the hypothalamus to terminate in the mamillary body (see Fig. 6.**8**).
- The **subthalamus**, which mainly consists of the subthalamic nucleus (corpus luysii, Fig. 6.**2**) and is located beneath the thalamus and dorsolateral to the mamillary body.

Thalamus

Nuclei

Flanking the third ventricle, on either side of the brain, there is a large, ovoid complex of neurons measuring about 3×1.5 cm in diameter. This complex, the thalamus, is not a uniform cluster of cells but rather a conglomerate of numerous, distinct nuclei, each with its own function and its own afferent and efferent connections. Each half of the thalamus (left and right) is divided into three major regions by sheetlike layers of white matter taking the form of a Y (the internal medullary laminae, Fig. 6.**3**). The **anterior nuclei** sit in the angle of the Y, the **ventrolateral nuclei** laterally, and the **medial nuclei** medially. The ventrolateral nuclei are further subdivided into *ventral* and *lateral nuclear groups*. The ventral nuclei include the *ventral anterior nucleus* (*VA*), the *ventral lateral nucleus* (*VL*), the *ventral posterolateral nucleus* (*VPL*), and the *ventral posteromedial nucleus* (*VPM*). The lateral nuclei consist of a *lateral dorsal nucleus* and a *lateral posterior nucleus*. Further caudally, one finds the **pulvinar**, with the **medial** and **lateral geniculate bodies** attached to its underside. There are a few small groups of neurons within the internal medullary laminae (the **interlaminar nuclei**), as well as one larger, centrally located cell complex, the **centromedian nucleus** (or *centre médian*). Laterally, the external medullary lamina separates the thalamus from the internal capsule; the **reticular nucleus of the thalamus** is a thin layer of cells closely applied to the external medullary lamina (Fig. 6.**2**).

The three major nuclear groups (anterior, ventrolateral, and medial) have been cytologically and functionally subdivided into about 120 smaller nuclei, the most important of which are shown in Fig. 6.**3**. There is still no uniform

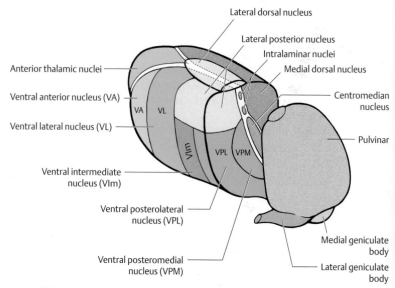

Fig. 6.**3 Thalamic nuclei.** The four major nuclear groups are shown: the **anterior group** (green), the **ventrolateral group** (various shades of blue), the **medial group** (red), and the **dorsal group,** consisting of the pulvinar (violet) and the geniculate bodies (shades of blue).

standard for the subdivision and nomenclature of the thalamic nuclei; the nomenclature followed in Fig. 6.**3** is that found in *Nomina Anatomica.*

Position of the Thalamic Nuclei in Ascending and Descending Pathways

In the preceding chapters, the pathways that ascend from the spinal cord, brainstem, and cerebellum to the cerebral cortex have been traced upward as far as the thalamus. The thalamus is the last major relay station for all ascending impulses (except olfactory impulses) before they continue, via thalamocortical fibers, to the cortex. Figure 6.**4** shows the termination of various afferent pathways in distinct thalamic nuclei, which then project to corresponding cortical areas (for further details, see below).

Like the spinal cord and brainstem (e. g., the medial lemniscus), the thalamic nuclei and the thalamocortical projections maintain a strict **point-to-point somatotopic organization.**

Specific and nonspecific projections. Thalamic nuclei that receive input from circumscribed areas of the body periphery and transmit impulses to the corresponding circumscribed cortical areas (primary projective fields) are called **specific thalamic nuclei** (or primary thalamic nuclei). Thalamic nuclei projecting to the unimodal and multimodal cortical association areas (secondary and tertiary thalamic nuclei) are also counted among the specific nuclei. The distinguishing feature of the specific nuclei is thus a *direct projection to the cerebral cortex.*

In contrast, **nonspecific thalamic nuclei** receive their afferent input from multiple, distinct sense organs, usually after an intervening synapse in the reticular formation and/or one of the primary thalamic nuclei. They project only indirectly to the cerebral cortex (e. g., by way of the basal ganglia), including the association fields.

Specific Thalamic Nuclei and Their Connections

Nuclei with Connections to Primary Cortical Areas

Ventral posterolateral nucleus (VPL) and ventral posteromedial nucleus (VPM). All somatosensory fibers ascending in the medial lemniscus, spinothalamic tract, trigeminothalamic tract, etc., terminate in a relay station in the ventroposterior nuclear complex of the thalamus. The ventral posterolateral nucleus is the *relay station for the medial lemniscus*, while the ventral posteromedial nucleus is the *relay station for trigeminal afferents*. These nuclei, in turn, project fibers to circumscribed areas of the somatosensory cortex (areas 3a, 3b, 1, and 2, Fig. 6.**4**).

Furthermore, *gustatory fibers* from the nucleus of the tractus solitarius terminate in the medial tip of the ventral posteromedial nucleus, which, in turn, projects to the postcentral region overlying the insula (Fig. 6.4).

Medial and lateral geniculate bodies. The medial and lateral geniculate bodies, too, are among the specific nuclei of the thalamus. The optic tract terminates in the lateral geniculate body, which relays *visual impulses* retinotopically, by way of the optic radiation, to the visual cortex (area 17). *Auditory impulses* are carried in the lateral lemniscus to the medial geniculate body and relayed tonotopically, by way of the auditory radiation, to the auditory cortex (transverse temporal gyri of Heschl, area 41) in the temporal lobe (Fig. 6.**5**).

Ventral oral nuclei and ventral anterior nucleus. The ventral oral posterior nucleus (V.o.p., a portion of the ventral lateral nucleus) receives input from the *dentate nucleus and red nucleus* by way of the dentatothalamic tract (Fig. 6.4) and projects to the *motor cortex* (area 4), while the ventral oral anterior nucleus

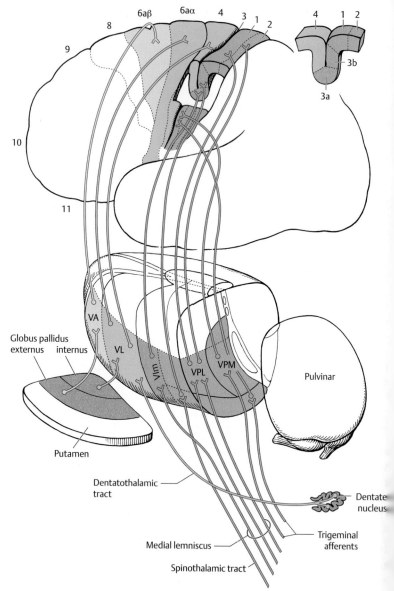

Fig. 6.**4 Afferent and efferent connections of the ventral nuclear group**

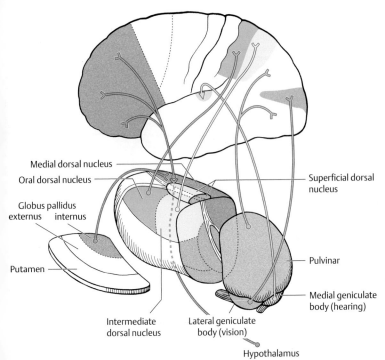

Medial dorsal nucleus
Oral dorsal nucleus
Globus pallidus
externus   internus
Putamen
Intermediate
dorsal nucleus
Lateral geniculate
body (vision)
Hypothalamus
Superficial dorsal
nucleus
Pulvinar
Medial geniculate
body (hearing)

Fig. 6.**5 Afferent and efferent connections of the medial** (red), **dorsal** (violet/blue), **and lateral** (blue) **nuclear groups**

(V.o.a.) and the ventral anterior nucleus (VA), both of which also belong to the ventral nuclear group, receive input from the *globus pallidus* and project to the *premotor cortex* (areas 6aα and 6aβ) (Fig. 6.**4**).

Nuclei Projecting to Association Areas of the Cerebral Cortex

The anterior nucleus, the medial nucleus, and the pulvinar are secondary and tertiary thalamic nuclei (Figs. 6.**5**, 6.**6**), i.e., specific thalamic nuclei projecting to the unimodal and multimodal cortical association fields (p. 384). These nuclei mostly receive their input not directly from the periphery but rather after a synaptic relay, which is usually located in one of the primary thalamic nuclei described above.

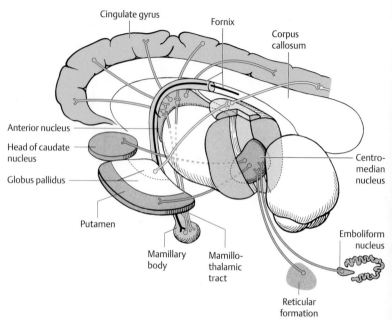

Fig. 6.6 **Afferent and efferent connections of the anterior nucleus** (green) **and the centromedian nucleus** (orange)

The **anterior nucleus** (Fig. 6.6) is reciprocally connected to the mamillary body and fornix through the mamillothalamic tract (of Vicq d'Azyr); it possesses bidirectional, point-to-point connections with the cingulate gyrus (area 24) and is thus an integral part of the limbic system, whose structure and function are described in Chapter 7.

The **medial nucleus** of the thalamus has bidirectional, point-to-point connections with the *association areas of the frontal lobe* and the *premotor region*. It receives afferent input from other thalamic nuclei (ventral and intralaminar nuclei), and from the hypothalamus, midbrain nuclei, and globus pallidus (Fig. 6.5).

Destruction of the medial nucleus by a tumor or other process causes a **frontal brain syndrome** with a change of personality (loss of self-representation, as described by Hassler), just as has been described after frontal leukotomy—a psychosurgical procedure, now rarely, if ever, performed, in which a lesion is made in the deep white matter of the frontal lobe. The visceral impulses that reach this nucleus by way of the hypothalamus exert an influence on the affective state of the individual, leading to a sense of well-being or uneasiness, good or bad mood, etc.

The **pulvinar** possesses reciprocal, point-to-point connections with the association areas of the parietal and occipital lobes (Fig. 6.**5**). These association areas are surrounded by the primary somatosensory, visual, and auditory cortices and thus probably play a major role in the binding of these different types of incoming sensory information. The pulvinar receives neural input from other thalamic nuclei, especially the intralaminar nuclei.

Lateral nuclei. The lateral dorsal nucleus and the lateral posterior nucleus do not receive any neural input from outside the thalamus and are connected only to other thalamic nuclei. They are thus known as integrative nuclei.

Nonspecific Thalamic Nuclei and Their Connections

Intralaminar nuclei. The intralaminar nuclei are the most important component of the nonspecific thalamic projection system. These nuclei are located within the internal medullary lamina, and the largest among them is the **centromedian nucleus**. These cell complexes receive their afferent input through ascending fibers from the brainstem *reticular formation* and the *emboliform nucleus* of the cerebellum, as well as from the *internal pallidal segment* and other thalamic nuclei. They project not to the cerebral cortex but rather to the *caudate nucleus*, *putamen*, and *globus pallidus* (Fig. 6.**6**). They probably also send efferent impulses diffusely to all nuclei of the thalamus, which then, in turn, project to widespread secondary areas of the cerebral cortex. The centromedian nucleus is an important component of the intralaminar cell complex, which constitutes the thalamic portion of the ascending reticular activating system (*ARAS* or *arousal system*, p. 271). Another portion of this arousal system probably involves the subthalamus and hypothalamus.

Functions of the Thalamus

The functions of the thalamus are highly complex because of the large number of nuclei it contains and their very diverse afferent and efferent connections.

- First of all, the thalamus is the largest subcortical **collecting point** for all exteroceptive and proprioceptive sensory impulses.
- Furthermore, it is a **relay station** for all impulses arising in cutaneous and visceral sensory receptors, for visual and auditory impulses, and for im-

pulses from the hypothalamus, cerebellum, and brainstem reticular formation, all of which are processed in the thalamus before being transmitted onward to other structures. The thalamus sends a small efferent component to the striatum, but most of its output goes to the cerebral cortex. All sensory impulses (other than olfactory impulses) must pass through the thalamus before they can be consciously perceived. Thus, the thalamus was traditionally called "the gateway to consciousness," though the conscious perception of smell implies that this conception is flawed and perhaps misleading.

- The thalamus, however, is not merely a relay station, but an important **center for integration and coordination,** in which afferent impulses of different modalities, from different regions of the body, are integrated and given an affective coloration. A neural substrate of certain elementary phenomena such as pain, displeasure, and well-being is already present in the thalamus before being transmitted upward to the cortex.

- Through its reciprocal connections (feedback loops) with the motor cortex, some of which pass through the basal ganglia and cerebellum, the thalamus **modulates motor function.**

- Some thalamic nuclei are also **components of the ascending reticular activating system** (ARAS), a specific arousal system originating in nuclei that are diffusely located throughout the brainstem reticular formation. Activating impulses from the ARAS are relayed by certain thalamic nuclei (ventral anterior nucleus, intralaminar nuclei [particularly the centromedian nucleus], reticular nuclei) to the entire neocortex. An intact ARAS is essential for normal consciousness.

Syndromes of Thalamic Lesions

The clinical manifestations of thalamic lesions depend on their precise location and extent because the functions of the individual thalamic nuclei are so highly varied.

Lesions of the ventral anterior and intralaminar nuclei. The ventral anterior (VA), intralaminar, and reticular nuclei are nonspecific "activating" nuclei. They project diffusely to the frontal lobes (ventral anterior nucleus, cf. Fig. 6.**4**, p. 266) and the entire neocortex (intralaminar nuclei), and they serve to modulate cortical responses. These pathways are components of the ascending reticular activating system (ARAS). Lesions in this area, particularly bilateral lesions, cause *disturbances of consciousness and attention*, and, if they extend to the midbrain tegmentum, **vertical gaze palsy.** Less commonly, paramedian lesions can cause agitation, dysphoria, or acute confusion. Isolated lesions of the ventral anterior nuclei with impaired frontal cortical activation have been reported to cause disturbances of voluntary behavior; right-sided lesions in this area have also been reported to cause more complex disturbances of mood, e. g., manic state and logorrhea, or, alternatively, delirium with confabulations and inappropriate behavior. Bilateral medial lesions can cause transient amnesia with or without anosognosia.

Lesions of the ventral nuclei. As described above, the **ventral posterior nuclei** are relay stations for specific sensory impulses, which are then sent onward to the corresponding primary cortical areas. Lesions of these nuclei produce specific deficits of one or more sensory modalities, as follows.

- Lesions of the **ventral posterolateral nucleus** produce *contralateral impairment of touch and proprioception,* as well as paresthesias of the limbs, which may feel as if they were swollen or abnormally heavy.
- Lesions affecting the **basal portion of the ventral posterolateral** and/or **posteromedial nucleus** can produce severe pain syndromes in addition to the sensory deficits just described ("thalamic pain," sometimes in anesthetic areas—*"anesthesia dolorosa"*; cf. Case Presentation 1).
- Lesions of the **ventral lateral nucleus** have mainly *motor* manifestations, as this nucleus is mainly connected to the primary and secondary motor areas of the cerebral cortex, and to the cerebellum and basal ganglia.
- **Acute lesions** of the ventral lateral nucleus and the neighboring subthalamic region can produce severe central "weakness," in which direct peripheral testing reveals no impairment of raw muscle strength (e. g., against resistance) ("thalamic astasia"). The patient falls to the side opposite the lesion and may be unable to sit unaided. Such manifestations appear either in isolation or in conjunction with transient thalamic neglect, in which both sensory and motor function is neglected on the side opposite the lesion. Thalamic neglect, due to involvement of thalamocortical fibers projecting to the parietal lobe, is usually short-lasting and almost always resolves completely.
- Lesions affecting the dentato-rubro-thalamic projections of the **ventral lateral nucleus** (V.o.p.) produce *contralateral hemiataxia* with action tremor, dysmetria, dysdiadochokinesia, and pathological rebound. Such findings may give the erroneous impression of a cerebellar lesion.

Case Presentation 1: *Thalamic Pain Syndrome after Hemorrhage in the Basal Ganglia*

This 51-year-old male schoolteacher was attending a friend's funeral when he suddenly fell and complained of nausea and a pulsatile headache. He had been standing in the hot sun during the eulogy, and the other funeral attendees at first thought he had simply fainted. When he was still unable to get up unaided and continued to complain of headache ten minutes later, they called an ambulance. The emergency physician on the scene found an arterial blood pressure of 220/120 mmHg and weakness of the left hand and the entire left lower limb, and the patient was transported to the hospital. Examination on admission revealed central-type left hemiparesis with increased deep tendon reflexes, as well as hypesthesia and hypalgesia near the midline, pallanesthesia, and a mild deficit of position sense on the left side of the body. A CT scan revealed an acute hemorrhage in the right basal ganglia. Over the next six months, the patient's hemiparesis and hemisensory deficit largely resolved, and he was able to resume playing tennis. In the same period of time, however, he began to experience repeated bouts of paroxysmal pain and dysesthesia in the previously hypesthetic areas on the left side of the body. These abnormal sensations were partly electric in character. An MRI scan of the head at this time revealed only a small remnant of the initial hemorrhage, with formation of a cyst in the right thalamus. The pain improved considerably on treatment with carbamazepine and amitriptyline but returned promptly as soon as the patient tried to stop taking these medications. They could finally be discontinued with a slow taper after a further three years.

Thalamic Vascular Syndromes

The thalamus is supplied by four arteries (p. 431). Interruption of the arterial blood supply in each of these distributions causes a characteristic syndrome, as described below in Chapter 11 on p. 468.

Epithalamus

The epithalamus consists of the **habenula** with its **habenular nuclei**, the **habenular commissure**, the **stria medullaris**, and the **epiphysis**. The habenula and the habenular nuclei constitute an important relay station of the olfactory system. Afferent olfactory fibers travel by way of the stria medullaris thalami to the habenular nuclei, which emit efferent projections to the autonomic (salivatory) nuclei of the brainstem, thus playing an important role in nutritional intake.

The **epiphysis (pineal gland)** contains specialized cells, called pinealocytes. Calcium and magnesium salts are deposited in the epiphysis from approximately age 15 years onward, making this structure visible in plain radiographs of the skull (an important midline marker before the era of CT and MRI). Epiphyseal tumors in childhood sometimes cause *precocious puberty*; it is thus presumed that this organ inhibits sexual maturation in some way, and that the destruction of epiphyseal tissue can remove this inhibition. In lower vertebrates, the epiphysis is a *light-sensitive organ* that regulates circadian rhythms. In primates, light cannot penetrate the skull, but the epiphysis still indirectly receives visual input relating to the light-dark cycle. Afferent impulses travel from the retina to the **suprachiasmatic nucleus** of the hypothalamus, from which, in turn, further impulses are conducted to the **intermediolateral nucleus** and, via postganglionic fibers of the cervical sympathetic chain, to the epiphysis.

Subthalamus

Location and components. The subthalamus is found immediately caudal to the thalamus at an early stage of embryological development and then moves laterally as the brain develops. It comprises the **subthalamic nucleus**, part of the **globus pallidus** (cf. p. 332), and various **fiber contingents** that pass through it on their way to the thalamus, including the medial lemniscus, the spinothalamic tract, and the trigeminothalamic tract. All of these tracts terminate in the ventroposterior region of the thalamus (Fig. 6.**4**, p. 266). The substantia nigra and red nucleus border the subthalamus anteriorly and posteriorly. Fibers of the dentatothalamic tract travel in the prerubral field H1 of Forel to terminate in the ventro-oral posterior nucleus of the thalamus (a part of the ventral lateral nucleus, VL); fibers from the globus pallidus travel in the lenticular fasciculus (Forel's fasciculus H2) to the ventro-oral anterior nucleus (another part of VL) and the ventral anterior nucleus (VA). These tracts are joined more rostrally by the ansa lenticularis. The subthalamus also contains the zona incerta, a rostral continuation of the midbrain reticular formation. The major connections of the putamen, pallidum, subthalamus, and thalamus are depicted in Fig. 6.**7**.

Function. The subthalamic nucleus (corpus Luysii) is, functionally speaking, a component of the basal ganglia and has reciprocal connections with the globus pallidus (p. 332). Lesions of the subthalamic nucleus produce contralateral *hemiballism* (p. 345 f.).

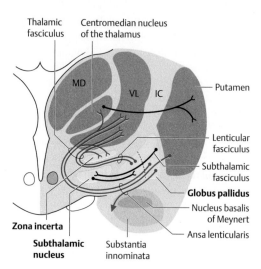

Thalamic fasciculus

Centromedian nucleus of the thalamus

MD

VL   IC

Putamen

Lenticular fasciculus

Subthalamic fasciculus

Globus pallidus

Nucleus basalis of Meynert

Ansa lenticularis

Zona incerta

Subthalamic nucleus

Substantia innominata

Fig. 6.**7 Fiber connections in the subthalamus.** MD = medial dorsal nucleus of the thalamus; VL = ventral lateral nucleus; IC = internal capsule.

Hypothalamus

Location and Components

The hypothalamus (Fig. 6.8) is composed of **gray matter in the walls of the third ventricle** from the hypothalamic sulcus downward and in the **floor of the third ventricle**, as well as the **infundibulum and the mamillary bodies**. The posterior pituitary lobe, or **neurohypophysis**, is also considered part of the hypothalamus; this structure is, in a sense, the enlarged caudal end of the infundibulum. The anterior pituitary lobe, on the other hand, is not derived from the neuroectoderm at all, but rather from Rathke's pouch, an outcropping of the rostral end of the primitive alimentary tract. The two pituitary lobes, though adjacent to each other, are not functionally connected. Remnants of Rathke's pouch in the sellar region can grow into tumors, e. g., craniopharyngioma.

The columns of the fornix, as they descend through the hypothalamus to the mamillary bodies on either side, divide the hypothalamus of each side into a **medial** and a **lateral segment** (Fig. 6.8). The lateral segment contains various groups of fibers, including the *medial forebrain bundle*, which runs from basal olfactory areas to the midbrain. It also contains the lateral tuberal nuclei (see

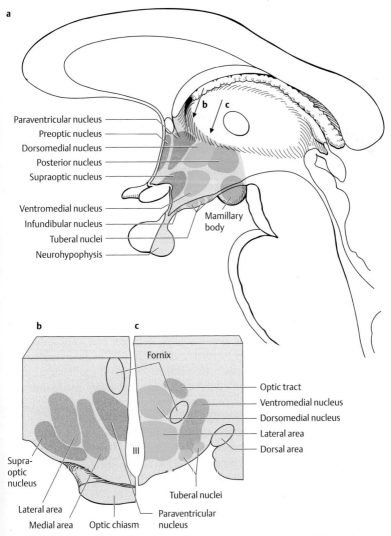

a

Paraventricular nucleus
Preoptic nucleus
Dorsomedial nucleus
Posterior nucleus
Supraoptic nucleus

Ventromedial nucleus
Infundibular nucleus
Tuberal nuclei
Neurohypophysis

Mamillary body

b   c

b   c

Fornix

Optic tract
Ventromedial nucleus
Dorsomedial nucleus
Lateral area
Dorsal area

III

Supra-optic nucleus

Lateral area
Medial area   Optic chiasm

Tuberal nuclei
Paraventricular nucleus

Fig. 6.**8 Hypothalamic nuclei. a** Lateral view. **b** and **c** Coronal sections in two different planes.

below). The medial segment, in contrast, contains a number of more or less clearly distinguishable nuclei (Fig. 6.**8a–c**), which are divided into an **anterior (rostral)**, a **middle (tuberal)**, and a **posterior (mamillary) nuclear group**.

Hypothalamic Nuclei

Anterior nuclear group. The important members of this group are the *preoptic*, *supraoptic*, and *paraventricular nuclei* (Fig. 6.**8**). The latter two nuclei project, by way of the supraoptico-hypophyseal tract, to the neurohypophysis (see Figs. 6.**10** and 6.**11**).

Middle nuclear group. The important members of this group are the *infundibular nucleus*, the *tuberal nuclei*, the *dorsomedial nucleus*, the *ventromedial nucleus*, and the *lateral nucleus* (or *tuberomamillary nucleus*) (Fig. 6.**8**).

Posterior nuclear group. This group includes the *mamillary nuclei* (the supramamillary nucleus, the mamillary nucleus, the intercalate nucleus, and others) and the *posterior nucleus* (Fig. 6.**8**). This area has been termed a dynamogenic zone (Hess), from which the autonomic nervous system can be immediately called into action, if necessary.

Afferent and Efferent Projections of the Hypothalamus

The neural connections of the hypothalamus (Figs. 6.**9** and 6.**10**) are multifarious and complex. In order to carry out its function as the coordinating center of all autonomic processes in the body (p. 282), the hypothalamus must communicate via afferent and efferent pathways with very many different areas of the nervous system. Information from the outside world reaches it through visual, olfactory, and probably also auditory pathways. The presence of cortical afferents implies that the hypothalamus can also be influenced by higher centers. The major connections of the hypothalamus are to the cingulate gyrus and frontal lobe, the hippocampal formation, the thalamus, the basal ganglia, the brainstem, and the spinal cord.

Some of the more important afferent connections (Fig. 6.**9**) will be described in the following section.

Afferent Pathways

The medial forebrain bundle originates in the basal olfactory areas and the septal nuclei and runs as a chain of neurons through the hypothalamus (lateral area) until it arrives in the midbrain reticular formation Along the way, it gives off collateral fibers to the preoptic nucleus, the dorsomedial nucleus, and the

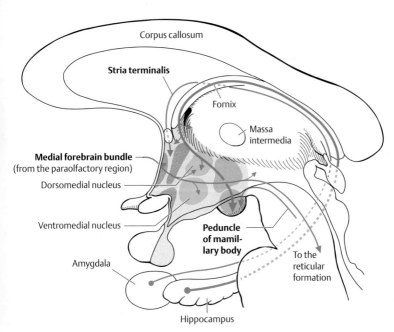

Fig. 6.**9 Major afferent connections of the hypothalamus** (schematic drawing)

ventromedial nucleus. The medial forebrain bundle constitutes a reciprocal connection between olfactory and preoptic nuclear areas and the midbrain. It has olfacto-visceral and olfacto-somatic functions.

The **striae terminales** originate in the amygdala in the temporal lobe, then form an arch over the thalamus, terminating in the preoptic area and to the anterior hypothalamic nuclei. These fiber bundles are thought to transmit olfactory information, as well as impulses relating to mood and drive.

The **fornix** transmits corticomamillary fibers originating in the hippocampus and subiculum and traveling to the mamillary body, with collaterals to the preoptic nucleus, the anterior nucleus of the thalamus, and the habenular nucleus. The fornix is an important pathway in the limbic system (p. 314). As it passes over the dorsal surface of the pulvinar, some of its fibers cross the midline to join the contralateral fornix (commissure of the fornices, psalterium).

At the level of the psalterium, the two fornices lie under the splenium of the corpus callosum, where they are usually not directly visible in an uncut brain

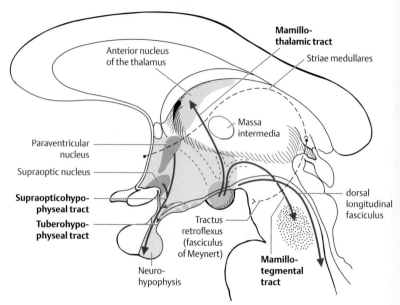

Fig. 6.10 Major efferent connections of the hypothalamus (schematic drawing)

specimen. Lesions in the area of the psalterium often affect both fornices, because these two thin structures are close together at this point. The serious functional deficits produced by bilateral limbic lesions are discussed below on p. 322 ff.

Ascending visceral impulses from the peripheral autonomic nervous system, and from the nucleus of the tractus solitarius (taste), reach the hypothalamus along various pathways: through relay nuclei in the brainstem reticular formation, from tegmental and interpeduncular nuclei, through reciprocal connections in the medial forebrain bundle, through the dorsal longitudinal fasciculus, and through the peduncle of the mamillary body (Figs. 6.**9** and 6.**10**). Somatosensory information from the erogenous zones (genitalia and nipples) also reach the hypothalamus by these pathways and induce autonomic reactions.

Finally, further afferent input comes to the hypothalamus from the medial nucleus of the thalamus, the orbitofrontal neocortex, and the globus pallidus.

Efferent Pathways

Efferent fibers to the brainstem. The most important efferent projections from the hypothalamus to the brainstem are the **dorsal longitudinal fasciculus** (of Schütz), which contains fibers traveling in both directions, and the **medial forebrain bundle** (Figs. 6.9 and 6.10). Hypothalamic impulses traveling in these pathways pass through multiple synaptic relays, mainly in the reticular formation, until they terminate in parasympathetic nuclei of the brainstem, including the oculomotor nucleus (miosis), the superior and inferior salivatory nuclei (lacrimation, salivation), and the dorsal nucleus of the vagus nerve. Other impulses travel to autonomic centers in the brainstem that coordinate circulatory, respiratory, and alimentary function (etc.), as well as to motor cranial nerve nuclei that play a role in eating and drinking: the motor nucleus of the trigeminal nerve (mastication), the nucleus of the facial nerve (facial expression), the nucleus ambiguus (swallowing), and the nucleus of the hypoglossal nerve (licking). Yet other impulses derived from the hypothalamus, relayed to the spinal cord through reticulospinal fibers, affect the activity of spinal neurons that participate in temperature regulation (shivering).

The mamillotegmental fasciculus (Fig. 6.10) runs from the mamillary body to the midbrain tegmentum, and then onward to the reticular formation.

The mamillothalamic tract (of Vicq d'Azyr) reciprocally connects the hypothalamus with the anterior nucleus of the thalamus, which, in turn, is reciprocally connected with the cingulate gyrus (Fig. 6.6). The anterior thalamic nucleus and the cingulate gyrus are important components of the limbic system. The main function of the limbic system is said to be the regulation of affective behavior so as to promote the survival of the individual and of the species (MacLean 1958; cf. p. 312).

The supraoptico-hypophyseal tract has already been mentioned as an efferent pathway to the neurohypophysis. Neurons in the supraoptic and paraventricular nuclei produce the hormones oxytocin and vasopressin (antidiuretic hormone), which are transported along the axons of the supraoptico-hypophyseal tract to the neurohypophysis, and are then released there, from the axon terminals, into the bloodstream (Figs. 6.10 and 6.11). The neurons in these nuclei are thus comparable to the hormone-producing cells of other organs, and are referred to as neurosecretory cells. Oxytocin and vasopressin mainly exert their effects on cells outside the nervous system: oxytocin induces contraction of the smooth muscle of the uterus and the mammary gland, while vasopressin induces water reuptake through the renal tubular epithelial cells (see also p. 283).

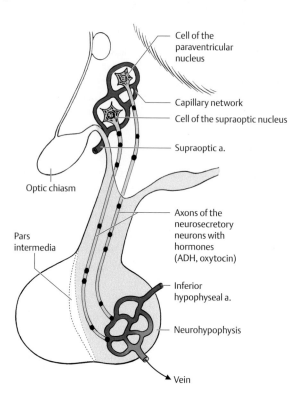

Fig. 6.**11 Posterior lobe of the pituitary gland** (neurohypophysis). Neurosecretory fibers reach the posterior lobe directly by way of the supraoptico-hypophyseal tract.

Labels in figure:
- Cell of the paraventricular nucleus
- Capillary network
- Cell of the supraoptic nucleus
- Supraoptic a.
- Optic chiasm
- Pars intermedia
- Axons of the neurosecretory neurons with hormones (ADH, oxytocin)
- Inferior hypophyseal a.
- Neurohypophysis
- Vein

Functional Connection of the Hypothalamus to the Adenohypophysis

There is no direct neural connection between the hypothalamic nuclei and the adenohypophysis. Nonetheless, it has long been recognized that the hypothalamus exerts a major influence on the adenohypophyseal endocrine cells. Fiber bundles from the tuberal nuclei carry *releasing factors* and *release-inhibiting factors* to the median eminence by intra-axonal transport; the median eminence, in turn, is connected to the adenohypophysis through a portal vascular network. The hypothalamus regulates adenohypophyseal hormone secretion by this mechanism (Fig. 6.**12**; cf. p. 284).

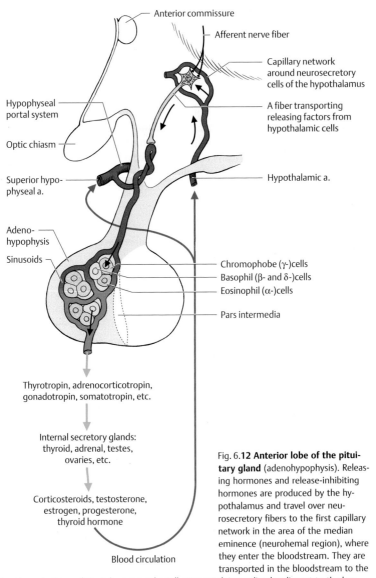

Anterior commissure

Afferent nerve fiber

Capillary network around neurosecretory cells of the hypothalamus

A fiber transporting releasing factors from hypothalamic cells

Hypophyseal portal system

Optic chiasm

Superior hypo-physeal a.

Hypothalamic a.

Adeno-hypophysis

Sinusoids

Chromophobe (γ-)cells
Basophil (β- and δ-)cells
Eosinophil (α-)cells

Pars intermedia

Thyrotropin, adrenocorticotropin, gonadotropin, somatotropin, etc.

Internal secretory glands: thyroid, adrenal, testes, ovaries, etc.

Corticosteroids, testosterone, estrogen, progesterone, thyroid hormone

Blood circulation

Fig. 6.**12 Anterior lobe of the pituitary gland** (adenohypophysis). Releasing hormones and release-inhibiting hormones are produced by the hypothalamus and travel over neurosecretory fibers to the first capillary network in the area of the median eminence (neurohemal region), where they enter the bloodstream. They are transported in the bloodstream to the adenohypophysis, reaching it by a second capillary network immediately adjacent to the hormone-producing glandular cells (hypophyseal portal system). Thus, hormone secretion by the anterior lobe of the pituitary gland is regulated by way of the bloodstream.

Functions of the Hypothalamus

The hypothalamus is the hierarchically uppermost regulatory organ ("head ganglion") of the autonomic nervous system. It plays the leading role in a wide variety of regulatory circuits for **vital bodily functions** such as temperature, heart rate, blood pressure, respiration, and food and water intake. These regulatory functions are carried out largely independently of any conscious thought on the part of the individual, i.e., autonomically. The hypothalamus also regulates important hormone systems through the hypothalamic-pituitary axis and coordinates the interaction of the endocrine and autonomic nervous systems. The elementary functions controlled by the hypothalamus will be described, briefly and individually, in this section.

Temperature Regulation

The *anterior preoptic hypothalamus* contains specific receptors for the maintenance of a constant internal temperature (*temperature homeostasis*). Physiological responses to *temperature changes* (vasoconstriction and shivering at low temperature, vasodilation and sweating at high temperature) are regulated by circuits in the *posterior hypothalamus.*

Disturbances of temperature regulation. Dysfunction of the anterior preoptic region of the hypothalamus (caused, for example, by traumatic brain injury or hemorrhage) can lead to **central hyperthermia**. Dysfunction of the posterior region can lead to **hypothermia** or **poikilothermia** (rapid fluctuations of body temperature by more than 2°C); the possible causative lesions here include hypothalamic tumors (craniopharyngioma, glioma), Wernicke's encephalopathy, and hydrocephalus.

Regulation of Heart Rate and Blood Pressure

The hypothalamus influences the autonomic nervous system directly through descending pathways that will be discussed below in the section on the autonomic nervous system (p. 289).

The *sympathetic* nervous system is regulated by the ventromedial and posterior portions of the hypothalamus (p. 292). Stimulation of these areas induces a rise in heart rate and blood pressure, dilatation of the pupils, vasoconstriction in the capillary beds, vasodilation in the skeletal musculature, and expressions of fear or rage.

The *parasympathetic* nervous system (p. 295), on the other hand, is regulated by the paraventricular and anterior or lateral portions of the hypothalamus. Stimulation of these areas induces a fall in heart rate and blood pressure and constriction of the pupils. Stimulation of posterior parasympathetic areas increases blood flow to the bladder and diminishes blood flow to skeletal muscle.

Regulation of Water Balance

The *hypothalamic osmoreceptors* are located in the *supraoptic* and *paraventricular nuclei*. They are stimulated either by intracellular dehydration, with an elevated intracellular sodium concentration, or by extracellular dehydration, with an elevated concentration of angiotensin II in the hypothalamic capillary blood; stimulation leads to the *secretion of ADH* (antidiuretic hormone, vasopressin). Conversely, an increase of intravascular volume stimulates peripheral volume receptors, ultimately leading to the inhibition of ADH secretion.

Disturbances of water balance. If 90 % or more of the neurons of the supraoptic and paraventricular nuclei are destroyed or rendered dysfunctional (e. g., by a granulomatous process, vascular lesion, trauma, or infection), then ADH is no longer secreted and **diabetes insipidus** results, manifested clinically by excessive thirst, polyuria, and polydipsia. The diagnosis is established by the demonstration of *hypo-osmolar polyuria*, i.e., the excretion of at least 3 liters of urine per day, with an osmolality between 50 and 150 mosm/l. ADH substitution is the treatment of choice. If the urine osmolality fails to rise by more than 50 % after the administration of 5 IU of ADH, then the patient is suffering from renal diabetes insipidus (inadequate response of the kidney to circulating ADH), in which substitution therapy is of no help.

Many types of hypothalamic lesion impair the thirst response, and can thus cause severe hyponatremia.

The syndrome of inappropriate ADH secretion (**SIADH** or **Schwartz-Bartter syndrome**), usually caused by abnormal ectopic secretion of ADH (e. g., by bronchial carcinoma or other malignant tumors), is manifested by hypervolemia, hyponatremia (< 130 mmol/l), low serum osmolarity (< 275 mosm/kg), and highly concentrated urine. The clinical manifestations include weight gain, weakness, nausea, and disturbances of consciousness, as well as epileptic seizures. SIADH is treated by eliminating the underlying cause, though it is often useful to treat the hypervolemia and hyponatremia symptomatically as well, by fluid restriction and correction of the sodium balance.

Regulation of Nutritional Intake

Lesions of the ventromedial hypothalamic nuclei may cause severe obesity through hyperphagia and poverty of movement. More lateral lesions can cause anorexia and abnormal weight loss.

Neurosecretion and Regulation of the Endocrine System

As mentioned above, the hypophysis (pituitary gland) has two components, the anterior lobe (adenohypophysis) and the posterior lobe (neurohypophysis). The hypothalamus controls each part differently.

Hormone secretion by the posterior lobe. Secretory neurons in the supraoptic and paraventricular nuclei produce oxytocin and ADH, which are transported intra-axonally to the neurohypophysis and released there into the bloodstream (neurosecretion). The functions of ADH have been described above. Oxytocin is secreted during the last few weeks of pregnancy; it induces the contraction of uterine smooth muscle as well as the secretion of milk from the mammary glands. Somatosensory stimulation (touching the nipple) produces afferent impulses that activate the neurosecretory neurons of the hypothalamus (by way of the thalamus and the cerebral cortex). The intimate connection between this regulatory circuit and emotion is illustrated by the fact that milk production decreases significantly when the mother suffers from fear or stress.

Hormone secretion by the anterior lobe. The parvocellular secretory neurons found in periventricular areas of the hypothalamus communicate with the adenohypophysis not by axonal connections (as in the case of the neurohypophysis) but rather through a portal vascular system (see above). These parvocellular neurons secrete the "**hypophysiotropic**" hormones gonadotropin-releasing hormone (GnRH), thyrotropin-releasing hormone (TRH), corticotropin-releasing hormone (CRH), growth-hormone-releasing hormone (GHRH), and factors regulating the secretion of melanocyte-stimulating hormone (MSH), namely MIF and MRF. All of these hormones, in turn, control the release of the corresponding pituitary hormones from the adenohypophysis, once they arrive there by way of the portal vascular network (cf. Fig. 6.**12** and Table 6.**1**). In the adenohypophysis, **acidophil cells** (α cells) secrete growth hormone (GH, also called somatotropic hormone or STH) and prolactin (PRL, also called luteotropic hormone or LTH). **Basophil cells** (β cells) secrete thyrotropin (thyroid-stimulating hormone, TSH), corticotropin (also called adrenocorticotropic hormone or ACTH), melanocyte-stimulating hormone (MSH), luteinizing hormone (LH), and follicle-stimulating hormone (FSH). **Chromophobe cells**

Tabelle 6.**1 Endocrine Regulation along the Hypothalamic—Pituitary Axis**

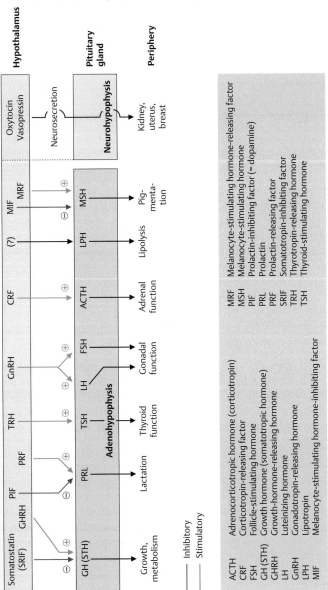

Hypothalamus								Pituitary gland		Periphery

Hypothalamus / **Pituitary gland** / **Periphery**

									Neurohypophysis	
Oxytocin Vasopressin	→ Neurosecretion →									Kidney, uterus, breast

Somatostatin (SRIF)	GHRH	PIF	PRF	TRH	GnRH	CRF	(?)	MIF MRF	

Adenohypophysis

GH (STH)	PRL	TSH	LH FSH	ACTH	LPH	MSH
Growth, metabolism	Lactation	Thyroid function	Gonadal function	Adrenal function	Lipolysis	Pigmentation

— Inhibitory

— Stimulatory

ACTH	Adrenocorticotropic hormone (corticotropin)
CRF	Corticotropin-releasing factor
FSH	Follicle-stimulating hormone
GH (STH)	Growth hormone (somatotropic hormone)
GHRH	Growth-hormone-releasing hormone
LH	Luteinizing hormone
GnRH	Gonadotropin-releasing hormone
LPH	Lipotropin
MIF	Melanocyte-stimulating hormone-inhibiting factor
MRF	Melanocyte-stimulating hormone-releasing factor
MSH	Melanocyte-stimulating hormone
PIF	Prolactin-inhibiting factor (= dopamine)
PRL	Prolactin
PRF	Prolactin-releasing factor
SRIF	Somatotropin-inhibiting factor
TRH	Thyrotropin-releasing hormone
TSH	Thyroid-stimulating hormone

(γ cells) are not known to secrete any hormones, but some authors state that they play a role in ACTH synthesis.

The hormones produced by the pituitary secretory cells enter the bloodstream and induce the respective peripheral endocrine organs to secrete hormones. These peripheral hormones circulate in the blood, and their concentrations, in turn, influence the secretion of the corresponding hypothalamic and pituitary hormones, in a negative feedback loop.

Hormonal Disturbances: Disturbances of the Hypothalamic–Pituitary Axis

The endocrine function of the hypophysis can be impaired by hormone-secreting tumors (e. g., pituitary adenoma) or by destruction of pituitary tissue by non-hormone-secreting tumors.

Panhypopituitarism. The most severe clinical syndrome consists of **loss of all functions of the hypophysis** and is clinically manifested by lack of drive, decline of physical performance, loss of weight, loss of libido, bradycardia, lessened skin pigmentation, loss of axillary and pubic hair, and, sometimes, diabetes insipidus (if the neurohypophysis is involved). This syndrome may be caused by large, hormonally inactive tumors of the hypophysis, infundibulum, or hypothalamus (e. g., adenoma, metastasis, glioma, or craniopharyngioma). The treatment of choice is surgical resection and hormone substitution. Hypopituitarism may also arise in the aftermath of trauma, or as a complication of neurosurgical procedures. Sudden loss of pituitary function with subsequent adrenal failure (addisonian crisis) is a life-threatening event.

Hormone-secreting pituitary tumors. A neoplasm arising from one of the cell types of the anterior pituitary lobe causes symptoms through an **excess of the corresponding hormone(s)**. If the tumor is large enough, the **suprasellar mass effect** will produce a characteristic visual field defect (usually bitemporal hemianopsia, because of compression of the optic chiasm; cf. p. 131).

Prolactinoma. Most pituitary adenomas (60-70%) secrete prolactin. In female patients, the resulting excess of circulating prolactin (hyperprolactinemia) causes **secondary amenorrhea** through the inhibition of gonadotropin-releasing hormone secretion (when the serum prolactin concentration rises above 40-100 ng/ml), as well as **galactorrhea** and, less commonly, hirsuitism. In male patients, hyperprolactinemia causes **impotence**, **gynecomastia**, and galactorrhea. Surgical resection (e. g., by the transsphenoidal route) is the treatment of choice for prolactinomas with mass effect; for smaller tumors with less severe manifestations, pharmacological treatment with a dopamine agonist such as bromocriptine can be tried. Dopamine agonists inhibit prolactin secretion.

Growth-hormone-secreting adenoma. Clinically, an excess of circulating growth hormone (> 5 ng/ml) causes **acromegaly**: increased growth of acral portions of the skeleton (hands, feet, head circumference), osteoporosis, hyperhidrosis, glucose intolerance, hypertension, hypertrophic cardiomyopathy, goiter, compressive neuropathies such as carpal tunnel syndrome, other types of neuropathy, proximal myopathy, sleep disturbances (hypersomnia, sleep apnea syndrome), and neuropsychiatric disturbances (depression, psychosis). The standard diagnostic test is an oral glucose tolerance test, with a characteristic overshoot in the reflex rise of growth hormone concentration. Surgical resection is the treatment of choice.

Case Presentation 2: *Pituitary Tumor/Prolactinoma*

This 40-year-old male office worker complained to his family physician of "peculiar" bodily changes that had been troubling him for some time. He had gained 50 kg in weight over the previous 2–3 years, and he now needed shoes two sizes larger than before. His hands also seemed to have become "rough." He had recently had an automobile accident caused by his failure to see another car approaching from the side, and a couple of days previously he had almost run over a pedestrian for the same reason. He could no longer trust himself to drive a car, both because of these occurrences and because he was always tired and could not concentrate. He had increasing difficulty on the job. He denied suffering from headache, loss of libido, or impotence.

The physician found his weight to be 132 kg (previously 82 kg), with an unchanged height of 193 cm. His hands and feet were disproportionately large (acromegaly), finger perimetry revealed severe bitemporal hemianopsia, and there was mild gynecomastia, though no galactorrhea could be induced. Laboratory testing revealed normal values of all thyroid parameters (T_3, T_4, basal TSH, and TRH test) as well as of ACTH and cortisol. The testosterone level, however, was very low (50 ng/ml) and the prolactin level extremely high (590 µg/dl). TRH administration caused the prolactin level to climb still further to 2020 µg/dl.

These findings suggested a prolactin-secreting adenoma of the pituitary gland with partial hypopituitarism affecting the anterior lobe hormones, particularly the gonadotropic axis.

A plain radiograph of the head revealed massive expansion of the sella turcica with partial destruction of the dorsum sellae and the sellar floor. An MRI scan revealed a tumor measuring 5 × 5 × 4 cm (Fig. 6.**13**), too large to be removed through a transsphenoidal approach. A frontotemporal craniotomy was performed. Intraoperatively, a firm, grayish-yellow tumor with some reddish areas was found; it was adherent to the floor of the middle cranial fossa, made contact with the terminal portion of the internal carotid artery, and compressed the optic chiasm. The histopathological finding was of a diffusely growing epithelial tumor, without lobular structure, in which the tumor cells occasionally showed a papillary organization. Immmunohistochemical study revealed an increased expression of prolactin in ca. 30–40 % of the tumor cells, while a few of them stained positive for ACTH, LH, or GH. Excessive GH secretion had presumably caused the patient's clinically evident acromegaly. Postoperatively, he had transient diabetes insipidus requiring treatment with desmopressin acetate. Anterior pituitary lobe insufficiency persisted in his subsequent course and he was treated with hydrocortisone and thyroxine substitution.

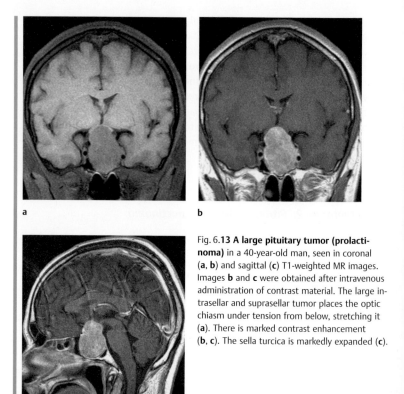

Fig. 6.**13 A large pituitary tumor (prolactinoma)** in a 40-year-old man, seen in coronal (**a, b**) and sagittal (**c**) T1-weighted MR images. Images **b** and **c** were obtained after intravenous administration of contrast material. The large intrasellar and suprasellar tumor places the optic chiasm under tension from below, stretching it (**a**). There is marked contrast enhancement (**b, c**). The sella turcica is markedly expanded (**c**).

ACTH-secreting adenoma causes **Cushing syndrome** with truncal obesity, moon facies, glucose intolerance, hypertension, edema, amenorrhea, impotence, a tendency to thromboembolism, polyuria, steroid myopathy, and neuropsychiatric disturbances. The diagnosis is made endocrinologically by the demonstration of an elevated amount of cortisol in a 24-hour urine collection. Surgical resection is the treatment of choice.

Peripheral Autonomic Nervous System

Fundamentals

The autonomic nervous system, working in concert with the endocrine system (see above) and various nuclei in the brainstem, regulates vital functions that are necessary for the maintenance of the internal environment (homeostasis), including respiration, circulation, metabolism, body temperature, water balance, digestion, secretion, and reproductive function. The designation "autonomic" is derived from the fact that these functions are controlled by unconscious (involuntary) mechanisms, as discussed above.

As already mentioned, the hypothalamus is the main regulatory center for the entire peripheral autonomic system. It exercises its control over many bodily functions partly through nerve impulses and partly through hormonal pathways, by means of the hypothalamic-pituitary system (see above and standard works on endocrinology, physiology, and anatomy).

The efferent arm of the autonomic nervous system is composed of two complementary systems, the **sympathetic** nervous system and the **parasympathetic** nervous system, whose effects are generally antagonistic to each other. The efferent fibers of both systems mainly innervate the smooth muscle of the viscera, blood vessels, and glands and are thus commonly called *visceral efferent (visceromotor) fibers*, to distinguish them from the sensory *visceral afferent fibers*. The latter, unlike the visceral efferent fibers, are not divided into two systems.

General scheme of the sympathetic and parasympathetic nervous systems. The final efferent pathway of both the sympathetic and the parasympathetic nervous systems consists of two neurons in series (Fig. 6.**14**). The cell body of the **first (preganglionic) neuron** lies within the central nervous system, while that of the **second (postganglionic) neuron** is found in a peripheral ganglion.

The first neurons of the sympathetic nervous system lie in the thoracic and lumbar segments of the spinal cord (intermediolateral cell column, T1-L2); for this reason, the sympathetic nervous system is sometimes called the **thoracolumbar system**. Some of the first neurons of the parasympathetic nervous system are found in the nuclei of cranial nerves III, VII, IX, and X (see below), while the remainder are found in the lateral horns of the sacral segments of the spinal cord (pelvic parasympathetic system, S2-S4). Thus, the parasympathetic nervous system is sometimes called the **craniosacral system.**

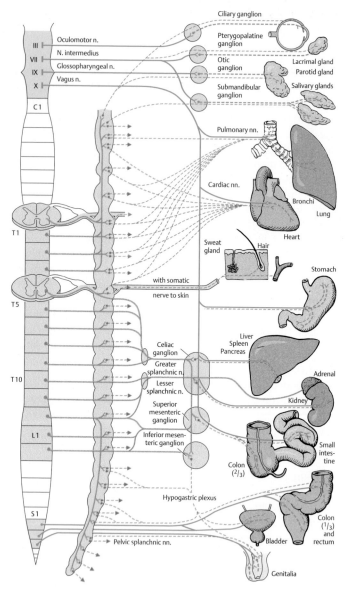

Fig. 6.14 The sympathetic and parasympathetic nervous system (schematic diagram). Yellow: sympathetic. Green: parasympathetic.

The second neurons of the sympathetic nervous system are arranged in prevertebral and paravertebral chains of ganglia (the sympathetic chains), while those of the parasympathetic nervous system generally lie in the walls of the innervated organs (intramural ganglia). The first neurons of both systems use acetylcholine as their neurotransmitter. The second neurons of the parasympathetic nervous system also use acetylcholine as their neurotransmitter (a further alternative name for the parasympathetic nervous system is, therefore, the **cholinergic system**). The neurotransmitter of the postganglionic sympathetic neurons, however, is norepinephrine (**adrenergic system**). The sweat glands are an exception to this rule: the second sympathetic neuron innervating them is cholinergic, like a second neuron in the parasympathetic nervous system.

Hypothalamic control of the sympathetic and parasympathetic nervous systems. Stimulation of the **rostral** hypothalamus induces **increased parasympathetic (trophotropic) activity**, including reduction of the cardiac minute volume, hypotonia, slowing of the heartbeat, reduction of the respiratory volume, lowering of the basal metabolic rate, vasodilatation, sweating, salivation, contraction of the bladder, reduced secretion of epinephrine, increased peristalsis, and pupillary constriction. Stimulation of the **caudal** hypothalamus, on the other hand, induces **increased sympathetic (ergotropic) activity**, including a rise in blood pressure, acceleration of the heartbeat, increased blood supply to the skeletal muscle and lungs, vasoconstriction in blood depots such as the capillary bed of the digestive tract, decreased blood supply to the abdominal viscera, increased respiratory volume, a rise in the blood glucose level, inhibition of peristalsis, urinary retention, increased secretion of epinephrine, widening of the palpebral fissure, and pupillary dilatation. A mass reaction thus occurs in the entire body, directed toward physical exertion and therefore enabling the whole organism to deal optimally with situations of attack and stress. While the sympathetic, ergotropic reaction is directed toward physical exertion, the parasympathetic, trophotropic reaction is directed toward rest and recovery. Despite these general principles, however, the distinction between parasympathetic and sympathetic activity is not always clear-cut.

Neural connections of the hypothalamus to the peripheral autonomic nervous system. The hypothalamus exerts its regulating and controlling functions over the sympathetic and parasympathetic nervous systems by means of descending pathways including the *medial forebrain bundle* (Fig. 6.**9**), the *mamillotegmental tract*, and the *dorsal longitudinal fasciculus* (of Schütz) (Fig. 6.**10**).

These three fiber pathways connect the hypothalamus to the *descending midbrain reticular system*, which, in turn, carries the central impulses to the various components of the parasympathetic and sympathetic nervous systems.

Sympathetic Nervous System

The sympathetic nervous system innervates the smooth musculature of the blood vessels, abdominal viscera, bladder, rectum, hair follicles, and pupils, as well as the cardiac muscle, the sweat glands, and the lacrimal, salivatory, and digestive glands. The smooth musculature of the abdominal viscera, bladder, rectum, and digestive glands is inhibited, while that of all other target organs is stimulated to contract.

The caliber of the body's arteries is mainly regulated by the sympathetic nervous system. Increased sympathetic activity leads to vasoconstriction, and decreased sympathetic activity to vasodilatation.

Anatomy. The origin of the preganglionic fibers from thoracic segments T1 through T12 and from the first two lumbar segments is shown in Fig. 6.**14**. Some of the preganglionic fibers terminate on second neurons in the right and left sympathetic chains (only the left sympathetic chain is depicted in the figure). The remainder pass through the sympathetic chain without a synapse and terminate on a second neuron in a prevertebral ganglion. In either case, the postganglionic fiber of the second neuron transmits the sympathetic impulses onward to the target organ.

Sympathetic chain. As shown in Fig. 6.**15**, the preganglionic fibers emerge from neurons in the lateral horn of the spinal cord (intermediolateral cell column) and then join the axons of the somatic motor neurons to exit from the spinal cord in the anterior root. At the level of the spinal ganglion, the autonomic fibers separate from the somatic fibers once again and enter the sympathetic chain by way of the *white ramus communicans*, which is white because its fibers are myelinated. Some preganglionic fibers already terminate on the second neuron in the pathway at the same segmental level, but others travel one or more levels up or down the sympathetic chain before making a synapse onto their second neuron. Yet other fibers traverse the sympathetic chain without making a synapse and then terminate on a second neuron in a prevertebral ganglion. In all cases, the unmyelinated postganglionic fibers leave the sympathetic chain in the *gray ramus communicans*, which rejoins the spinal nerve at the same segmental level, so that its fibers travel to the corresponding cutaneous dermatome. In the skin, the autonomic fibers innervate the cutaneous vessels, the piloerector muscles, and the sweat glands.

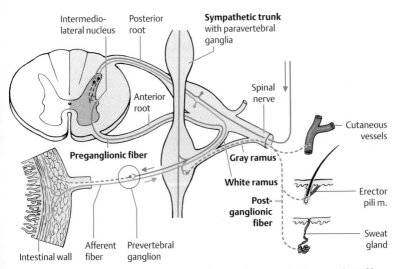

Fig. 6.**15 The sympathetic trunk and the preganglionic and postganglionic sympathetic fibers** (schematic diagram)

Sympathetic innervation of the head and neck. As mentioned above, some postganglionic fibers reach their targets in the periphery by way of the segmental spinal nerves, but others do so by traveling along the blood vessels and their branches, particularly in the head and neck. The cervical spinal cord contains no sympathetic nuclei; thus, the sympathetic innervation of the head and neck is derived from the intermediolateral cell column of the upper four or five thoracic segments. Postganglionic fibers from these segments ascend in the sympathetic chain, and terminate in three ganglia at its rostral end: the *superior cervical ganglion*, the *middle cervical ganglion*, and the *cervicothoracic (stellate) ganglion*. These ganglia are the sites of the synaptic relay onto the second neurons, which emit the postganglionic fibers. Some of these fibers travel with the spinal nerves to the cervical cutaneous dermatomes. Other, unmyelinated fibers from the superior cervical ganglion form the *external carotid plexus*, which accompanies the external carotid artery and its branches to the head and the face, innervating the sweat glands, the smooth muscles of the hair follicles, and the blood vessels. Yet other fibers accompany the internal carotid artery as the *internal carotid plexus*, which innervates the eye (dilator pupillae muscle, orbitalis muscle, and tarsal muscle) as well as the lacrimal and salivary glands (Figs. 4.**27** and 4.**28** [p. 158 f.] and 6.**14**).

Sympathetic innervation of heart and lungs. Postganglionic fibers from the cervical and upper four or five thoracic ganglia run in the *cardiac nerves* to the *cardiac plexus*, which innervates the heart. *Pulmonary nerves* innervate the bronchi and lungs (Fig. 6.**14**).

Sympathetic innervation of the abdominal and pelvic organs. Preganglionic fibers arise in thoracic segments T5 through T12 and travel, by way of the *greater* and *lesser splanchnic nerves*, to the unpaired prevertebral ganglia (the *celiac, superior mesenteric*, and *inferior mesenteric ganglia*), which are located along the aorta at the levels of origin of the correspondingly named aortic branches. Within these ganglia, the splanchnic fibers make synapses onto the second sympathetic neurons, which, in turn, emit the postganglionic fibers for the abdominal and pelvic viscera. In contrast to the parasympathetic fibers, the sympathetic postganglionic fibers are very long and form various plexuses before reaching their target organs (Fig. 6.**14**).

Adrenal medulla. The adrenal medulla occupies a special position in the sympathetic nervous system. It is analogous to a sympathetic ganglion, in that it is directly innervated by preganglionic fibers. These fibers form synapses onto modified second neurons within the adrenal medulla, which, rather than possessing an axon, secrete epinephrine and norepinephrine into the bloodstream (Fig. 6.**14**). Sympathetic activation induces the adrenal medulla to secrete epinephrine and norepinephrine, which then exert sympathetic effects in the periphery. This is particularly important under conditions of stress.

Clinical Symptoms of Sympathetic Lesions

Horner syndrome. As mentioned in Chapter 4 (p. 157 ff.), lesions affecting the ciliospinal center, the cervical sympathetic chain (cervicothoracic ganglion), or the autonomic plexuses along the blood vessels of the head and neck cause ipsilateral Horner syndrome. This consists of the clinical triad of a constricted pupil/**miosis** (due to loss of contraction of the dilator pupillae muscle), a hanging eyelid/**ptosis** (due to loss of contraction of the tarsal muscle), and an inwardly sunken globe/**enophthalmos** (due to loss of contraction of the orbitalis muscle). There is also loss of sweating (**anhidrosis**) and **vasodilatation** (due to loss of the vasoconstrictive effect of the sympathetic nerves) on the ipsilateral half of the face, which therefore appears dry and reddened.

Causes of Horner syndrome. Interruption of the sympathetic pathway to the head and neck at any point can cause Horner syndrome. One common cause is a bronchial carcinoma at the apex of the lung (**Pancoast tumor**) impinging on the cervical sympathetic chain. Such tumors may present with Horner syndrome before becoming otherwise symptomatic.

Dissection of the internal carotid artery is another important cause of Horner syndrome. When the intima of the artery is torn, blood enters the vessel wall and the lumen is narrowed or occluded; rupture of the artery with pseudoaneurysm formation is rare. Carotid dissection has many possible etiologies; dissection may be *traumatic* or due to an *intrinsic abnormality* of the tissue of the vessel wall, e. g., fibromuscular dysplasia, which predisposes to the development of an intimal tear. In most cases, however, the etiology of carotid dissection cannot be determined.

The pathogenesis of sympathetic dysfunction in carotid dissection is not yet fully understood. According to one current hypothesis, *compression* of the sympathetic nerve branches by an intramural hematoma leads to nerve injury and dysfunction. According to another hypothesis, *ischemia* of the sympathetic nerve branches is the major cause of their dysfunction, as these nerve branches are supplied by small perforating branches of the internal carotid artery, which can be displaced or occluded by the dissection. Neither hypothesis is fully satisfactory.

Horner syndrome also arises as a result of brainstem lesions affecting the central sympathetic pathway, as in Wallenberg syndrome (p. 226 ff.)

Vasomotor phenomena in sympathetic dysfunction. The vasodilatation that follows a sympathetic lesion can be exploited therapeutically: *sympathectomy* is sometimes performed to increase regional blood flow, e. g., in Raynaud disease.

The vasodilatation due to a sympathetic lesion is also evident after interruption of the splanchnic nerves, which leads to a large increase of intravascular volume in the blood vessels of the bowel, i.e., to pooling of blood in the splanchnic area, with the risk of internal hemorrhage.

Parasympathetic Nervous System

In contrast to the sympathetic nervous system, the parasympathetic nervous system does not evoke any systemic responses, but instead produces its effects in individual, circumscribed areas, as reflected in the fact that its second (postganglionic) neurons lie near their target organs. Furthermore, acetylcholine, which is released as a neurotransmitter at the parasympathetic nerve terminals, is rapidly broken down by cholinesterases, and its effect is thus relatively short-lived.

The preganglionic fibers of the parasympathetic nervous system are long (unlike the short preganglionic fibers of the sympathetic nervous system).

They emerge from nuclei in the brainstem and sacral spinal cord (S2, S3, S4) (Fig. 6.**14**).

Cranial Portion of the Parasympathetic Nervous System

Parasympathetic innervation of the head. The cell bodies of the preganglionic neurons lie in various *brainstem nuclei*, and their axons are found in *cranial nerves III, VII, IX, and X.* (The anatomy and course of these nerves was described in Chapter 4.) The preganglionic fibers travel to a number of ganglia that lie very close to their respective end organs (the *ciliary, pterygopalatine, submandibular,* and *otic ganglia*). These ganglia are relay stations in which the preganglionic fibers form synapses onto the second (postganglionic) neurons. The parasympathetic postganglionic fibers in the head are short, as they have only a short distance to travel before they reach their end organs. Like the sympathetic postganglionic fibers, they innervate smooth muscle, sweat glands, and lacrimal and salivary glands (Fig. 6.**14**). The smooth muscle of the blood vessel walls receives no parasympathetic innervation.

Parasympathetic innervation of the thoracic and abdominal organs. The parasympathetic portion of the *vagus nerve* (Fig. 4.**49**, p. 199) originates in the *dorsal nucleus of the vagus nerve* and carries preganglionic fibers for the innervation of the heart, lungs, and abdominal viscera down to the distal third of the transverse colon (Fig. 6.**14**). The second (postganglionic) neurons are found in autonomic plexuses located immediately adjacent to their end organs, or else within the bowel wall (myenteric plexus of Auerbach, submucosal plexus of Meissner).

Sacral Portion of the Parasympathetic Nervous System

Parasympathetic innervation of the pelvic organs and genitalia. The sacral portion of the parasympathetic nervous system carries impulses in the *pelvic splanchnic nerves* and the *superior and inferior hypogastric (pelvic) plexuses* to ganglia in the muscular wall of the colon (from the distal third of the transverse colon onward), rectum, bladder, and genitalia (Fig. 6.**14**). In the pelvic area, the parasympathetic nervous system is responsible for the emptying of the rectum and bladder. It also brings about penile erection, while sympathetic fibers are responsible for ejaculation, which occurs through contractions of the ductus deferens and the seminal vesicles.

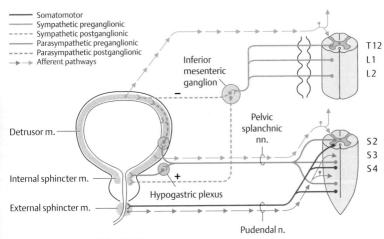

Fig. 6.**16 Innervation of the bladder**

Autonomic Innervation and Functional Disturbances of Individual Organs

The sympathetic and parasympathetic innervation of individual organs is summarized in Table 6.**2**. The innervation of the pelvic organs will be discussed in greater detail in the following sections, because the function of these organs is commonly impaired in disturbances of the autonomic nervous system. Bladder dysfunction is the most important problem of this type.

Innervation of the Bladder

Parasympathetic innervation. The motor innervation of the urinary bladder is mostly parasympathetic. The pelvic splanchnic nerves, derived from segments S2, S3, and S4, travel to parasympathetic ganglia in the bladder wall and to the smooth muscle of the internal urethral sphincter (Figs. 6.**14** and 6.**16**). Parasympathetic stimulation induces contraction of the smooth detrusor muscle of the bladder wall and simultaneous relaxation of the internal urethral sphincter. Micturition results.

Sympathetic innervation. The sympathetic fibers innervating the bladder are derived from neurons in the intermediolateral cell column of the lower thoracic and upper lumbar spinal cord (segments T12, L1, and L2). These fibers

Tabelle 6.2 The Sympathetic and Parasympathetic Nervous System

Organ	Sympathetic			Parasympathetic		
	Preganglionic neuron	Postganglionic neuron	Activity	Preganglionic neuron	Postganglionic neuron	Activity
Eye	T1–T2	Superior cervical ganglion	Mydriasis	Edinger–Westphal nucleus (accessory oculomotor nucleus)	Ciliary ganglion	Miosis, contraction of the ciliary muscle (accommodation)
Lacrimal, sublingual, and submandibular glands	T1–T2	Superior cervical ganglion	Vasoconstriction Secretion (viscous)	Superior salivatory nucleus	Pterygopalatine ganglion	Lacrimation, salivation (watery), vasodilation
Parotid gland	T1–T2	Superior cervical ganglion	Vasoconstriction Secretion	Inferior salivatory nucleus	Otic ganglion	Salivation
Heart	T1–T4 (T5)	Superior, middle, and inferior cervical ganglia and upper thoracic ganglia	Acceleration Dilation of coronary arteries	Dorsal nucleus of the vagus nerve	Cardiac plexus	Bradycardia, constriction of coronary arteries
Small intestine and ascending colon	T6–T10	Celiac ganglion, superior mesenteric ganglion	Inhibition of peristalsis and secretion	Dorsal nucleus of the vagus nerve	Myenteric plexus (of Auerbach), submucosal plexus (of Meissner)	Peristalsis, secretion, vasodilation
Pancreas	T6–T10	Celiac ganglion	—	Dorsal nucleus of the vagus nerve	Periarterial plexus	Secretion

	Sympathetic			Parasympathetic		
Descending colon and rectum	L1–L2	Inferior mesenteric ganglion, hypogastric ganglion	Inhibition of peristalsis and secretion	S2–S4	Myenteric plexus (of Auerbach), submucosal plexus (of Meissner)	Secretion, peristalsis, evacuation
Kidney Bladder	L1–L2	Celiac ganglion, renal and hypogastric plexuses	Activation of internal sphincter muscle, vasoconstriction	S2–S4	Hypogastric plexus (vesical plexus)	Relaxation of the internal sphincter muscle, contraction of the detrusor muscle, vasodilation
Adrenal gland	T11–L1	Adrenal cells	Secretion (norepinephrine, epinephrine)	—	—	—
Male genitalia	L1–L2 (pelvic splanchnic nerves)	Superior and inferior hypogastric plexuses (pelvic plexus)	Ejaculation Vasoconstriction	S2–S4	Hypogastric plexus (pelvic plexus)	Erection, vasodilation, secretion
Skin of head and neck	T2–T4	Superior and middle cervical ganglia	Vasoconstriction Sweating Piloerection	—	—	—
Arms	T3–T6	Inferior cervical ganglion and upper thoracic ganglia		—	—	—
Legs	T10–L2	Lower lumbar and upper sacral ganglia		—	—	—

travel through the caudal portion of the sympathetic chain and the inferior splanchnic nerves to the inferior mesenteric ganglion. Postganglionic sympathetic fibers then travel, by way of the inferior hypogastric plexus, to the bladder wall (tunica muscularis) and to the smooth muscle of the internal urethral sphincter (Fig. 6.**14** and 6.**16**).

Sensory innervation. Afferent fibers originate in nociceptors and proprioceptors of the bladder wall, which respond to stretch. As the bladder fills, there is a reflexive increase in muscle tone in the bladder wall and internal sphincter, which is mediated by the sacral segments (S2-S4) and the pelvic splanchnic nerves Increasing tension on the bladder wall is consciously perceived, as some of the afferent impulses travel centrally, by way of the posterior columns, to the so-called pontine micturition center, which lies in the reticular formation near the locus ceruleus. From the micturition center, impulses travel onward to the paracentral lobule on the medial surface of the cerebral hemispheres, and to other brain areas.

Regulation of Bladder Function: Continence and Micturition

The bladder performs its two major functions, the **continent storage of urine** and **periodic**, **complete emptying**, as follows.

Urinary continence is achieved by *activation of the internal and external urethral sphincters*, and, in women, mainly by activation of the *muscles of the pelvic floor*. Sympathetic efferent fibers from T11-L2 activate alpha-receptors of the internal sphincter and are also thought to inhibit the detrusor muscle by a mechanism that has not yet been determined. The external urethral sphincter is a striated muscle that, like the muscles of the pelvic floor, receives its somatic innervation through efferent fibers of the pudendal nerve (S2-S4, see above).

As the bladder is filled and the tension on the bladder wall increases, involuntary reflex contraction of the detrusor muscle is effectively countered by activation of the external sphincter by the sacral somatic motor neurons. At the same time, lumbar sympathetic activation induces closure of the internal sphincter as well as relaxation of the detrusor muscle.

Micturition. The most important stimulus for micturition is *stretching of the bladder wall*, which excites visceral sensory afferent neurons, induces the urge to void, and, with the cooperation of higher nervous centers, leads to *contraction of the detrusor muscle*. This hollow muscle receives its parasympathetic innervation from the sacral spinal cord by way of the pelvic nerve. Bladder emptying is further promoted by somatic, voluntarily controlled *abdominal* *pressing* and by *simultaneous relaxation of the internal and external urethral sphincters.*

At a supraspinal level, micturition is controlled by the *pontine micturition center*, which projects descending efferent fibers in the medial and lateral reticulospinal tracts to coordinate the simultaneous relaxation of the internal and external sphincters and contraction of the detrusor muscle. The neurotransmitter glutamate may play a role in this pathway. The pontine micturition center is anatomically poorly characterized. It can be inhibited through afferent fibers from higher centers, including the frontal cortex, cingulate gyrus, paracentral lobule, and basal ganglia.

Bladder Dysfunction

As discussed in the last section, the regulation of continence and micturition requires the perfect functional cooperation of numerous anatomical structures, some of which are very distant from others. Lesions at many different sites in the central or peripheral nervous system can have far-ranging deleterious effects on bladder function.

Bladder dysfunction may be due to structural/anatomical lesions of the bladder or urethra (**bladder dysfunction of urological origin**: vesical tumors, infravesical obstruction by urethral stricture or prostatic hypertrophy), or it may be due to a lesion of the neural structures innervating the bladder (**neurogenic bladder dysfunction**). The responsible neural lesion may lie in the peripheral nerve pathways, the autonomic plexuses, the spinal cord, or higher centers.

Impairment of supraspinal control mechanisms frequently causes bladder dysfunction in patients with multiple sclerosis, for example. Disturbances of the interaction between the pontine micturition center and other, higher centers that modulate it play an important role in the types of neurogenic bladder dysfunction seen in neurodegenerative diseases, including Parkinson disease.

Neurogenic Bladder Dysfunction

Typical manifestations of neurogenic bladder dysfunction include *urinary frequency and urgency, incontinence, difficult and incomplete bladder emptying, and recurrent urinary tract infections.*

The first step toward the successful treatment of neurogenic bladder dysfunction is a correct clinical diagnosis. Various aspects of urinary function must be taken into account, including the answers to the following questions: When and how frequently is the bladder emptied? Is it emptied completely? Is the urge to void normal, diminished, or abnormally severe (urinary urgency)? Has a urinary tract infection been ruled out? Is the patient continent?

Detrusor instability and detrusor hyperreflexia are characterized by premature detrusor contractions during the vesical filling phase. The term "instability" refers to a lack of the normal inhibition of detrusor contraction; the term "hyperreflexia" implies that a neurological disease is causing the bladder emptying disorder. Thus, clinical entities such as uninhibited neurogenic bladder, automatic bladder, and motor instability of the bladder all belong within the etiological category of detrusor hyperreflexia. In such cases, *the lesion lies above the sacral spinal cord* and impairs the function of suprasacral inhibitory projections to the detrusor muscle. The major symptom of isolated detrusor hyperreflexia is **imperative urinary urgency with urge incontinence and low residual volume**. The more common causes are multiple sclerosis, cerebrovascular diseases, normal pressure hydrocephalus, Parkinson disease, spinal cord trauma, and trauma or tumor affecting the frontal lobes of the brain.

Detrusorsphincter dyssynergia is defined as involuntary detrusor contraction without relaxation of the external urethral sphincter. The lesion lies *between the sacral spinal cord and the pontine micturition center*. The major symptom is **imperative urinary urgency with incomplete emptying of the bladder**. Detrusor-sphincter dyssynergia causes complications (in particular, ascending urinary tract infections) more frequently in men than in women, because women have a lower bladder outlet resistance than men. The more common causes are multiple sclerosis, cervical myelopathy, spinal tumors, vascular malformations, and trauma. This entity should be distinguished from the rare *functional obstruction of the bladder neck*, a disorder of unknown etiology that is associated with increased residual volume and can impair renal function.

Detrusor areflexia results from deficient afferent or efferent innervation of the detrusor muscle. Afferent and efferent disturbances hardly ever occur in isolation, presumably because both afferent and efferent impulses travel through the pelvic parasympathetic nerves and the sacral spinal segments, so that any lesion impairing one type of impulses necessarily impairs the other. The clinical manifestations of detrusor areflexia are **reduced urge to void**, **inability to initiate micturition**, **and overflow incontinence** with an increased bladder volume (up to 2000 ml). *The lesion lies within the sacral spinal cord or the peripheral nerves that enter and emerge from it.* Causes include tumors involving the conus medullaris and/or cauda equina, lumbar spinal stenosis and disk herniation, polyradiculitis (including Guillain-Barré syndrome), diabetic or alcoholic polyneuropathy, tabes dorsalis, pelvic surgery and radiation therapy, myelodysplasia, and tethered cord syndrome.

Detrusor areflexia due to sacral spinal cord dysfunction is found in 20-30% of patients with multiple sclerosis. Most of these patients have markedly elevated residual volumes because the attempt to urinate is further thwarted by lack of relaxation of the external urethral sphincter.

Case Presentation 3: *Tethered Cord Syndrome*

This previously healthy 27-year-old nurse complained to her family physician of difficulty urinating. She had trouble initiating the flow of urine, needed to strain to urinate, and felt that her bladder was still full afterward. At other times, she passed small amounts of urine involuntarily. Finally, she had also had a single episode of stool incontinence. She was very worried and embarrassed, was afraid to leave the house, and had stopped going to work. She denied having pain or any history of trauma.

Neurological examination revealed hypesthesia in the sacral dermatomes (saddle hypesthesia), normal strength in the lower limbs, and markedly diminished sphincter tone. An MRI scan was ordered to rule out a mass compressing the conus medullaris or cauda equina

(Fig. 6.**17**). This study revealed a developmental anomaly in the lumbosacral spinal canal, in which the conus medullaris lay at an abnormally low level (tethered cord syndrome).

In this disorder, the conus, because it lies immediately under the dorsal dura mater and adheres to it, cannot ascend normally to the L1–2 level over the course of development. The resulting neurological deficits may not arise until later in life, and their pathogenesis remains incompletely understood. Because of her progressive neurological deficits, the patient presented here was treated neurosurgically, with an operative detachment of the conus from the dura mater. Her deficits resolved completely thereafter.

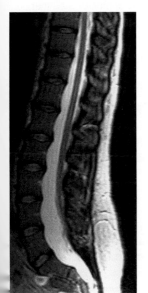

Fig. 6.**17 Tethered cord syndrome. a** The sagittal T2-weighted image shows an enlarged lumbar spinal canal with the conus medullaris lying at an abnormally low position (L4) immediately underlying the dorsal dura mater. In this case, there were no associated anomalies such as a dermal sinus, lipoma, or meningomyelocele. **b, c** The T2-weighted axial sections through the spinal canal at T12 (**b**) and L2 (**c**) reveal spinal cord at both levels. Even at the L2 level, the cord has a greater diameter than the cauda equina. It adheres to the dorsal dura mater.

Figs. 6.**17 b, c** ▷

a

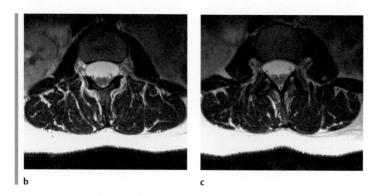

b   c

Genuine stress incontinence is said to be present when detrusor function is normal and stress incontinence is due solely to deficient activation of the external urethral sphincter. Genuine stress incontinence, the most common type of bladder emptying disorder in women, occurs mainly after hysterectomy and in multiparous women with uterine prolapse. Its incidence rises with age. It also occurs as a manifestation of various neurogenic bladder emptying disorders, including detrusor hyperreflexia and detrusor-sphincter dyssynergia.

Nonneurogenic Bladder Dysfunction

Infravesical obstruction usually occurs in men, often as the result of benign prostatic hyperplasia, and manifests itself clinically with urinary urgency, pollakiuria, nocturia, urinary retention, and overflow incontinence.

Dysfunction of the external urethral sphincter, preventing adequate relaxation of the sphincter muscle, has been found to be a common cause of obstructive bladder emptying disturbances in young women. It is characterized by myotoniform discharges in the EMG. Electromyographic study is necessary to distinguish this disorder from two important alternative diagnoses in young women with bladder emptying disturbances, namely, multiple sclerosis and psychogenic bladder dysfunction.

Enuresis is defined as bedwetting, by day or night, in individuals over the age of 4 years, in the absence of any demonstrable causative lesion. Enuresis is thus, by definition, not a neurogenic disturbance. The important differential diagnoses include *organic* neurological and urological causes of bedwetting, including epilepsy, spina bifida occulta, and malformations of the urogenital tract. A 24-hour EEG recording is indicated in some cases.

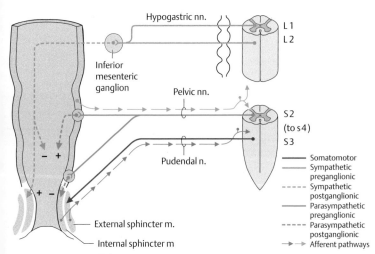

Fig. 6.**18 Innervation of the rectum**

Innervation of the Rectum

Emptying of the rectum is analogous to emptying of the bladder in many respects (Fig. 6.**18**).

Filling of the rectum activates stretch receptors in the rectal wall, which transmit impulses by way of the inferior hypogastric plexus to segments S2 through S4 of the sacral spinal cord. Afferent impulses then ascend the spinal cord to higher control centers, which are probably located in the pontine reticular formation and the cerebral cortex.

Rectal peristalsis is induced by parasympathetic activation from segments S2 through S4, which also induces relaxation of the internal sphincter. The sympathetic nervous system inhibits peristalsis. The external sphincter consists of striated muscle and is under voluntary control.

Rectal emptying is mainly accomplished voluntarily by abdominal pressing.

Rectal Emptying Disorders

Fecal retention. Transection of the spinal cord above the lumbosacral centers for defecation leads to fecal retention. Interruption of the afferent arm of the reflex pathway for defecation deprives higher centers of information about the filling state of the rectum, while interruption of descending motor fibers im-

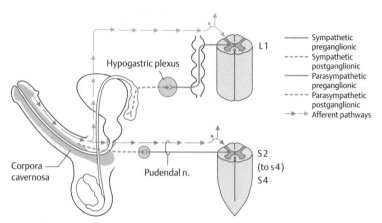

Fig. 6.**19 Innervation of the male genitalia** (erection and ejaculation)

pairs voluntary abdominal pressing. Sphincter closure is often inadequate because of spastic weakness.

Fecal incontinence. Lesions of the sacral spinal cord (S2-S4) abolish the anal reflex and produce fecal incontinence. If the stool is watery, involuntary loss of stool occurs.

Innervation of the Male Genitalia

Efferent sympathetic fibers from the upper lumbar spinal cord travel by way of a periarterial nervous plexus (the hypogastric plexus) to the seminal vesicles, prostate, and ductus deferentes. Stimulation of the plexus causes ejaculation (Fig. 6.**19**).

Parasympathetic fibers from segments S2 through S4 travel through the pelvic splanchnic nerves (the nervi erigentes) to the corpora cavernosa. Parasympathetically induced vasodilatation in the corpora cavernosa brings about penile erection (Fig. 6.**19**). The urethral sphincter and the ischiocavernosus and bulbospongiosus muscles are innervated by the pudendal nerve.

Genital function is ultimately under the control of hypothalamic centers, which exert their effects partly through neural connections (reticulospinal fibers) and partly by humoral means (hormones).

Genital Dysfunction

Spinal cord transection at a thoracic level causes impotence. Reflex priapism may occur, and occasional ejaculation is also possible. Paraplegia has been reported to be associated with testicular atrophy.

Lesions of the sacral spinal cord from S2 to S4 also cause impotence. In these cases, neither erection nor ejaculation is possible.

Visceral and Referred Pain

Afferent autonomic fibers participate in a large number of autonomic regulatory circuits. Most of the impulses traveling in these fibers do *not* rise to consciousness.

Visceral pain. The individual *can*, however, consciously perceive the filling state of the hollow viscera, which is reported to the central nervous system through afferent autonomic fibers arising from pressure or stretch receptors in the visceral wall. Overfilling of a hollow viscus is perceived as pain. Moreover, irritation of the wall of a viscus can cause reflex spasm of smooth muscle, which also gives rise to pain (biliary colic due to gallstones, renal colic due to kidney stones). Visceral inflammation or ischemia is also painful, e. g., angina pectoris.

Pain originating in the internal organs is diffuse and poorly localizable. Furthermore, the patient may report feeling pain not in the organ itself but in a related zone of the body surface (these are the zones of Head, cf. Fig. 6.**20**).

Referred pain. The cell bodies of the afferent autonomic fibers, like those of the somatic afferent fibers, are located in the spinal ganglia. The autonomic fibers enter the spinal cord through the posterior root together with the somatic afferent fibers from the myotome and dermatome of each segmental level. Thus, each individual segment of the posterior horn receives converging afferent input, both from the internal organs and from the related myotome and dermatome. Activation from either set of afferent fibers (visceral or somatic) is transmitted centrally by the same fibers of the lateral spinothalamic tract (Fig. 6.**21**). It is therefore understandable that pain arising in a particular viscus is sometimes felt elsewhere, namely, in the dermatome or myotome represented by the same spinal segment. This phenomenon is called referred pain. It may be accompanied by a certain degree of hypersensitivity to somatosensory stimulation in the dermatome to which pain is referred. The abdominal wall may also become rigid. The exact mechanism by which referred pain arises has not yet been conclusively explained, though there are a number of hypotheses.

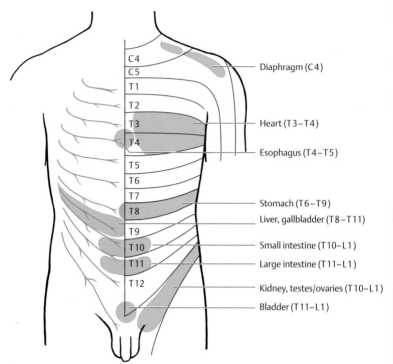

C4
C5
T1
T2
T3
T4
T5
T6
T7
T8
T9
T10
T11
T12

Diaphragm (C4)

Heart (T3–T4)

Esophagus (T4–T5)

Stomach (T6–T9)
Liver, gallbladder (T8–T11)

Small intestine (T10–L1)

Large intestine (T11–L1)

Kidney, testes/ovaries (T10–L1)

Bladder (T11–L1)

Fig. 6.**20 The zones of Head**

Pain of cardiac origin, for example, is often referred elsewhere. The upper thoracic segments on the left side receive somatic afferent fibers from the left side of the chest and the left arm, as well as visceral afferent fibers from the heart. Cardiac disease, particularly ischemia, often produces pain in one of these dermatomes (angina pectoris). The particular zones to which pain is referred from the individual internal organs are very important in physical diagnosis and are called the zones of Head (Fig. 6.20). It is also the case, however, that impulses arising from the skin can be projected (referred) to the internal organs. Clearly, the somatic afferent fibers are interconnected with visceral reflex arcs within the spinal cord. This may explain how therapeutic measures at the body surface (such as the application of warmth or heat, compresses, rubbing, etc.) often relieve pain arising from the autonomically innervated viscera.

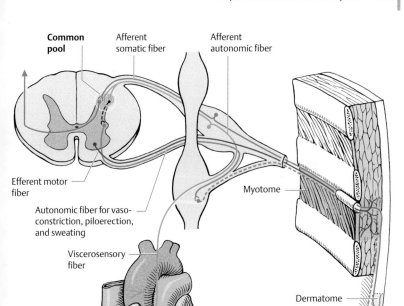

Common pool

Afferent somatic fiber

Afferent autonomic fiber

Efferent motor fiber

Autonomic fiber for vaso-constriction, piloerection, and sweating

Viscerosensory fiber

Myotome

Dermatome

Fig. 6.**21 The viscerocutaneous reflex arc** with myotome, dermatome, and enterotome. Viscerosensory and somatosensory impulses converge at the level of the posterior horn onto a common neuron, which transmits further impulses centrally along a single common pathway. Thus, afferent signals from the internal organs can be "misinterpreted" as having arisen in the corresponding cutaneous or muscular areas (dermatome or myotome). This is the mechanism of referred pain.

7 Limbic System

7   Limbic System

The limbic system is composed of both **neocortical** and **phylogenetically older cortical areas** (portions of the archicortex and paleocortex) and a number of **nuclei**. The cellular architecture of the archicortex and paleocortex differs from that of the neocortex. The major structures of the limbic system are the hippocampal formation, the parahippocampal gyrus and entorhinal area, the cingulate gyrus, the mamillary body, and the amygdala. These structures are interconnected in the **Papez circuit** and also make extensive connections with other regions of the brain (neocortex, thalamus, brainstem). The limbic system thereby enables communication between mesencephalic, diencephalic, and neocortical structures.

Through its connection with the hypothalamus, and thus with the autonomic nervous system, the limbic system participates in the **regulation of drive and affective behavior.** Its main function, teleologically speaking, is said to be the generation of behavior that promotes the survival of the individual and of the species. Moreover, the hippocampus plays a very important role in **learning and memory.** Lesions of the hippocampal formation, or of other structures that are functionally associated with it, produce an **amnestic syndrome.** Different disturbances of memory can arise, depending on the site of the lesion.

Anatomical Overview

Broca, in 1878, described the ring of brain convolutions surrounding the corpus callosum, diencephalon, and basal ganglia, naming it the "grand lobe limbique" (great limbic lobe, from the Latin *limbus*, ring). In some respects, this complex of structures can be considered a zone of transition between the brainstem and the neocortex. The cortical areas within it are composed of **archicortex** (hippocampus and dentate gyrus), **paleocortex** (piriform cortex), and **mesocortex** (cingulate gyrus). Further limbic structures are the entorhinal and septal areas, the indusium griseum, the amygdala, and the mamillary bodies (Fig. 7.**1**). The extensive fiber connections linking all of these structures led Papez, in 1937, to propose that a loop, or circuit, of neural activation (the Papez circuit, see Fig. 7.**2**) might be the anatomical substrate of emotional feeling and expression and of affective states corresponding to instinctual drive. This theory received support from the studies of Klüver and Bucy (Klüver-Bucy syndrome). Growing

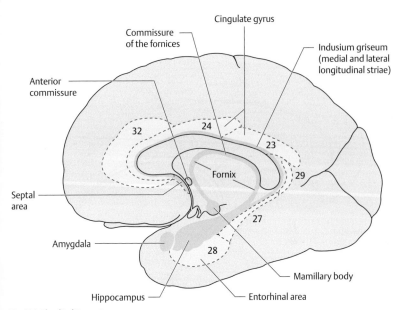

Fig. 7.**1 The limbic cortex**

evidence of the anatomical and functional linkage of the various limbic structures led MacLean to coin the term "limbic system."

More recently, however, the concept of the limbic system as a discrete functional unit has come into question, as further studies have shown that the limbic structures possess important neural connections not just with each other but with outside structures as well. Thus, the limbic system cannot be regarded as a *closed* system in either an anatomical or a functional sense. The functions associated with the limbic system, such as instinctual and affective behavior, motivation, and drive, as well as learning and memory (see below), should not be thought of as the preserve of the limbic system alone. These functions depend on an intact cooperation of the limbic system with many other areas of the brain.

Once this has been understood, there is no further objection to the use of the term "limbic system," particularly because the anatomical connections between the various limbic structures, which originally motivated this term, are indeed present, robust, and functionally important. No uniform alternative terminology has yet come into general use. Pathological changes of the limbic structures are still described, in the clinical setting, as lesions of the limbic system.

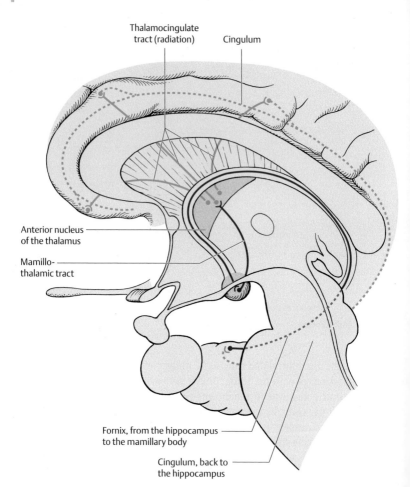

Thalamocingulate
tract (radiation)

Cingulum

Anterior nucleus
of the thalamus

Mamillo-
thalamic tract

Fornix, from the hippocampus
to the mamillary body

Cingulum, back to
the hippocampus

Fig. 7.**2 The Papez circuit** (hippocampus – fornix – mamillary body – anterior nucleus of the thalamus – cingulate gyrus – cingulum – hippocampus)

Internal and External Connections

Papez Circuit

A group of limbic structures, including the hippocampus, are connected to one another in the so-called Papez circuit, which contains a number of neural relay stations arranged in a circuit or loop. Beyond the basic wiring diagram of the

Papez circuit, as originally described, much further information has come to light regarding additional connections and the particular neurotransmitters used at various points in the circuit.

The Papez circuit runs as follows. From the *hippocampus* (Ammon's horn), impulses travel through the great arch of the *fornix* to the *mamillary body.* This nucleus, in turn, is the site of origin of the *mamillothalamic tract* (of Vicq d'Azyr), which conveys impulses to the *anterior nucleus of the thalamus.* The anterior nucleus projects to the *cingulate gyrus* by way of the *thalamocingulate radiation.* From the cingulate gyrus, impulses travel by way of the *cingulum* back to the hippocampus, completing the circuit (Fig. 7.**2**).

Connections to Other Areas of the Brain

The mamillary body occupies a key position in the Papez circuit because it connects the limbic system with the *midbrain* (nuclei of Gudden and Bekhterev) and the *reticular formation.* The mamillotegmental tract and the peduncle of the mamillary body (see Figs. 6.**9** and 6.10, p. 277 f.) form a regulatory circuit of their own. Impulses arising in the limbic system can travel by way of the anterior nucleus of the thalamus to the cingulate gyrus, but also, via association fibers, to the *neocortex.* Furthermore, impulses from the autonomic nervous system can travel through the hypothalamus and the medial dorsal nucleus of the thalamus to reach the *orbitofrontal cortex.*

Major Components of the Limbic System

Hippocampus

The hippocampal formation is the central structure of the limbic system. Its structure and neural connections and the clinical changes observed in patients with hippocampal lesions form the subject of this section.

Microanatomy of the Hippocampal Formation

The hippocampal cortex consists of *archicortex*, a phylogenetically old type of cerebral cortex, which possesses only **three layers** instead of the usual six. Because of this different structure, the hippocampus and a few other cortical areas are called *allo*cortex (as opposed to the six-layered *iso*cortex). The hippocampus proper (Ammon's horn or *cornu Ammonis*) is distinct from the dentate gyrus (*fascia dentata,* Fig. 7.**3a** and **b**). The principal cell type in the hippocampus is the **pyramidal cell.** There are different types of pyramidal cells in the in-

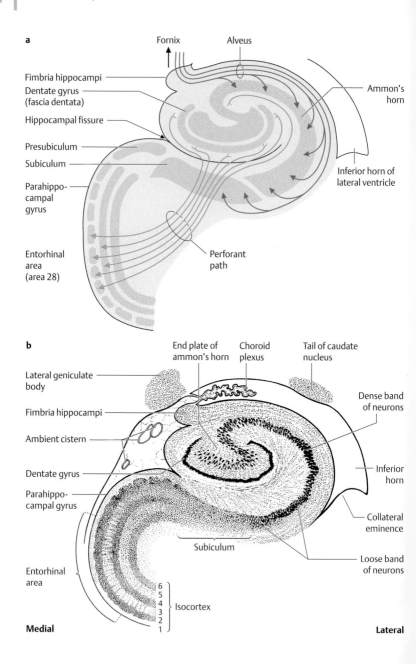

a

Fornix

Alveus

Fimbria hippocampi

Dentate gyrus
(fascia dentata)

Ammon's
horn

Hippocampal fissure

Presubiculum

Subiculum

Inferior horn of
lateral ventricle

Parahippo-
campal
gyrus

Entorhinal
area
(area 28)

Perforant
path

b

End plate of
ammon's horn

Choroid
plexus

Tail of caudate
nucleus

Lateral geniculate
body

Dense band
of neurons

Fimbria hippocampi

Ambient cistern

Inferior
horn

Dentate gyrus

Parahippo-
campal gyrus

Collateral
eminence

Subiculum

Loose band
of neurons

Entorhinal
area

6
5
4
3
2
1

Isocortex

Medial

Lateral

c

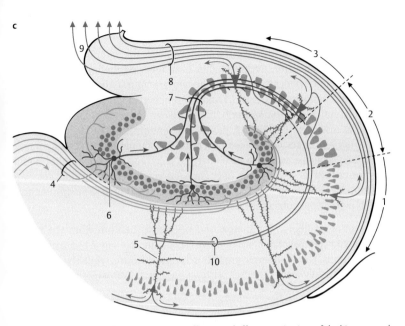

Fig. 7.**3 The hippocampal formation**. **a** Major afferent and efferent projections of the hippocampal formation: the perforant path and the fornix, respectively. The perforant path penetrates the subiculum to link the entorhinal area with the dentate gyrus. **b** Cytoarchitecture of the hippocampal formation. **c** Diagram of the various cell types of the hippocampal formation and their connections. **13**, Ammon's horn regions CA1 through CA3. **4**, Perforant path. **5**, Pyramidal cells. **6**, Granule cells of the dentate gyrus. **7**, Mossy fibers. **8**, Alveus. **9**, Fimbria hippocampi. **10**, Recurrent Schaffer collaterals of the CA3 pyramidal cells, which form synapses with the dendrites of the CA1 pyramidal cells. Fig. 7.**3c** from: Kahle W and Frotscher M: Taschenatlas der Anatomie, vol. 3, 8th ed., Thieme, Stuttgart, 2002.

dividual regions of Ammon's horn, designated **CA1**, **CA2**, and **CA3** ("CA" stands for cornu Ammonis) (Fig. 7.**3c**); some authors also describe a further CA4 region adjacent to the hilus of the dentate gyrus. The principal cells of the dentate gyrus are the granule cells, which connect the dentate gyrus with the hippocampus proper (CA4/CA3) through their axons, called mossy fibers. In addition to the principal cell types (pyramidal cells and granule cells) constituting the principal cell layers, the hippocampus and dentate gyrus also contain **GABAergic interneurons** that are not restricted to any particular cellular layer. These cells contain not only the inhibitory neurotransmitter GABA but also various neuropeptides and calcium-binding proteins.

Neural Connections of the Hippocampal Formation

Entorhinal afferent fibers. Like the hippocampus, the *entorhinal area*, too, is composed of allocortex. Recent studies have revealed the importance of this brain area, which is located lateral to the hippocampus in the parahippocampal gyrus (Brodmann area 28, Figs. 7.**1** and 7.**3**) and borders the amygdala rostrally. The collateral sulcus marks the border between the entorhinal area and the temporal isocortex (see Fig. 9.**9**, p. 357). The entorhinal area receives *afferent fibers from very widespread neocortical areas*. It is thought to serve as a *gateway to the hippocampus,* which in turn analyzes incoming neocortical information with respect to its novelty. The fiber connection from the entorhinal cortex to the hippocampus is massive. Most of these fibers belong to the *perforant path,* which pierces the subiculum (Fig. 7.**3a**).

Septal afferent fibers. Cholinergic and GABAergic neurons from the medial septum and the diagonal band of Broca (septal area, cf. Fig. 7.**1**) project to the hippocampus. The cholinergic projection is rather diffuse, while the GABAergic fibers specifically form synapses with hippocampal GABAergic neurons.

Commissural afferent fibers. Axons of the CA3 pyramidal cells and certain neurons in the hilar region of the dentate gyrus (mossy cells) connect the two hippocampi with each other, terminating on the proximal dendritic segments of the pyramidal and granule cells of the contralateral hippocampus.

Afferent fibers from the brainstem. Various brainstem nuclei send catecholaminergic fibers to the hippocampus, mostly in diffuse fashion.

Spread of Activation in the Hippocampus

As mentioned above, the projection from the entorhinal cortex is the major afferent pathway to the hippocampus. The entorhinal fibers are glutamatergic and terminate on the distal dendritic segments of the granule and pyramidal cells. The following **trisynaptic main pathway of excitation** has been proposed (Fig. 7.**3c**): entorhinal cortex → granule cells of the dentate gyrus (*first synapse*) → mossy fiber system → CA3 pyramidal cells (*second synapse*) → recurrent Schaffer collaterals of the CA3 pyramidal cell axons → CA1 pyramidal cells (*third synapse*). At all three relay stations, the forward transfer of excitation is regulated by GABAergic inhibitory interneurons. GABAergic synapses onto the neurons of the main excitatory pathway are found either on the cell body (basket cells), at the initial segment of the pyramidal and granule cell axons (axo-axonal cells or chandelier cells), or at the dendrites.

The CA1 neurons project onward to the *subiculum*, whose efferent fibers, in turn, form the *fimbria* and *fornix*, the major efferent bundle of the hippocampal formation (Fig. 7.**3**c). The fornix arches over the diencephalon to terminate in the mamillary body. The fornix is the main connection of the hippocampus with the hypothalamus, and thus with the autonomic nervous system (Fig. 7.**2**).

Amygdala

The amygdala is made up of several distinct components, some of which are functionally more closely related to the olfactory system, while others (the medial and central zones) are considered to belong to the limbic system. The amygdala is the nucleus of origin of the *stria terminalis* (Fig. 6.**9**, p. 277), which forms a large arch upward and forward in the groove between the thalamus and the caudate nucleus until it reaches the level of the interventricular foramen, where it divides into several separate fiber bundles. Some of its fibers continue to the *septal area*, others to the *rostral portion of the hypothalamus*, and a few others by way of the stria medullaris to the *habenular nucleus*. Furthermore, the amygdala is thought to make connections to the *midbrain* and, particularly, to the *medial dorsal nucleus of the thalamus*, which, in turn, projects to the *orbitofrontal cortex*. The two amygdalae are also connected to each other.

Experimental stimulation of the amygdala has been found to produce *affective activation.* Emotional reactions, such as rage and aggression, arise and are accompanied by autonomic reactions such as a rise in blood pressure, heart rate, and respiratory rate. Alterations of attention, of nutritional intake, and of sexual behavior occur, depending on which nuclear subdivision of the amygdala is stimulated.

Functions of the Limbic System

As explained above, the entorhinal cortex receives afferent input from widespread regions of the neocortex and transmits this information through the perforant path to the hippocampus. Neural processing at these levels involves the testing of incoming information for its novelty. This, in turn, implies that the hippocampus must play an important role in the processes of **learning and memory.** Such a role has been abundantly confirmed by clinical observation.

Properly functioning memory depends not only on an intact hippocampus but also on intact fiber connections linking the hippocampus and amygdala to other regions of the brain. The following fiber pathways are particularly important for memory (more specifically, for so-called declarative memory, see below):

- **Projections from the hippocampus** by way of the fornix
  - to the septal nuclei and
  - to the mamillary bodies and onward to the anterior nucleus of the thalamus and cingulate gyrus (Papez circuit)
- **Projections from the amygdala** to the dorsomedial nuclear region of the thalamus and onward to the orbitofrontal cortex.

Types of Memory

Short-term and long-term memory. A few basic concepts of neuropsychology will be introduced here as important background knowledge for an understanding of the functioning of the limbic system with respect to memory. William James, a founding father of modern neuropsychology, divided memory into two types, which he called "**primary memory**" and "**secondary memory.**" The contents of primary memory are held in consciousness for a short time after the sensory impressions that produced them are no longer present (**short-term memory**). Secondary memory, on the other hand, enables the individual to call up earlier events or states that have "disappeared from consciousness" in the meantime (**long-term memory**). The distinction between short-term memory (STM) and long-term memory (LTM) is now an empirically well-founded model in neuropsychology. Certain illnesses or lesions of the brain can impair these two memory systems to different extents. Both systems must function normally to enable normal cognitive performance. Dysfunction of either system can be revealed by standardized testing.

Neural substrates of short-term and long-term memory. Hebb, in the 1940s, postulated that the two forms of memory just described have different neural substrates. Hebb thought of STM as a circulating activation in a pool of neurons, and of LTM as the product of long-lasting structural changes at the level of synaptic connections. According to the hebbian model, a process of consolidation, taking minutes or hours, is required for this structural adaptation to take place. Later neuropsychological studies in patients with memory disorders revealed that the hippocampus indeed plays a crucial role in the consolidation of conscious memories.

Diagnostic tests of STM and LTM. A commonly used test of STM is performed as follows. The subject (or patient) is asked to listen to, and repeat, spoken sequences of numbers of increasing length. A normal individual can repeat seven, plus or minus two, numbers presented in this way. These memory traces are very rapidly lost and fail to enter LTM. LTM, on the other hand, can be tested by presenting certain stimuli (e. g., a list of terms or a set of objects) and asking the subject to take note of them over a defined interval of time, and then to recognize or reproduce them some time later. This is a test of voluntary recall of conscious memories.

Subtypes of LTM. There are two distinct subtypes (subsystems) of LTM, called **episodic** and **semantic memory.** Episodic memory deals with data that belong to a particular spatial and temporal setting, i.e., memories of personal experiences (a trip, concert, sporting event, etc.). Semantic memory, on the other hand, deals with facts belonging to general fields of knowledge (medicine, physics, etc.).

Part of LTM can influence behavior without the subject's conscious knowledge. A basic distinction is drawn between **explicit** (**declarative**) and **implicit** (**nondeclarative**) memory. The former deals with *conscious and verbally communicable memories*, as already described, while the latter deals with *nonverbal memory traces*, such as those that must be learned and recalled during the performance of a motor task. Implicit memory is also responsible for classical conditioning (as demonstrated in Pavlov's well-known experiment with the dog), as well as for perceptual and cognitive skills, and for the *priming effect*: information presented in one context can be processed later more efficiently in another context, even if the subject does not consciously remember the earlier presentation. The type of memory involved in the priming effect is stored and recalled "unconsciously," so to speak, and can only be recalled during the performance of the relevant tasks.

Complex patterns can also be stored in implicit memory. Thus, chess players can remember a particular pattern of chessmen on a chessboard better than can nonplayers, but only if the pattern has been drawn from a real chess game; they perform no better than control subjects who do not play chess if the pattern to be remembered has been generated at random.

In summary, memory is not a single functional entity, but rather possesses multiple distinct components.

Squire's taxonomy of memory. Squire (1987) proposed a classification scheme for the subtypes of memory. In addition to **explicit** and **implicit memory structures,** this scheme recognizes other subtypes of memory that are required to perform **metacognitive tasks,** such as evaluating one's own memory performance or generating strategies to organize information storage and recall. Strategies of the latter type are called **frontal-lobe-type memory functions,** because they apparently depend on intact functioning of the frontal lobes. During the process of memory storage, there seems to be a transition from the concrete to the abstract: for example, one might be able to remember the approximate appearance of the school one attended as a child, without being able to sketch it in detail. Yet, while memory storage suppresses some aspects of experience, it accentuates others. The "memories" laid down by the storage process thus bear less resemblance to a documentary film than to a subjectively colored reconstruction of events. In summary, LTM should be thought of as a dynamic process, which changes over the years and often becomes increasingly abstract, but nonetheless remains capable of storing vivid and detailed traces of certain experiences, particularly those that are of personal importance.

Case Presentation 1: **Amnesia after Bilateral Resection of Medial Temporal Structures**

The famous and historic case of H.M. illustrates the vitally important role that medial temporal structures play in memory. In the decades since this case was described, the various subtypes of memory described have been characterized in detail, and a large number of specific neuropsychological tests have been developed to study them.

Medically intractable epilepsy is sometimes treated by neurosurgical resection of the area or areas of the brain from which the seizures arise. Often, the tissue to be resected is in the temporal lobe. In 1953, H.M., a patient with intractable epilepsy, underwent resection of the medial portions of the temporal lobe on both sides. (This procedure is no longer performed bilaterally, in large part because of adverse sequelae like those described in H.M.'s case.) Postoperatively, H.M. manifested severe disturbances of memory, which have persisted to the present day with hardly any improvement (he is still alive as this book is being written). Ever since the operation, he has been unable to lay down new memories, even though his general level of intelligence, as measured by standardized tests, is normal.

Shortly after the operation, for example, when H.M. conversed with the doctor, his cognitive ability appeared to be unimpaired, and he had no trouble answering questions about how he felt. Yet, if the doctor left the room and returned a few minutes later, H.M. completely forgot ever having seen him and complained about having to talk to a new doctor each time. His short-term memory was preserved, that is, he could still retain new information for periods of up to about one minute: he could, for example, correctly reproduce sequences of numbers or pictures that were presented to him, but only immediately after their presentation. Thus, his deficit involved the consolidation of newly laid down memories from short-term into long-term memory.

H.M.'s nondeclarative memory was not impaired: for example, his performance on tasks involving the completion of word or image sequences improved over time just as much as that of normal subjects. This implies that H.M. was able to learn and retain certain problem-solving strategies, even though, a short time later, he could no longer remember ever having performed the task. He was still able to acquire new motor skills postoperatively, and his metacognitive functions were also intact, at least in part: he was aware, for example, that his memory was deficient.

This remarkable case history shows that the medial temporal lobe is necessary for the storage of new information, as well as for the recall of information that has already been stored. The medial temporal lobe—specifically, the hippocampus—can apparently be thought of as a kind of intermediate or working storage system, in which explicit memory traces are held for a short time before they are transferred to long-term storage or sent on to other neural centers for further cognitive processing.

Memory Dysfunction—the Amnestic Syndrome and Its Causes

As already mentioned on p. 320, normally functioning memory, particularly of the declarative type, depends above all on the integrity of the hippocampus and its fiber connections. Fiber projections from the amygdala to the orbitofrontal cortex also play an important role.

Lesions or illnesses of the brain involving these important structures and regulatory circuits can produce an amnestic syndrome.

General definition of the amnestic syndrome. A patient is said to be suffering from an amnestic syndrome when there is a specific (i.e., isolated or predominant) impairment of the ability to lay down new memories and to recall information stored before the onset of the problem (**anterograde** and **retrograde amnesia,** respectively). In an isolated (pure) amnestic syndrome, other mental abilities, such as language, logical thinking, and problem-solving behavior, are not impaired. Amnestic syndromes mainly affect LTM and largely spare STM, as can be demonstrated by testing the patient's digit or block span; procedural memory, i.e., the learning of behavioral sequences, also remains essentially intact. Amnestic syndromes are commonly accompanied by personality changes or abnormalities of drive, e. g., in the context of Korsakoff syndrome, or after bilateral thalamic infarction (cf. Case Presentation 3, p. 326).

The differential diagnosis of the amnestic syndrome from dementia is of major clinical importance, e. g., with respect to Alzheimer disease, a common cause of dementia. Dementia involves not only amnesia but also additional focal neuropsychological deficits, such as aphasia and agnosia, as well as an overall decline in cognitive performance, which is typically reflected by worsening IQ scores.

Causes of the amnestic syndrome. Memory disturbances can arise either acutely or slowly and progressively, depending on the nature of the underlying brain illness.

Memory can be impaired by *traumatic brain injury, hemorrhage, ischemia, degenerative processes* such as Alzheimer disease, and various types of *metab-*

olic encephalopathy, including the Wernicke-Korsakoff syndrome. Memory impairment may also be iatrogenic, arising, for example, after a neurosurgical procedure in the temporal lobe as treatment for medically intractable epilepsy, or after electroconvulsive therapy for severe depression.

It has been convincingly shown that unilateral damage of the structures and regulatory circuits subserving memory can produce "lateralized" memory deficits: left-sided lesions impair verbal memory, right-sided lesions impair visual memory, and bilateral lesions impair both. When the two major fiber pathways involved in memory (cf. p. 320) are simultaneously interrupted in experimental animals, severe and persistent amnesia results. If only one of them is interrupted, the ensuing amnesia has been reported to be relatively mild and transient.

Posttraumatic amnesia. Amnesia after a traumatic brain injury usually consists of both anterograde amnesia (the inability to remember events that took place *after* the injury) and retrograde amnesia (the inability to remember events that took place *before* it). Anterograde and retrograde amnesia affect variable periods of time after and before the injury, and they can also be incomplete, leaving so-called *islands of memory* in between amnestic memory gaps. Persons suffering from retrograde amnesia usually have better recall for events that took place in the distant past. Organic disturbances of memory, unlike psychogenic disturbances, usually have both anterograde and retrograde components, which can improve to a variable extent, and sometimes even recover fully. Anterograde and retrograde amnesia may be accompanied by other neuropsychological abnormalities, depending on their underlying cause.

Other diseases causing amnesia. In principle, any brain illness or injury that affects the structures subserving memory bilaterally will produce an amnestic syndrome. The following conditions are of particular clinical importance:

- *Herpes simplex encephalitis*, which preferentially involves limbic structures and usually produces bilateral lesions of the mesiobasal temporal lobes and cingulate gyri
- *Thalamic infarction,* which, because of the nature of the thalamic blood supply, is often bilateral
- *Hemorrhage or infarction of the septal nuclei* after rupture and/or neurosurgical treatment of a saccular aneurysm of the anterior cerebral artery
- *Lesions of the splenium of the corpus callosum* (either traumatic or ischemic), which commonly also involve the immediately underlying commissure of the fornices (psalterium)

Three of these conditions are illustrated in Case Presentations 2, 3, and 4 below.

Case Presentation 2: *Bilateral Medial Temporal Dysfunction due to Viral Infection*

This 11-year-old girl suffered from increasingly severe headaches, nausea, and vomiting for two weeks, and then became confused. At times, she could no longer find her way around the apartment in which she lived; she spoke little, and, when she spoke, she made no sense. Her pediatrician referred her to the hospital, and she was admitted.

On admission, the patient could not remember any new information for more than a few minutes. She was thus suffering from severe an-

terograde amnesia. No other focal neurological deficits were noted. The initial magnetic resonance images revealed edema of the temporal lobes and cingulate gyri bilaterally (Fig. 7.**4**). Later images additionally revealed hemorrhages in these areas. Serological testing showed the cause of the amnestic syndrome to be a herpes simplex infection of the brain. The patient's memory impairment improved slowly after antiviral treatment, but she nonetheless had to repeat the sixth grade.

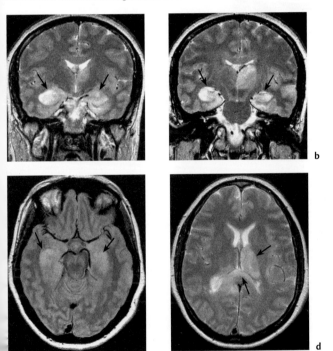

Fig. 7.4 An 11-year-old girl with herpes simplex encephalitis. a and **b** The coronal T2-weighted images reveal bilateral hyperintense signal abnormalities in the medial portions of the temporal lobes. The hippocampal formations are swollen bilaterally. The pathological process also extends into the left thalamus, lateral temporal cortex, and insula.

c and **d** The axial proton-density-weighted and T2-weighted images reveal bilateral medial temporal signal abnormalities, as well as very unusual-appearing abnormalities in the left thalamus (**c**) and splenium of the corpus callosum (**d**).   Fig. 7.**4e** ▷

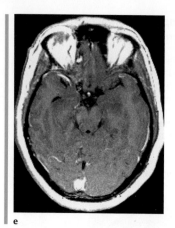

Fig. 7.**4e** The contrast-enhanced axial T1-weighted image reveals an intact blood–brain barrier, as is typically found in the early stage of herpes simplex encephalitis.

e

Case Presentation 3: *Bilateral Thalamic Infarction*

When this 54-year-old businessman and his wife returned home from a celebration they had attended with friends, she was surprised to find him sleepy and abnormally indifferent. He also seemed to have suddenly "forgotten" that it was late at night, repeatedly mumbling questions such as, "Do I have to get up now?" He asked her where he was, even though he was sitting in his own living room. He could no longer remember any individual details of the evening, or even that a celebration had taken place. He did not remember having made a speech. At first, his wife attributed his strange behavior to the influence of a moderate amount of alcohol, combined with an oncoming cold. In the morning, however, finding that the problem had only worsened overnight, she took him to the hospital.

On admission, the most remarkable immediate findings were the patient's apathy and lack of drive. It was very difficult to get him to undress for the examination or perform tasks of any other kind. He also fell asleep several times while being examined. He could give no more than cursory information about his person, and was not oriented at all to time or place.

The magnetic resonance images revealed bilateral hyperintense lesions in the dorsomedial thalamus, indicating ischemia in the territory of the thalamotuberal arteries (arteries of Percheron) bilaterally; these arteries often arise from a common, unpaired trunk (Fig. 7.5). The patient's neurological deficits resolved relatively rapidly, and he was able to return to work a few months later.

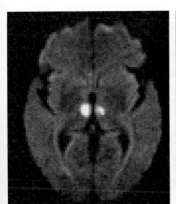 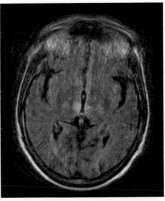

b

Fig. 7.**5 Bilateral thalamic infarction. a** The diffusion-weighted MR image reveals two acute ischemic lesions in the medial rostral portion of the thalamus on both sides. **b** The T2-weighted image with FLAIR sequence still reveals the ischemic lesions, though much less clearly than the diffusion-weighted image. The patient was confused and moved during the study. A diffusion-weighted image can be obtained in 4 seconds, but a T2-weighted image takes 3–5 minutes.

Case Presentation 4: Bilateral Lesions Involving the Septal Nuclei and the Frontobasal Cortex

This 61-year-old housewife had prepared lunch for herself and her husband as usual. After the meal, she suddenly began acting strangely: she could no longer carry on a coherent conversation with him, continually changed the subject, and asked him three times whether he had already had his midday nap. She seemed to take no regard of his answers, or to forget them at once. When he tested her by asking her the date, she could not give the correct day of the week or the correct month, or even remember what year it was. She also seemed to have undergone a change of personality, at times reacting aggressively when he approached her in a friendly way, and at times seeming totally apathetic. Furthermore (he reported), she began making coffee again and again, at brief intervals, even after he objected, each time, that she had just had her coffee a few minutes before. When he confronted her about her unusual behavior and her apparent deficits, she said, in stereotypic fashion, "What do you want from me? I'm perfectly all right." He succeeded with difficulty in bringing her to the hospital, over her objections.

The admitting physician diagnosed an amnestic syndrome, an affective disturbance with alternating aggressiveness and apathy, and a lack of insight into the illness (anosognosia). A further finding, on neurological examination, was marked perseveration (i.e., the involuntary and apparently purposeless repetition of actions and behaviors): while being examined, for example, the patient could not stop combing her hair in front of a mirror.

Magnetic resonance imaging (Fig. 7.6) and subsequent cerebral angiography revealed the acute infarction of part of the corpus callosum as well as of the fornices, left basal ganglia, and frontal cortex, caused by occlusion of perforating branches of the anterior communicating artery.

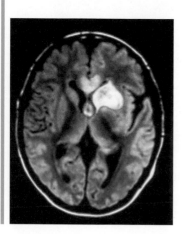

Fig. 7.6 **Bilateral lesions involving the septal nuclei.** This proton-weighted MR image reveals signal abnormalities in the anterior portion of the corpus callosum and in both fornices. There is also a large signal abnormality in the left basal ganglia.

8 Basal Ganglia

8 Basal Ganglia

The basal ganglia are a part of the motor system. The principal nuclei of the basal ganglia are the **caudate nucleus**, the **putamen**, and the **globus pallidus**, all of which lie in the subcortical white matter of the telencephalon. These nuclei are connected to each other, and to the motor cortex, in complex regulatory circuits. They exert both excitatory and inhibitory effects on the motor cortex. They play an important role in the **initiation** and **modulation of movement** and in the **control of muscle tone.** Lesions of the basal ganglia, and of other, functionally related nuclei, such as the substantia nigra and the subthalamic nucleus, can produce either an excess or a deficiency of movement-related impulses, and/or pathological alterations of muscle tone. The most common disease of the basal ganglia is Parkinson disease, which is characterized by the clinical triad of rigidity, akinesia, and tremor.

Preliminary Remarks on Terminology

The hierarchically uppermost center for the control of movement is the cerebral cortex, whose signals are transmitted by the pyramidal pathway to the motor cranial nerve nuclei and to the anterior horn cells of the spinal cord (**pyramidal system**). A number of other structures in the central nervous system participate in the initiation and modulation of movement. The most important of these "accessory motor centers" are the basal ganglia, a set of subcortical nuclei located within the deep white matter of the telencephalon. The pyramidal system was long regarded as the "major" system for the control of movement as it provides the most direct and most rapid connection between the cortex and the motor neurons of the brainstem and spinal cord. All other structures playing a role in movement were relegated to the so-called "**extrapyramidal system.**" This term is misleading, however, because the pyramidal and extrapyramidal systems do not, in fact, operate separately. Rather, they are subunits of a *single*, integrated motor system and, as such, are closely linked to each other both structurally and functionally. Thus, there are extensive connections, for example, between the motor cortex and the striatum, an important nucleus within the basal ganglia. The term "extrapyramidal system" is now obsolete and will be used only rarely in this book. Instead, we will speak of normal and abnormal function of the basal ganglia.

The Role of the Basal Ganglia in the Motor System: Phylogenetic Aspects

The corpus striatum is an important control center for the motor system. We will briefly consider its phylogenetic development in this section in order to make its function and anatomical connections easier to understand.

The phylogenetically oldest motor centers in the central nervous system are the spinal cord and the primitive apparatus of the reticular formation in the midbrain tectum. Over the course of phylogeny, the paleostriatum (*globus pallidus*) developed next, and then the neostriatum (*caudate nucleus* and *putamen*), which enlarged in parallel with the cerebral cortex. The neostriatum is particularly well developed in higher mammals, including humans. As the phylogenetically more recent structures grew larger, the older structures came under their influence to an increasing extent. In phylogenetically older species, the older neural centers are primarily responsible for the maintenance of normal muscle tone and for the more or less automatic control of locomotion.

As the cerebral cortex developed, the phylogenetically older motor centers (paleostriatum and neostriatum) came increasingly under the control of the new motor system, i.e., the pyramidal system. While most mammals, including the cat, can still walk without much difficulty after the cerebral cortex is removed, humans are entirely dependent on an intact pyramidal system. Human phylogenetic development has reached the point that the older neural centers can no longer compensate for the functional loss of the new ones. Yet, even in humans, a spastically paralyzed limb can still be seen to make certain involuntary movements, called associated movements, which are generated by the older motor centers.

Components of the Basal Ganglia and Their Connections

Nuclei

The basal ganglia include all of the functionally interrelated nuclei *within* the deep white matter of the telencephalon that are embryologically derived from the ganglionic eminence (anterior portion of the telencephalic vesicle). The major nuclei of the basal ganglia are the *caudate nucleus*, the *putamen*, and part of the *globus pallidus* (Figs. 8.1 and 8.2); other nuclei that are considered part of the basal ganglia on embryological grounds are the *claustrum* (Figs. 8.5 and 8.6) and the *amygdala* (Figs. 8.1 and 8.2). The amygdala has already been discussed in connection with the limbic system (p. 319). Like the claustrum, whose function is not precisely known, the amygdala has no direct functional connection to the remainder of the basal ganglia. These two structures will not be discussed any further in this chapter.

The caudate nucleus forms part of the wall of the lateral ventricle and, like it, has an arched shape, due to the rotation of the telencephalon during embryonic development (cf. p. 352). The head of the caudate nucleus forms the lateral wall of the lateral ventricle; its tail forms the roof of the inferior horn of the lateral ventricle in the temporal lobe, extending as far forward as the amygdala, which lies at the anterior end of the inferior horn (Fig. 8.2). The caudate nucleus can therefore be seen in two separate locations on some coronal sections (cf. Figs. 8.3-8.8, especially Fig. 8.7), in the lateral wall of the body of the lateral ventricle as well as in the roof of the inferior horn. The rostral portion (head) of the caudate nucleus is continuous with the putamen.

The putamen lies lateral to the globus pallidus (or pallidum, so called because of its relatively pale coloration), covering it like a shell and extending somewhat beyond it both rostrally and caudally. The putamen and globus pallidus are separated by a thin layer of white matter called the medial medullary lamina.

The caudate nucleus and putamen are connected by numerous small bridges of gray matter, which are seen as stripes in anatomical sections. These two nuclei together have, therefore, been given the alternative name **corpus striatum** (striped body), or *striatum* for short (Fig. 8.2). The striation arises during development, when the fibers of the internal capsule grow through the originally uniform basal ganglion.

Globus pallidus. The third major nucleus of the basal ganglia is made up of an internal and an external segment (pars interna and pars externa). Because the

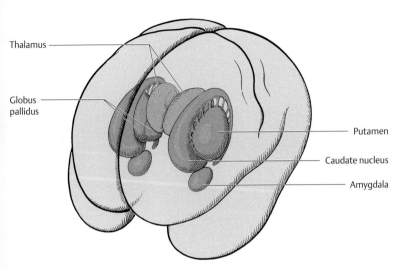

Thalamus

Globus
pallidus

Putamen

Caudate nucleus

Amygdala

Fig. 8.**1 Topographical relationships of the basal ganglia (in red)**

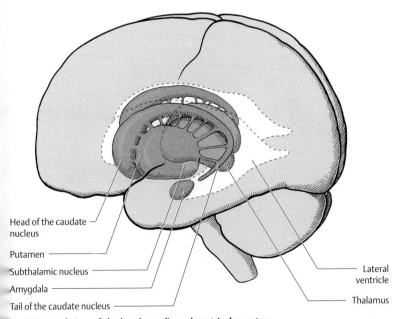

Head of the caudate
nucleus

Putamen

Subthalamic nucleus

Amygdala

Tail of the caudate nucleus

Lateral
ventricle

Thalamus

Fig. 8.**2 Lateral view of the basal ganglia and ventricular system**

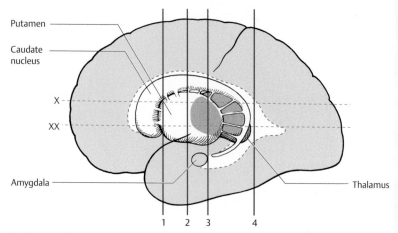

Fig. 8.**3 Lateral view of the basal ganglia.** X, XX: horizontal planes of section for Fig. 8.**4**. **1–4**: coronal planes of section for Figs. 8.**5**–8.**8**.

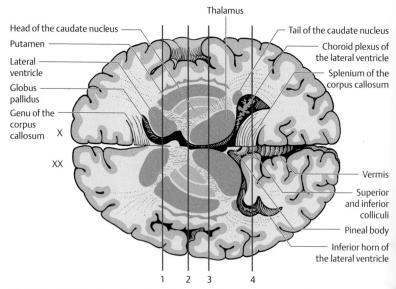

Fig. 8.**4 Two horizontal sections through the basal ganglia** (for planes of section, see. Fig. 8.**3**)

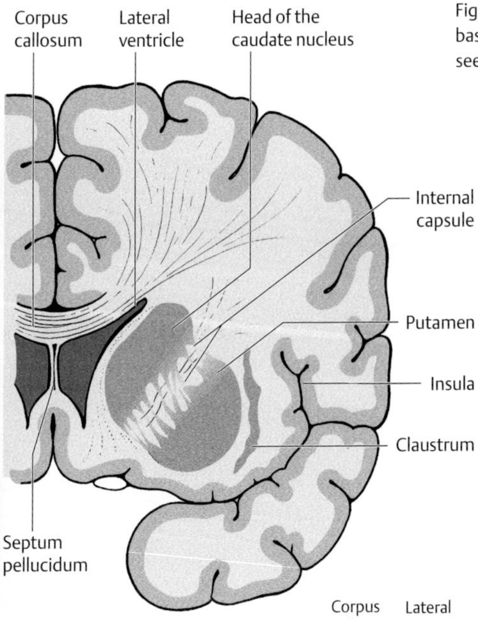

Fig. 8.**5 Coronal section 1** through the basal ganglia (for planes of section, see. Figs. 8.**3** and 8.**4**)

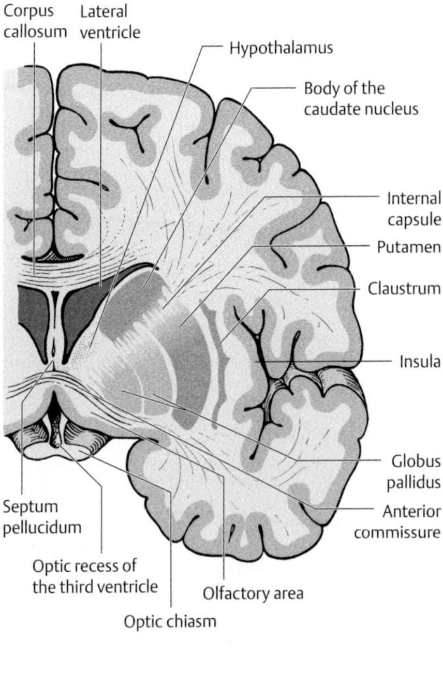

Corpus callosum

Lateral ventricle

Head of the caudate nucleus

Internal capsule

Putamen

Insula

Claustrum

Septum pellucidum

Corpus callosum

Lateral ventricle

Hypothalamus

Body of the caudate nucleus

Internal capsule

Putamen

Claustrum

Insula

Globus pallidus

Anterior commissure

Septum pellucidum

Optic recess of the third ventricle

Olfactory area

Optic chiasm

Fig. 8.**6 Coronal section 2** through the basal ganglia (for planes of section, see Figs. 8.**3** and 8.**4**)

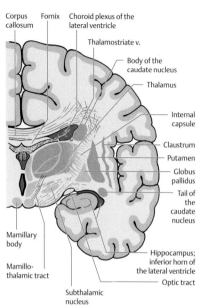

Corpus callosum
Fornix
Choroid plexus of the lateral ventricle
Thalamostriate v.
Body of the caudate nucleus
Thalamus
Internal capsule
Claustrum
Putamen
Globus pallidus
Tail of the caudate nucleus
Mamillary body
Mamillo-thalamic tract
Subthalamic nucleus
Hippocampus; inferior horn of the lateral ventricle
Optic tract

Fig. 8.**7 Coronal section 3** through the basal ganglia (for planes of section, see Figs. 8.**3** and 8.**4**)

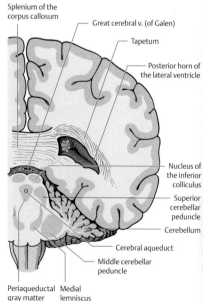

Splenium of the corpus callosum
Great cerebral v. (of Galen)
Tapetum
Posterior horn of the lateral ventricle
Nucleus of the inferior colliculus
Superior cerebellar peduncle
Cerebellum
Cerebral aqueduct
Middle cerebellar peduncle
Periaqueductal gray matter
Medial lemniscus

Fig. 8.**8 Coronal section 4** through the basal ganglia (for planes of section, see Figs. 8.**3** and 8.**4**)

globus pallidus is phylogenetically older than the other nuclei, it is also called the paleostriatum. Part of it is, embryologically speaking, a component of the diencephalon. The putamen and globus pallidus are collectively termed the **lentiform** or **lenticular nucleus** (lens-shaped nucleus).

Associated nuclei. Further nuclei that are closely functionally related to the basal ganglia include two midbrain nuclei—the **substantia nigra** (reciprocally connected to the striatum) and the **red nucleus**—and one diencephalic nucleus, the **subthalamic nucleus** (reciprocally connected to the globus pallidus). The globus pallidus caudally borders the rostral portion (red zone) of the substantia nigra. The pallidum, substantia nigra, and red nucleus contain large amounts of iron. The dark pigmentation of the substantia nigra ("black substance") is due to its high melanin content.

Connections of the Basal Ganglia

The neural connections of the basal ganglia with one another and with other regions of the brain are not yet completely understood. The major afferent and efferent pathways will be described in this section.

Afferent Pathways

Afferent pathways to the corpus striatum. The corpus striatum receives afferent input from extensive areas of the cerebral cortex, particularly the **motor areas of the frontal lobe**, i.e., Brodmann areas 4, 6aα, and 6aβ. These cortical afferents are derived from projection neurons of the cerebral cortex (pyramidal cells of the fifth layer of the cortex), are *glutamatergic*, run *ipsilaterally*, and are *topically organized*. There are probably no reciprocal fibers running from the corpus striatum back to the cortex. A further point-to-point afferent input to the corpus striatum is derived from the **centromedian nucleus of the thalamus**, and is probably excitatory. This afferent pathway transmits impulses from the cerebellum and the midbrain reticular formation to the striatum. The **substantia nigra** sends *dopaminergic* afferent fibers to the striatum, whose loss is the cause of Parkinson disease (see below). Finally, the striatum also receives a *serotonergic* input from the **raphe nuclei.**

Other afferent pathways. The globus pallidus derives its major afferent input from the corpus striatum and receives no direct afferent fibers from the cerebral cortex. Cortically derived afferent fibers do, however, travel to the substantia nigra, red nucleus, and subthalamic nucleus.

Efferent Pathways

Efferent pathways of the corpus striatum. The major efferent projections of the corpus striatum go to the **external** and **internal segments of the globus pallidus**. Further efferent fibers travel to the pars compacta and pars reticulata of the **substantia nigra**. The cells of origin of the striatal efferent fibers are GABAergic spiny neurons, the most common cell type in the striatum.

Efferent pathways of the globus pallidus. The major contingent of efferent fibers runs to the **thalamus**, which, in turn, projects to the cerebral cortex, completing a feedback loop.

The **functional interpretation** of the afferent and efferent projections of the basal ganglia requires consideration of the particular neurotransmitter substances and receptors involved, and of the types of neurological deficit that are produced when certain pathways cease to function normally. Thus, Parkinson disease is characterized by degeneration of the dopaminergic neurons of the substantia nigra that project to the corpus striatum. The clinical deficits observed in Parkinson disease provide a clue to the probable functions of the nigrostriatal system in normal individuals.

Participation of the Basal Ganglia in Regulatory Circuits

The basal ganglia and their afferent and efferent connections are integral parts of complex regulatory circuits that excite and inhibit the neurons of the motor cortex. Neural transmission within these circuits can be characterized in terms of the anatomical course along which the impulses travel, as well as the particular neurotransmitters and receptors that are involved at each synapse. One of the more important circuits conveys impulses along two separate paths from the cortex, via the corpus striatum, to the globus pallidus, and then to the thalamus and back to the cortex (Fig. 8.**9**). In addition to this major regulatory circuit, there are other feedback loops that will not be explicitly described in this book.

Cortico-striato-pallido-thalamo-cortical pathway. The motor and sensory cortex sends a topographically organized projection to the *striatum* that uses the excitatory neurotransmitter, glutamate. Beyond the striatum, the basal ganglionic circuit splits into two parts, which are known as the direct and indirect pathways.

Direct pathway. The direct pathway is GABAergic and runs from the striatum to the *internal pallidal segment*. Substance P is used as a co-transmitter. From the pallidum, the pathway proceeds to the glutamatergic projection neurons of the *thalamus*, which complete the loop *back to the cerebral cortex* (Fig. 8.**9**).

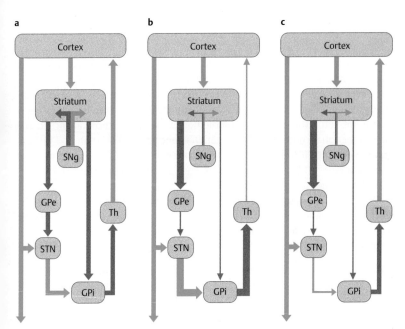

Fig. 8.**9 The direct and indirect basal ganglia pathways. a** The normal situation (green = excitation, red = inhibition). GPe = globus pallidus, external segment. STN = subthalamic nucleus. GPi = globus pallidus, internal segment. Th = thalamus. SNg = substantia nigra. **b** The situation in Parkinson disease (untreated). **c** The situation in Parkinson disease during treatment with subthalamic stimulation (i.e., blockage of neural activity in the STN).

Indirect pathway. The indirect pathway, which uses the neurotransmitters GABA and enkephalin, runs from the striatum to the *external pallidal segment.* From this point, a further GABAergic projection proceeds to the *subthalamic nucleus,* which, in turn, sends a glutamatergic projection to the *internal pallidal segment.* The further course of the indirect pathway is identical to that of the direct pathway, i.e., *from the thalamus back to the cerebral cortex* (Fig. 8.**9**).

It follows from the combination of inhibitory and excitatory neurotransmitters used by these two pathways that the overall effect of stimulation of the direct pathway on the cerebral cortex is excitatory, while that of stimulation of the indirect pathway is inhibitory (Fig. 8.**9**). The dopaminergic projection from the substantia nigra (pars compacta) plays a modulating role in this system.

Function and Dysfunction of the Basal Ganglia

Normal functions of the basal ganglia. The basal ganglia participate in many motor processes, including the expression of emotion, as well as in the integration of sensory and motor impulses and in cognitive processes. The basal ganglia carry out their motor functions indirectly through the influence they exert on the premotor, motor, and supplementary areas of the cerebral cortex. The major functional roles of the basal ganglia concern the **initiation** and **facilitation** of voluntary movement, and the simultaneous suppression of unwanted or involuntary influences that might disturb the smooth and effective execution of movement.

Moreover, the basal ganglia apparently use proprioceptive feedback from the periphery to compare the movement patterns or programs generated by the motor cortex with the movements that are actually initiated, so that movement is subject to ongoing refinement by a continuous servo-control mechanism.

Typical deficits. Lesions of the basal ganglia can produce complex movement disorders and cognitive disturbances of various types depending on their site and extent.

- Clinical disorders involving the basal ganglia may present with a deficiency of movement (**hypokinesia**) or
  - an excess of movement (**hyperkinesia, chorea, athetosis, ballism**).
- **Abnormalities of muscle tone** commonly accompany abnormalities of the above two types,
  - but can also be the predominant or sole manifestation of basal ganglia dysfunction (**dystonia**).

Wilson disease is a good example of a basal ganglia disorder, where a combination of all of the above manifestations can be seen (cf. Case Presentation 4, p. 347) because of variable and diffuse affection of the different nuclei and subsystems. In the remainder of this chapter, we will discuss the major disorders that mainly affect one particular subsystem of the basal ganglia.

Clinical Syndromes of Basal Ganglia Lesions

Parkinsonism

Etiology and pathogenesis. In **idiopathic Parkinson disease**, the dopaminergic nigrostriatal projection degenerates (see above). Consequently, the GABAergic activity of the striatal neurons is enhanced, and there is thus an excess of activity in the indirect basal ganglia loop. At the same time, the subthalamic nucleus also shows increased activity and thus excessively inhibits the glutamatergic neurons of the thalamus. The overall effect is *net inhibition at the output of the basal ganglia loop* (Fig. 8.**9b**) and, therefore, *reduced activation of cortical motor areas.*

A characteristic neuropathological hallmark of the disease is intracytoplasmic inclusion bodies called *Lewy bodies.* A major component of Lewy bodies is α-synuclein. It is not yet known what role this protein plays, if any, in the pathogenesis of sporadic (idiopathic) Parkinson disease. However, in **familial forms** of Parkinson disease, which represent a small minority of cases, mutations in several different genes have been found to cause disease. Interestingly, mutations are also found in α-synuclein, suggesting a direct pathological role in the degeneration of dopaminergic neurons. Familial forms usually show earlier onset of disease and specific clinical symptoms, which are listed in Table 8.**1**.

Table 8.1 Familial forms of Parkinson Disease

Locus	Chromosomal Localization	Gene Product	Inheritance	Lewy Body Pathology	Specific Clinical Symptoms
PARK 1	4q21	α-Synuclein	AD	Yes	Dementia
PARK 2	6q25.2–27	Parkin	AR	No	Early onset, L-dopa-induced dyskinesias, improvement during sleep, foot dystonia
PARK 3	2p13		AD	Yes	Dementia
PARK 4	4p15	α-Synuclein	AD	Yes	Dementia, postural tremor
PARK 5	4p14	UCH-L1	AD	Unknown	Not described
PARK 6	1q35–36	PINK-1	AR	Unknown	Early onset, tremor dominant
PARK 7	1q36	DJ-1	AR	Unknown	Early onset, dystonia, psychiatric alterations
PARK 8	12cen	LRRK 2	AD	Unknown	Unknown
PARK 9	1p32		AR (?)	Unknown	Late onset
PARK 10	1p32		? (susceptibility gene)	Unknown	Late onset

In addition to idiopathic Parkinson disease, a neurodegenerative condition, there are also **symptomatic forms of parkinsonism** that are caused by structural/inflammatory lesions of the central nervous system, or by toxic influences. Parkinsonism can thus be produced, for example, by medications (neuroleptics, antiemetics, calcium antagonists, reserpine-containing antihypertensive agents) as well as by encephalitis, ischemic lesions, intoxications, and metabolic disturbances.

If typical parkinsonian manifestations are seen together with other neurological deficits suggesting dysfunction of other central nervous structures beyond the basal ganglia, a **Parkinson-plus syndrome** is said to be present. There are a number of distinct Parkinson-plus syndromes. For example, parkinsonism, vertical gaze palsy, and marked nuchal rigidity make up the characteristic clinical triad of *Steele-Richardson-Olszewski syndrome*, also known as *progressive supranuclear palsy*. On the other hand, severe autonomic dysfunction, postural instability, and deficits involving other components of the central nervous system (e. g., pyramidal tract signs) are seen in *multiple system atrophy*.

Clinical manifestations. Loss of dopaminergic afferents in the striatum leads to reduced voluntary movements (**hypokinesia**), continually elevated, waxy muscle tone (**rigidity**), and oscillating movements at a frequency of 4-6 Hz when the limbs are held at rest (resting **tremor**) (see Case Presentation 1, p. 343).

Parkinson disease has **three clinical subtypes** that are defined by the motor manifestations that predominate in each type:

- Patients with the **akinetic-rigid** type of Parkinson disease can be recognized at an early stage by their increasing poverty of movement, including a *lack of accessory movements of the arms*, slow shuffling gait, a lack of facial expression (*hypomimia*), and a characteristic *stooped posture*. Some patients initially complain of shoulder stiffness ("frozen shoulder"), which may prompt erroneous referral to an orthopedist before the progressive course of the disease has revealed the true diagnosis.
- Patients with **tremor-dominant** Parkinson disease suffer mainly from the low-frequency rest tremor, which—like the other motor manifestations—is often unilateral at the onset of disease. Parkinsonian tremor is often of the pill-rolling type (see Case Presentation 1).
- Patients with **mixed-type** Parkinson disease show a more or less equal manifestation of akinesia, rigidity, and tremor.

Case Presentation 1: **Idiopathic Parkinson Disease**

A 59-year-old bank teller first realized while counting banknotes that he could not use his right hand normally. On repeated occasions, he counted off several notes at once instead of a single note, so that the tally was incorrect. Meanwhile, his handwriting gradually became smaller and less legible, so that he could no longer perform his job effectively. He complained of right shoulder pain and cramps in the right arm and was treated unsuccessfully by an orthopedist for presumed arthritis of the shoulder. As time went on, his facial expression became sparse (hypomimia) and a resting tremor of the right hand developed, at a frequency of about 8 Hz. None of the patient's relatives had ever suffered from similar problems.

His family physician referred him to a neurologist, whose examination revealed cog-wheel rigidity of the limbs, worst in the right arm, a mildly stooped posture, and a small-stepped gait with reduced arm swing on the right. The patient took an excessive number of steps while turning around. There were no autonomic deficits, and his mental status was normal.

A CT scan with intravenous contrast and an EEG were normal. The patient was given the diagnosis of idiopathic Parkinson disease of mixed type.

Pharmacotherapy with L-dopa and a dopamine agonist brought a marked improvement in the patient's rigidity, though his tremor remained essentially unchanged. He was able to return to work at the bank, taking up the same job as before.

Some four years after the onset of symptoms, the movement disorder took a turn for the worse, despite an increase in the dose of medication. The patient now had difficulty turning in bed and began to suffer from seborrhea.

Two years later, he began to experience fluctuations in the effectiveness of L-dopa. The duration of the effect after each dose became shorter, and he occasionally had involuntary excessive movements (dyskinesia). A change of medications to controlled-release preparations of L-dopa and dopamine agonists with longer half-life brought no more than a transient benefit. The patient finally underwent neurosurgical treatment, with stereotactic implantation of deep brain electrodes for chronic stimulation of the subthalamic nucleus. This resulted in a marked improvement of rigor and hypokinesia and a definite, but less than complete, improvement of tremor. These improvements persisted even after the dose of L-dopa was significantly reduced.

Chorea—Huntington Disease

Etiology and pathogenesis. This disorder of autosomal dominant inheritance is caused by an expansion of CAG trinucleotides within the huntingtin gene on chromosome 4. Its histopathological hallmark is degeneration of the medium-sized spiny enkephalinergic/GABAergic neurons of the striatum. Loss of these neurons leads to inhibition of the indirect basal ganglia pathway at its initial stage. The ensuing increased inhibition of the subthalamic nucleus leads to reduced inhibition of the thalamic glutamatergic neurons, so that the final result is net increased activation of cortical motor neurons.

Clinical manifestations. Huntington disease is clinically characterized by short-lasting involuntary movements that affect multiple muscle groups, seemingly at random (**chorea** or **choreiform hyperkinesia**). The patient at first tries to incorporate these rapid movements into voluntary motor behavior, such that observers may not realize that these are truly involuntary and may, instead, perceive the patient as merely clumsy or fidgety. As the disease progresses, however, hyperkinesia becomes increasingly severe and difficult to suppress. Facial twitching appears in the form of a grimace, and the patient finds it ever more difficult to keep the limbs at rest, or to keep the tongue protruded for more than a few seconds (so-called chameleon or trombone tongue). These problems are accompanied by progressively severe dysarthria and dysphagia (Case Presentation 2). The disturbing involuntary movements become more pronounced with emotional stress and stop only during sleep.

At later stages of the disease, the hyperkinesia decreases and gives way to a rigid and, in some cases, dystonic **elevation of muscle tone**. The patient's cognitive ability also declines; i.e., there is progressive **dementia** (Case Presentation 2).

Case Presentation 2: **Huntington Disease**

At the age of 34 years, this skilled worker first noticed uncontrollable motor restlessness affecting all four limbs. His co-workers made fun of him for dropping objects repeatedly, and eventually suspected him of being an alcoholic. Within a year, he developed dysarthria: his speech became abnormally soft, slurred, and hard to understand. He paid less attention to his surroundings and lost interest in his regular daily activities, which became increasingly slow and cumbersome. Ultimately, he no longer took notice of even the simplest things, and forgot tasks that had been assigned to him just minutes before. He was fired from his job and remained unemployed thereafter. Three months later, at his wife's urging, he consulted a medical specialist.

Taking the family history, the specialist learned that the patient's father had suffered from a similar movement disorder from age 40 onward. The disease progressed until he became totally dependent on nursing care and finally died at age 54. No diagnosis was ever made.

The most prominent finding on neurological examination was involuntary movement of all parts of the body, particularly around the shoulder girdle and in the face. The patient's speech was soft, somewhat slurred, and monotonous. His sensation and reflexes were normal. Ancillary studies were performed to rule out a metabolic disorder or other systemic cause of symptomatic involuntary movements. Magnetic resonance imaging of the head (Fig. 8.**10**) revealed a loss of volume of the head of the caudate nucleus on both sides, reflecting neuronal atrophy in this area. Moreover, global brain atrophy was apparent, to a degree that would not be expected at the patient's age.

The diagnosis of Huntington disease was established by a molecular-genetic study, which showed an expansion of CAG trinucleotide repeats in one allele of the huntingtin gene; 51 repeats were found (normal up to 38).

Pharmacotherapy with neuroleptic agents brought a transient improvement of the motor manifestations, attributable to inhibition of dopaminergic neurotransmission. The disease continued to progress, however, so that the patient remained unable to work and depended increasingly on nursing care.

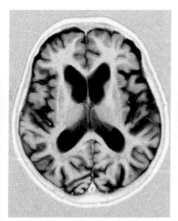

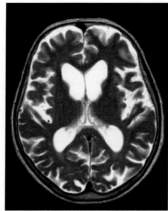

a

b

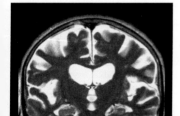

Fig. 8.**10 Huntington disease.** The axial T1-
weighted (**a**), axial T2-weighted (**b**), and coronal
T2-weighted (**c**) magnetic resonance images reveal
not only global brain atrophy (dilatation of the internal and external CSF spaces), but also a reduction of the volume of the basal ganglia (i.e., the
putamen, globus pallidus, and caudate nucleus).
The ventricles in **c** therefore have a boxlike shape,
characteristic of Huntington disease. Although
atrophic, the basal ganglia are of normal signal intensity (in contrast to Wilson disease, cf.
Fig. 8.**12**).

c

Ballism and Dystonia

Ballism. This rare movement disorder is caused by lesions of the subthalamic nucleus. It leads to large-amplitude flinging/throwing movements of the limbs,
proceeding from the proximal joints. In the vast majority of cases it arises on one
side only (hemiballism) contralateral to the lesion. (See Case Presentation 3.)

Dystonia is characterized by involuntary, long-lasting muscle contractions that
produce bizarre movements and contorted postures of the limbs. Like many
other types of movement disorders caused by basal ganglia disease, dystonia
worsens with mental concentration or emotional stress and improves during
sleep. During the intervals when dystonia is absent, the muscle tone on passive
movement of the affected limbs tends to be decreased.

There are different varieties of dystonia. Dystonia restricted to a single muscle group is called **focal dystonia**: examples include blepharospasm, an involuntary forced closure of the eyes due to contractions of the orbicularis oculi muscle, and spasmodic torticollis, i.e., dystonic wry neck. **Generalized dystonias**, of which there are multiple types, affect all muscle groups of the body to varying degrees. Patients suffering from generalized dystonia are often most severely disturbed by the dysarthria and dysphagia that usually form part of the syndrome: the patient's speech is hurried, and often barely intelligible.

The precise nature of the functional abnormality in the basal ganglia that gives rise to dystonia is poorly understood at present.

Case Presentation 3: *Hemiballism*

One evening, while watching television, this 63-year-old retired mason suddenly could no longer hold his beer bottle and spilled its contents on the carpet. When he tried to stand up, he developed uncontrollable flinging movements of the left arm and leg. He and his wife were very concerned about this disturbance, which hit him like a bolt from the blue, and called a physician on call for emergencies, who arranged admission to the hospital.

The admitting neurologist observed flinging, choreiform movements of the left arm and leg. The patient was very distressed by these uncontrollable, excessive movements, which rendered him unable to stand or walk unaided. He was given a variety of objects to hold and dropped all of them on the floor. The neurologist diagnosed hemiballism.

The patient's past medical history was notable for medically controlled arterial hypertension,

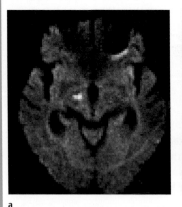
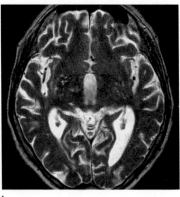

a   b

Fig. 8.**11 Small infarct in the right subthalamic nucleus causing acute hemiballism.** The diffusion-weighted image (**a**) reveals the lesion well. The T2-weighted image (**b**) shows a hyperintensity at the same location, which, however, is not clear enough to make the diagnosis. The other areas of hyperintensity in the basal ganglia are dilated perivascular spaces (Virchow–Robin spaces), not infarcts. The brain is markedly atrophic.

type II diabetes, and obesity. An imaging study revealed the cause of the acute hemiballism, a fresh ischemic lesion in the right subthalamic nucleus. In view of the multiple cardiovascular risk factors, the lesion was considered most likely to be a lacunar (microangiopathic) infarct (Fig. 8.**11**).

Symptomatic treatment with a neuroleptic agent was followed by complete regression of the movement disorder within a few days.

Case Presentation 4: *Wilson Disease*

This 17-year-old electrician's apprentice complained of progressive clumsiness of the hands, which had been troubling him for three years and was getting in the way of his work. He could no longer write cursively and had to resort to a "printed" handwriting. His hands had also been trembling for a year, the right hand worse than the left. The tremor became worse whenever he tried to grasp an object. His speech had become slow and ridden with errors.

On neurological examination, the ocular pursuit movements were mildly saccadic, but there were no other cranial nerve abnormalities. Although the muscles of mastication and facial expression were of normal strength and bulk, marked hypomimia was evident. The patient's speech was slow and labored. He had a fine,

high-frequency tremor in both hands. His gait was somewhat clumsy, and he had trouble hopping on one leg (either right or left). He tended to fall in all directions when his tandem gait was tested, or when he walked with his eyes closed. Nonetheless, he performed finger-pointing tests accurately. He had bradykinesia and dysdiadochokinesia, left worse than right, as well as bilateral marked impairment of fine motor control of the hands and feet. His deep tendon reflexes were normal and symmetric, and there were no pyramidal tract signs or sensory abnormalities. His mental status was normal. Split-lamp corneal examination distinctly revealed a Kayser–Fleischer ring.

T2-weighted magnetic resonance images of the brain (Fig. 8.**12**) revealed marked symmetric

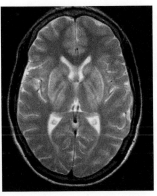 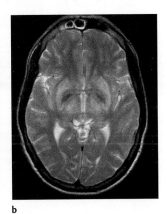

a   b

Fig. 8.**12 Wilson disease.** T2-weighted magnetic resonance images in axial (**a–c**) and coronal (**d**) planes. The axial images are at the level of the frontal horns (**a**), the anterior commissure (**b**), and the red nucleus and substantia nigra (**c**). The basal ganglia, lateral thalami, and midbrain gray matter appear much brighter than usual (hyperintense compared to normal brain tissue), probably because of parenchymal injury caused by the elevated serum copper concentration. The internal part

(Continued) ▷

signal changes in the basal ganglia and thalami (Fig. 8.**12a,b,d**), the midbrain (Fig. 8.**12c,d**), and the cerebellum (Fig. 8.**12d**). The MR signal was bright in the putamen, particularly laterally, but dark in the globus pallidus on both sides (Fig. 8.**12b**). Moderate signal abnormalities were also seen in the caudate nucleus, the lateral thalamus, the midbrain (especially the red nucleus) (Fig. 8.**12c**), and the middle cerebellar peduncle on both sides (Fig. 8.**12d**).

This combination of findings on history, physical examination, and MRI suggested the diagnosis of Wilson disease, which was confirmed by further tests: the patient's urinary copper excretion was markedly elevated and his serum ceruloplasmin concentration was low.

The MR signal increases in the basal ganglia, lateral thalami, midbrain, and cerebellar peduncles represent toxic changes of the brain parenchyma caused by the elevated serum copper concentration. The signal decreases in the globus pallidus, on the other hand, are probably due to local copper deposition.

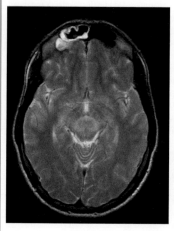 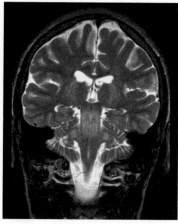

c   **d**

of the globus pallidus, however, is hypointense, probably because of local copper deposition. The white matter of the anterior commissure has normal signal characteristics but is seen more distinctly than usual because of the abnormal structures surrounding it. The coronal image (**d**) reveals the signal abnormalities in the midbrain and the middle cerebellar peduncles.

9 Cerebrum

9 Cerebrum

Macroscopically, the cerebrum is made up of the cerebral cortex, the **subcortical white matter**, and the **basal ganglia**, which were discussed in Chapter 8. The gross structure of the cerebrum can be understood best with reference to its embryological development. Its most impressive feature is the immense expansion of the cortex, which causes folding (gyration) of the brain surface. The individual cortical areas are connected to each other, and to deeper brain structures, by the numerous fiber pathways that make up the subcortical white matter.

Histologically, most of the **cerebral cortex** possesses a six-**layered cellular architecture**. This basic histological pattern undergoes characteristic variations from one location in the cortex to another, giving rise to numerous, **cytoarchitecturally distinct cortical areas**. The early neuroanatomists proposed that the specific cellular structure of each area corresponded to the specific task that it carried out. It has, indeed, been possible to assign a single, concrete function to a number of areas, the so-called **primary cortical fields**. Yet the greater part of the cerebral cortex consists of **association areas**, whose function apparently consists of higher-level processing of information derived from, or traveling to, the primary fields. Higher cortical functions such as language, in particular, cannot be localized to a single cortical area but depend instead on a complex interaction of multiple areas.

Development

The cerebrum or endbrain (telencephalon) develops from the paired telencephalic vesicles at the front end of the neural tube, the so-called **prosencephalon**. The enormous growth of the telencephalic vesicles makes the endbrain envelop the brainstem like a cloak (pallium) and leads to the development of the lateral ventricles, with their characteristic anatomical subdivisions, from outpouchings of the fluid-filled lumen of the neural tube. The **semicircular extension** that characterizes the growth of the telencephalon (Fig. 9.**1**) and the lateral ventricles can also be seen in the developing fiber projections, in the fornices, and in the corpus callosum, the great fibrous connection between the two hemispheres. A few more details of telencephalic development will be presented here as a useful aid to the understanding of cerebral anatomy.

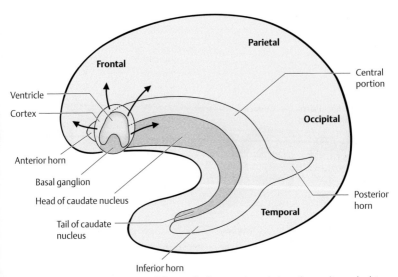

Fig. 9.**1 Ontogenetic development of the cerebral cortex.** Lateral view of an earlier and a later developmental stage of the telencephalon. The telencephalic vesicle expands massively (arrows) in the form of an arch, resulting in simultaneous, archlike expansion of the cerebral cortex (yellow), ventricle (blue), and basal ganglion (orange).

Evolution of the endbrain. In the telencephalon, as elsewhere in the central nervous system, the neural tube consists of two parts, ventral and dorsal. The **ventral part** gives rise to the septal region medially and the basal ganglion laterally. The basal ganglion, in turn, gives rise to the caudate ("tailed") nucleus, putamen, claustrum, and amygdala. The cortex derived from the **dorsal part** becomes differentiated over the course of phylogenetic development into the more laterally lying **paleocortex**, the oldest portion of cerebral cortex, and the more medially lying and phylogenetically younger **archicortex**.

The spatial arrangement of paleocortex and archicortex is preserved unchanged in amphibians. In reptiles, however, the **neocortex** arises in a lateral position between the paleocortex and the archicortex. The neocortex takes on an enormous size in higher organisms, pushing the paleocortex and archicortex far apart. In humans, the paleocortex is ultimately displaced to the base of the brain, where it makes up various components of the phylogenetically ancient *olfactory system* (olfactory bulb, tract, and trigone, anterior perforated substance, and lateral olfactory stria; cf. p. 128 f.). Meanwhile, the archicortex is displaced medially; the semicircular growth of the telencephalic vesicle

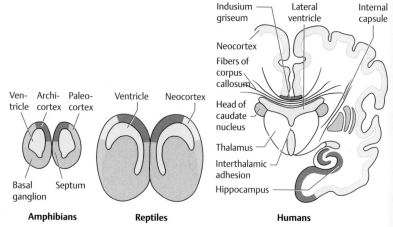

Fig. 9.**2 Phylogenetic development of the cerebral cortex** (coronal sections). The neocortex (yellow) arises between the archicortex (red) and paleocortex (blue). It expands markedly in higher organisms; in humans it displaces the paleocortex to the base of the brain (olfactory cortex, not shown) and the archicortex to a medial position overlying the corpus callosum (indusium griseum). The hippocampal formation (archicortex) in the floor of the inferior horn of the lateral ventricle reaches its basal position through the archlike expansion of the telencephalon (cf. Fig. 9.**1**).

pushes it into the inferior horn of the lateral ventricle, where it makes up the massive *hippocampal formation.* Only a thin layer of archicortex is found medio-dorsally on the outer surface of the corpus callosum: this is the *indusium griseum*, with its medial and lateral longitudinal striae. By far the greatest part of the human cerebral cortex is of neocortical origin (Fig. 9.**2**).

Inside-out stratification of the cerebral cortex. The neurons of the cerebral cortex, as of all parts of the central nervous system, are initially formed in the **ventricular zone**, i.e., near the fluid-filled lumen (ventricle) of the neural tube. The cells formed earliest make up the so-called **preplate**, which is later subdivided into the **marginal zone** and the **subplate**. The **cortical plate** proper, consisting of six cellular layers, develops between these two structures. The cortical neurons that are formed first occupy the deeper layers (layers 5 and 6), and those formed later migrate upward into the more superficial layers ("inside-out" arrangement). Thus, the later neurons must travel past their precursor cells to get to the subpial cortical layers (Fig. 9.**3**), passing from the ventricular zone to the cortical plate along *radial glial fibers.* The six cortical layers are numbered topographically from outside in (the traditional system, as used in this book), or, alternatively, in the order of their formation, as has lately been

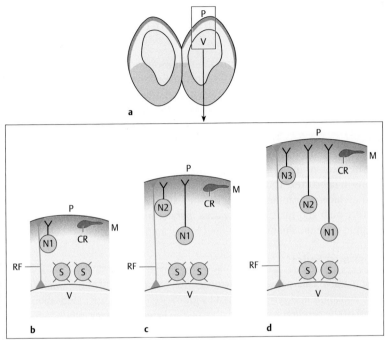

Fig. 9.**3 Inside-out lamination of the cerebral cortex.** The earliest neurons form the so-called pre-plate, which soon divides into the marginal zone (M), with its Cajal−Retzius cells (CR), and the "sub-plate" with its subplate neurons (S). The neurons of the cortical plate are deposited in the interven-ing space (N1−N3). Early cortical neurons (N1) migrate upward, from the vicinity of the ventricle (V), along radial glial fibers (RF) to the marginal zone of the cerebral cortex, where it is thought that they are stopped by reelin (brown), a protein of the extracellular matrix produced by the Cajal−Ret-zius cells. As the cortex thickens, later cortical neurons (N2, N3) must travel longer distances to reach the reelin-containing marginal zone. As a result, the neurons that are laid down earliest form the deeper layers of the cerebral cortex, while those that are laid down later form its more superfi-cial layers. P = brain surface with pia mater.

proposed (Marin-Padilla, 1998). According to the findings of recent studies, normal neuronal migration, leading to the characteristic inside-out cortical layering, depends crucially on the participation of the *Cajal-Retzius cells* of the marginal zone. These cells secrete a protein called *reelin*, which apparently directs neuronal migration along the radial glial fibers (Fig. 9.**3**). Abnormalities of neuron formation, migration, or separation from the radial glial fibers are collectively called *neuronal migration disorders*.

Gross Anatomy and Subdivision of the Cerebrum

The **cerebral longitudinal fissure** (interhemispheric fissure) separates the two hemispheres down to the corpus callosum. Each hemisphere possesses lateral, medial, and basal surfaces; the transitional area between the (dorso-)lateral and medial surfaces is called the **parasagittal region**. Each hemisphere is also divided into **four lobes**, namely, the *frontal, parietal, occipital,* and *temporal lobes* (Figs. 9.**4**-9.**6**). The **insula** is sometimes counted as a fifth lobe. The massive enlargement of the mammalian neopallium (= neocortex) achieves its greatest extent in humans, enveloping the phylogenetically older cortical regions in neocortex. Thus, most of the structures derived from the paleocortex and archicortex cannot be seen on the external surface of the brain (the olfactory bulb and tract, olfactory area, paraterminal gyrus, fasciolar gyrus, indusium griseum, dentate gyrus, and hippocampal formation).

Gyri and Sulci

The massive enlargement of the neocortex causes folding of the brain surface into convolutions (gyri) separated by grooves (sulci, fissures). Only about one-third of the cerebral cortex is visible on the external surface, while two-thirds are hidden in the sulci (Figs. 9.**7**-9.**9**).

Only a few sulci have a relatively unchanging anatomical position. The **lateral sulcus** (sylvian fissure) separates the temporal lobe from the frontal and parietal lobes. Unlike other named sulci, the lateral sulcus does not merely form the border between two adjacent gyri. It extends deep under the surface of the brain, widening out into a broad, flat space containing cerebrospinal fluid, the sylvian cistern, which is not visible from the outside. The sylvian cistern is usually very narrow, almost a virtual space, except in markedly atrophic brains. Its medial wall is the insula (island of Reil; cf. Figs. 9.**10** and 9.**11**), sometimes called the buried or central lobe of the brain. The lateral wall of the sylvian cistern is called the operculum ("lid"), because it covers the cistern like a lid; it consists of buried portions of the three lobes of the brain lying around it, which are called the temporal, frontal, and parietal opercula. A buried portion of the superior temporal gyrus contains the transverse gyri of Heschl (primary auditory cortex, Fig. 9.**10**).

Among the other relatively invariant sulci, the **central sulcus** (rolandic fissure) defines the border between the frontal and parietal lobes. The *precentral gyrus*, which lies in front of the central sulcus and is therefore in the frontal lobe, contains the primary motor cortex; the *postcentral gyrus*, which lies be-

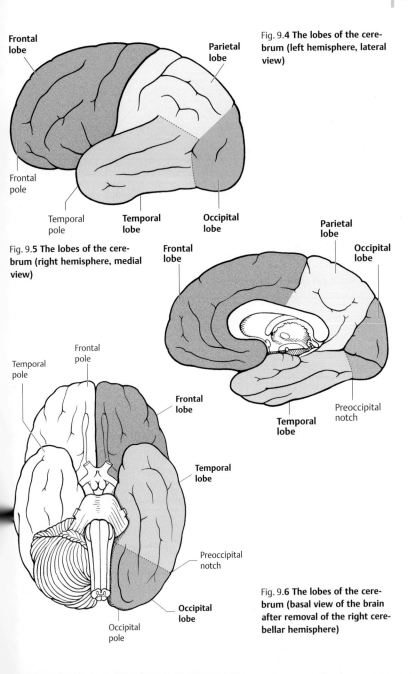

Fig. 9.4 The lobes of the cerebrum (left hemisphere, lateral view)

Frontal lobe

Parietal lobe

Frontal pole

Temporal pole

Temporal lobe

Occipital lobe

Fig. 9.5 The lobes of the cerebrum (right hemisphere, medial view)

Frontal lobe

Parietal lobe

Occipital lobe

Frontal pole

Temporal pole

Temporal lobe

Preoccipital notch

Temporal pole

Frontal pole

Frontal lobe

Temporal lobe

Preoccipital notch

Occipital lobe

Occipital pole

Fig. 9.6 The lobes of the cerebrum (basal view of the brain after removal of the right cerebellar hemisphere)

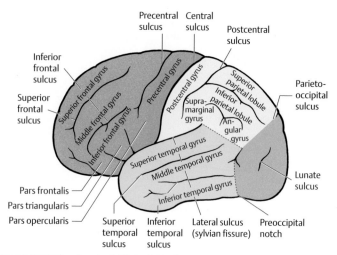

Fig. 9.**7 Cortical gyri and sulci (lateral view)**

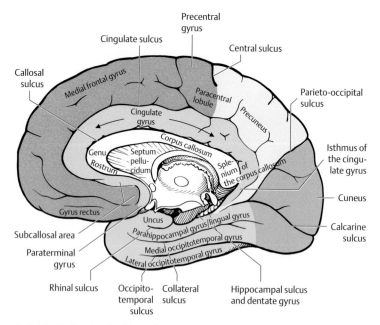

Fig. 9.**8 Cortical gyri and sulci (medial view)**

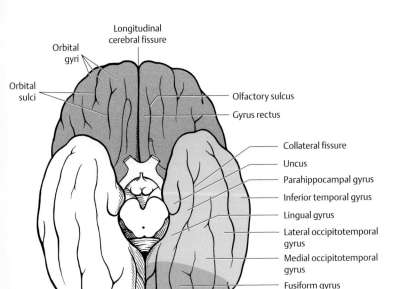

Fig. 9.9 Cortical gyri and sulci (basal view)

hind it and is therefore in the parietal lobe, contains the primary somatosensory cortex. On the medial surface of the hemisphere, the **parieto-occipital sulcus** forms the border between the parietal and occipital lobes. Its inferior end joins the anterior end of the **calcarine sulcus**, which lies entirely in the occipital lobe and runs backward toward the occipital pole. Most of the primary visual cortex is located in the depths of this sulcus, and the remainder in the gyri on either side of it. Finally, the **cingulate sulcus** separates the neocortex from the mesocortex of the cingulate gyrus.

The borders of the occipital lobe are incompletely defined by the **parieto-occipital sulcus** and the preoccipital notch (Figs. 9.7 and 9.8).

The portion of the lateral surface of the frontal lobe that lies anterior to the precentral gyrus is divided into the superior, middle, and inferior frontal gyri. For the names and locations of all gyri mentioned in this section, and a few others, as well as the names of the sulci that lie between them, see Figs. 9.7–9.9. The anatomy of many of the gyri and sulci varies greatly from one individual to another, and even between the two hemispheres of the same individual.

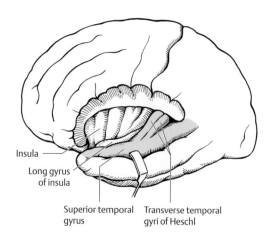

Fig. 9.**10 The transverse gyri of Heschl on the superior aspect of the superior temporal gyrus**

Insula

Long gyrus of insula

Superior temporal gyrus

Transverse temporal gyri of Heschl

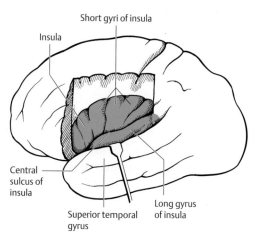

Fig. 9.**11 The insula (revealed by dissection)**

Short gyri of insula

Insula

Central sulcus of insula

Superior temporal gyrus

Long gyrus of insula

Histological Organization of the Cerebral Cortex

The folded surface of the brain is made up of the gray matter of the cerebral cortex, which is gray because of the very high density of neurons within it. The cortex varies in thickness from 1.5 mm (visual cortex) to 4.5–5 mm (precentral gyrus); it is generally thicker on the crown of a gyrus than in the depths of the neighboring sulci.

Laminar Architecture

The laminar structure of the cerebral cortex is visible to the naked eye in only a few cortical areas, most clearly in the visual cortex, where an anatomical section perpendicular to the brain surface reveals the white stripe of Gennari (or of Vicq d'Azyr) within the cortical gray matter. Microscopic examination of most cortical areas reveals the **basic six-layered structure** that typifies the cerebral cortex (neocortex), as described by Brodmann. Cortical areas possessing this structure are called **isocortex** (after O. Vogt), as opposed to the phylogenetically older **allocortex**, which, in turn, is divided into the *paleocortex* and the *archicortex*. The paleocortex includes the olfactory area, while the archicortex includes the fasciolar gyrus, hippocampus, dentate gyrus, and parahippocampal gyrus.

The internal structure of the six-layered isocortex is depicted in Fig. 9.**12**. In an anatomical section perpendicular to the brain surface, the following layers can be distinguished, from outside to inside (i.e., from the pial surface to the subcortical white matter).

1. **Molecular layer (zonal layer).** This layer is relatively poor in cells. In addition to the distal dendritic trees (*apical tuft*) of lower-lying pyramidal cells and the axons that make synaptic contact with them, this layer contains mostly small neurons (*Cajal-Retzius cells*), whose dendrites run tangentially within the layer. The Cajal-Retzius cells play an essential role in the development of the cortical laminar pattern. Some of them degenerate once this development is complete.

2. **External granular layer.** This layer contains many *granule cells* ("nonpyramidal cells") and a few pyramidal cells whose dendrites branch out both within the external granular layer and upward into the molecular layer. The nonpyramidal cells are mostly GABAergic inhibitory neurons, while the pyramidal cells are excitatory and use glutamate as their neurotransmitter.

3. **External pyramidal layer.** As its name implies, this layer contains many *pyramidal cells*, which, however, are smaller than those of the deeper cortical layers. These cells are oriented with their bases toward the subcortical white matter. The axon of each pyramidal cell arises from the cell base and travels down into the white matter. The axon already receives a myelin sheath within the external pyramidal layer. It may function as a projection fiber or, more commonly, as an association or commissural fiber (p. 366 ff.). A dendrite emerging from the apex of the pyramidal cell travels upward into the external granular and molecular layers, where it divides into its terminal branches (apical tuft).

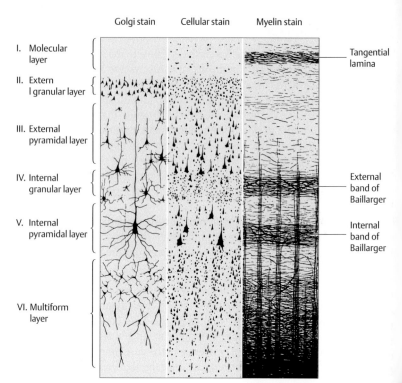

| Golgi stain | Cellular stain | Myelin stain |

I. Molecular layer — Tangential lamina

II. Extern l granular layer

III. External pyramidal layer

IV. Internal granular layer — External band of Baillarger

V. Internal pyramidal layer — Internal band of Baillarger

VI. Multiform layer

Fig. 9.**12 Cytoarchitecture of the human cerebral cortex** as revealed by three different staining techniques. (Diagram after Brodmann, from Rauber-Kopsch: Lehrbuch und Atlas der Anatomie des Menschen, 19th ed., vol. II, Thieme, Stuttgart, 1955.)

4. Internal granular layer. Like the external granular layer, this layer contains many nonpyramidal cells. These *granule cells* mainly receive afferent input from thalamic neurons by way of the thalamocortical projection. The fibers lying in the external pyramidal layer are mostly radially oriented, but those of the internal granular layer are overwhelmingly tangential, forming the *external band of Baillarger*.

5. Internal pyramidal layer. This layer contains medium-sized and large pyramidal cells. The largest cells of this layer (Betz cells) are found only in the region of the precentral gyrus. The especially thickly myelinated neurites of these cells form the corticonuclear and corticospinal tracts. This layer also contains many tangentially oriented fibers (*internal band of Baillarger*).

6. Multiform layer. This layer of polymorph cells is subdivided into an inner, less dense layer containing smaller cells, and an outer layer containing larger cells.

Types of Neurons in the Cerebral Cortex

The cerebral cortex thus contains two major types of neurons: the excitatory projection neurons (**pyramidal cells**) and the other **nonpyramidal cells** (granule cells or interneurons), which are more commonly inhibitory and tend to make local rather than long-distance connections. But this dichotomy is over-simplified. The interneurons, for example, come in a number of subtypes, such as *basket cells*, *chandelier cells* (axo-axonal cells), and *double bouquet cells*. Furthermore, the pyramidal cells also participate in local regulatory circuits (recurrent inhibition: backward-running local collaterals of the pyramidal cells activate GABAergic inhibitory interneurons, which, in turn, inhibit the py-ramidal cells).

The pyramidal cells of the fifth cortical layer give rise to the *projection path-ways* (Fig. 9.**13**), which travel through the subcortical white matter and the in-ternal capsule to the thalamus, striatum, brainstem nuclei, and spinal cord. The *association and commissural fibers* traveling to other ipsilateral and con-tralateral cortical areas, respectively, are derived from the pyramidal cells of the third cortical layer (numbered **4** in Fig. 9.**13**). The granule cells of the sec-ond and fourth cortical layers, as well as the pyramidal cells, receive projection fibers from the thalamus (**1**), as well as association and commissural fibers from other cortical areas (**2**).

Variations of the Laminar Pattern

The six-layered laminar pattern just described is called the **homotypical** pat-tern. In some cortical areas, however, the full pattern of six layers is barely dis-cernible; these areas are called **heterotypical**.

In the receptive cortical fields, such as the visual, auditory, and soma-tosensory cortices, the density of granule cells is increased, while that of py-ramidal cells is decreased ("*granulization*"; "**granular** cortex"). In the motor cortical fields, on the other hand, there are relatively more pyramidal cells ("*pyramidalization*"; "**agranular** cortex").

Cytoarchitectural cortical fields. As we have seen, cortical areas vary not only in thickness but also in histological structure. The heterogeneous distribution of various types of neurons across cortical areas, and the resulting variations in the cortical laminar pattern, led the neuroanatomists Brodmann, O. Vogt, and

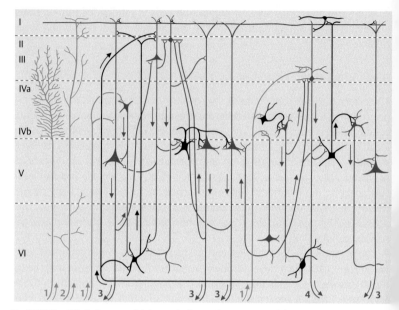

Fig. 9.13 Simplified diagram of intracortical neural connections (after Lorente de Nó and Larsell). Efferent neurons/neurites are red, afferent ones are blue, and interneurons are black. For details, cf. text, p. 361.

von Economo to subdivide the cerebral cortex into a large number of cytoarchitectural fields. **Brodmann's cytoarchitectural map of the cerebral cortex**, which is somewhat simpler than von Economo's, is now in general use as a system for naming cortical areas. Agranular cortex is found in Brodmann areas 4 and 6 (primary and secondary motor cortical fields, p. 372); the inner granular layer of these areas is rich in pyramidal cell components. Granular cortex (koniocortex), on the other hand, is found in Brodmann areas 3, 1, 2, 41, and especially 17 the striate cortex (primary receptive cortical areas, p. 380). As shown in Fig. 9.14, the cytoarchitectural fields do not coincide with the gyral pattern of the brain surface. They partly overlap with one another and vary across individuals in their shape and extent.

It is possible to subdivide the cerebral cortex histologically, not only according to cytoarchitectural criteria but also on the basis of local variations in myelinated fibers, glial cells, or blood vessels (i.e., according to its *myeloarchitecture*, *glioarchitecture*, or *angioarchitecture*). More recent brain maps have also exploited variations in neurotransmitters, neurotransmitter-related enzymes

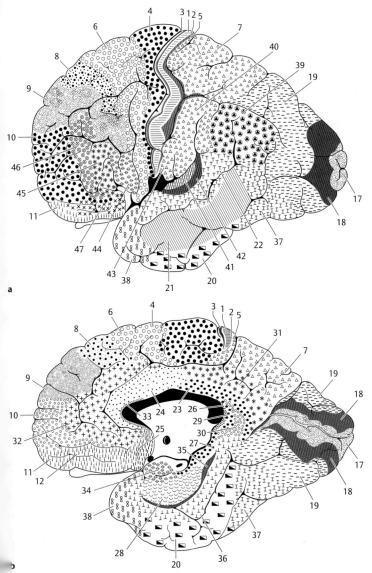

Fig. 9.14 Cytoarchitectural fields of the human cerebral cortex. a Lateral view of left hemisphere. **b** Medial view of right hemisphere. The cortical fields are numbered. (After Brodmann, from Bargmann W: Histologie und Mikroskopische Anatomie des Menschen, 6th ed., Thieme, Stuttgart, 1967.)

neuropeptides, and calcium-binding proteins, as revealed by immunohisto-chemical studies using specific antibodies against these substances.

Plasticity of cortical architecture. The microscopic structure of the cerebral cortex is not strictly genetically determined, nor is it immutable. Much current research concerns the question of how environmental influences, by activating specific groups of neurons, can decisively affect the structural differentiation of cortical areas over the course of ontogenetic development. A further question is whether, and by what mechanisms, long-lasting changes in neuronal activity in the mature brain (e. g., through perturbations of the external environment or loss of a sensory organ) can actually bring about changes in the microarchitecture of the cortex, including a changed anatomy of synaptic connections.

Many studies of this kind have been performed on the **visual system**, because the environmental conditions affecting it (visual stimuli) are relatively easy to manipulate. It has been found that certain "elementary components" of visual stimuli, including their color, orientation, and localization on the retina, are processed separately by distinct groups of neurons, which are distributed over the visual cortex in small, interspersed areas. These specialized cortical areas take on different characteristic shapes, depending on the elementary aspect of visual processing with which they are concerned: color is processed in so-called "blobs," while the spatial localization and orientation of the stimulus are dealt with by ocular dominance and orientation columns (cf. p. 380 f.). Experimental manipulation of a given type of elementary stimulus, for a sufficiently long period of time, can be shown to produce morphological changes in the corresponding processing units.

Input-specific differentiation of cortical microstructures can be demonstrated in other areas as well. The **cortical barrels** of the rodent somatosensory cortex, composed of annular collections of cells, are a well-known example: each barrel represents a single whisker of the animal.

Thus, a large number of recent studies permit the following general conclusions: (1) Certain cortical areas contain a topical representation of the sensory stimuli that they process. (2) This representation can undergo plastic change.

The diversity of histological structure among cortical fields immediately implies that they must have correspondingly diverse functions. For well over a hundred years, much research has focused on the assignment of function to different cortical fields. The knowledge that has been gained is of vital clinical importance. We will discuss functional localization in detail in the section after next (Section 9.5), but first, as a necessary prerequisite, the fiber connections of the cerebral cortex will be presented in Section 9.4.

Cerebral White Matter

Each hemisphere contains a large amount of subcortical white matter, which is composed of **myelinated nerve fibers** of varying thickness and **neuroglia** (mainly oligodendrocytes, the cells that form myelin sheaths).

The subcortical white matter is bounded by the cerebral cortex, the lateral ventricles, and the striatum. Its nerve fibers are of three types:

1   Projection fibers
2   Association fibers
3   Commissural fibers

Projection Fibers

Projection fibers connect different parts of the central nervous system with each other over long distances.

Efferent fibers from the cerebral cortex traverse the subcortical white matter and then come together to form the internal capsule. As discussed in Chapter 3, these are the corticonuclear, corticospinal, and corticopontine fibers, as well as the fibers that link the cerebral cortex with the thalamus, striatum, reticular formation, substantia nigra, subthalamic nucleus, midbrain tectum, and red nucleus. The long efferent corticospinal fibers arise mainly in areas 4, 3, 1, and 2, and also in area 6, while fibers to other destinations, such as the corticopontine and corticothalamic fibers, arise from larger association areas of the cortex.

Afferent fibers travel from the thalamus to extensive areas of the cerebral cortex. These include fibers of all somatosensory modalities, which travel to areas 3, 1, 2, and 4, as well as other fibers carrying impulses from the cerebellum, globus pallidus, and mamillary body by way of the thalamus to the cerebral cortex. The thalamus is the last major relay station that sensory impulses must traverse before reaching their specific primary cortical areas and is therefore sometimes called the "gateway to consciousness." Olfactory fibers are the only exception to this rule: they reach the cortex directly, without any thalamic relay.

Thalamocortical reciprocity. Most thalamocortical projections are reciprocal (i.e., there are fibers running in both directions). The cerebral cortex is thus presumed to modulate its own input by means of a feedback loop between the cortex and the thalamus. These massive thalamocortical and corticothalamic projections make up the large white matter tracts known as the anterior, superior, posterior, and inferior thalamic peduncles, which are usually collectively termed the *corona radiata*. The topical organization of the thalamic projections is their most important feature.

Association Fibers

The association fibers (Figs. 9.**15** and 9.**16**) make up most of the subcortical white matter. These fibers connect neighboring distant cortical areas of the *same* hemisphere with each other. The cerebral cortex is able to carry out its diverse associative and integrative functions only because all of its functionally important areas are tightly interconnected and neural impulses can travel easily from one cortical area to another. These extensive fiber connections between cortical areas may also be an important anatomical substrate for the partial recovery of function often seen in the aftermath of cortical injury (e. g., after trauma or stroke). Over time, as the individual practices the impaired activities, performance may improve because the corresponding neural impulses have been redirected along the remaining, intact pathways.

The **superior longitudinal fasciculus** runs dorsal to the insula and connects the frontal lobe with large parts of the parietal, occipital, and temporal lobes. An extension of it, the *arcuate fasciculus*, winds around the posterior end of the lateral sulcus (sylvian fissure) in the depths of the subcortical white matter. This fiber bundle connects the frontal and temporal language areas (of Broca and Wernicke, p. 387) with each other. Lesions of the arcuate fasciculus produce conduction aphasia (p. 389). The **inferior longitudinal fasciculus** connects the temporal lobe with the occipital lobe. The **uncinate fasciculus** travels around the anterior end of the lateral sulcus like a hook, connecting the orbital frontal gyri with the anterior portion of the temporal lobe.

Other important bundles of association fibers are the *superior and inferior occipitofrontal fasciculi* and the *vertical occipital fasciculus*. The *cerebral arcuate fibers*, also called U fibers, connect neighboring as well as distant gyri. Nerve fibers that travel exclusively within the cerebral cortex are called **intracortical** fibers, in contrast to the **subcortical** fibers that make up the cerebral white matter.

The **cingulum** is an association bundle of the limbic system. It runs from the subcallosal area to the parahippocampal gyrus (entorhinal area).

Commissural Fibers

Fibers linking cortical regions with their counterparts in the opposite cerebral hemisphere are called commissural fibers (Fig. 9.**16c, d**) and are found in the **corpus callosum** and the **anterior commissure**. The fibers of the corpus callo-

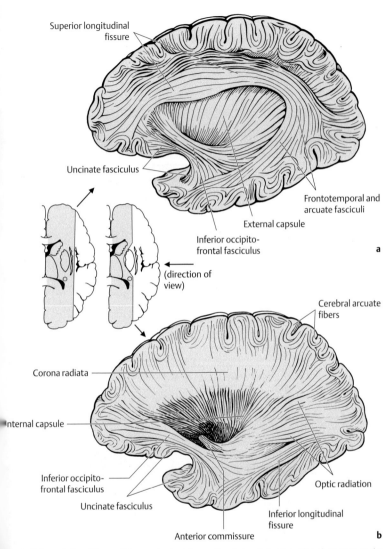

Superior longitudinal fissure

Uncinate fasciculus

Frontotemporal and arcuate fasciculi

External capsule

Inferior occipito-frontal fasciculus

a

(direction of view)

Cerebral arcuate fibers

Corona radiata

Internal capsule

Inferior occipito-frontal fasciculus

Uncinate fasciculus

Optic radiation

Inferior longitudinal fissure

Anterior commissure

b

Fig. 9.**15 Association fibers of the cerebral white matter (lateral view). a** After dissection to the depth of the external capsule. **b** After removal of the striatum to expose the internal capsule.

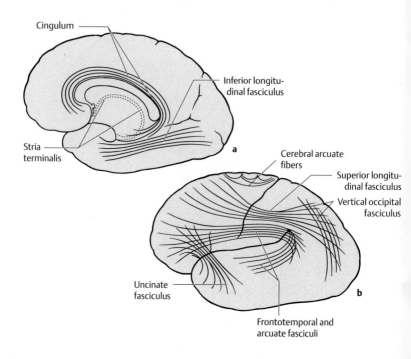

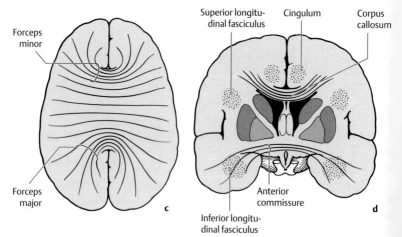

Fig. 9.**16 The major tracts of association fibers and commissural fibers** (diagram)

sum are derived from very extensive areas of the cerebral cortex; a midline section of the brain shows them tightly bundled in the corpus callosum. Once they have crossed over to the opposite hemisphere, the callosal fibers fan out again, in the so-called *callosal radiation*, to reach the cortical locations that correspond, in mirror-image fashion, to their sites of origin. This symmetrical linkage of homotopic cortical areas by commissural fibers is absent only in the primary visual cortex (area 17) and in the hand and foot areas of the somatosensory cortex.

The commissural fibers are interspersed in the subcortical white matter with the fibers of the corona radiata and the association bundles. As the corpus callosum is shorter than the hemispheres, the fibers at its anterior end (rostrum, genu) or posterior end (splenium) take a U-shaped course to link mirror-symmetric cortical areas at the frontal or occipital poles. These curving fibers form the *forceps minor* (for the frontal pole) and the *forceps major* (for the occipital pole).

Functional Localization in the Cerebral Cortex

The earliest clinical neurologists and neuroscientists were already deeply interested in the question whether individual functions of the brain could be localized to particular brain areas. From the mid-nineteenth century onward, researchers answered this question through the painstaking study of brain lesions found at autopsy in patients who, during their lives, had suffered from particular types of neurological deficit. This *patho-anatomically oriented functional analysis* of cortical structures was supplemented, from 1870 onward, by experiments with direct electrical or chemical *stimulation* of the cerebral cortex, both in animals and in humans. Later techniques, including *stereotaxy*, *electroencephalography*, and *microelectrode recording* of potentials from individual neurons and nerve fibers, yielded ever more detailed functional "maps" of the brain (cf. Fig. 9.**17**). The original idea of the "localizability" of brain function remains valid after a century and a half of study, especially with respect to the primary cortical areas, which we will describe further below.

In the last 20 years, however, basic neurobiological research on the localization of cortical function has been largely transformed by the emergence of newer, more powerful techniques of investigation, particularly functional neuroimaging. Current thinking has turned away from the parceling out of functions to individual anatomical structures (as derived from the important studies of Brodmann, Penfield, and many others) and toward the concept of

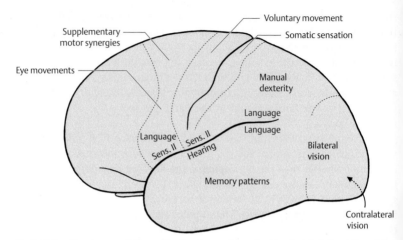

Fig. 9.**17 Functional areas of the cerebral cortex** as determined by electrical stimulation of the cortex during neurosurgical procedures. (From: Penfield W and Rasmussen T: The Cerebral Cortex of Man, Macmillan, New York, 1950.)

functional neural networks. It is now clear that cortical functions, particularly higher ones like language, cognition, and the control of specific patterns of behavior, cannot always be assigned to a single cortical location. Rather, individual components of these complex functions are subserved by separate parts of the neocortex, which must then interact with each other in manifold ways to produce the corresponding functional competence.

In the past, the study of functional localization in the cerebral cortex relied on examination of the sick or injured brain (the "lesional approach"), and on nonphysiological experiments involving brain stimulation. In contrast, researchers now try to understand the physiological basis and complexity of cortical functions by means of images of the entire *normal* brain, obtained while these functions are being carried out.

The major techniques of functional neuroimaging that are used in this type of research are magnetoencephalography (MEG), positron emission tomography (PET), and functional magnetic resonance imaging (fMRI).

Magnetoencephalography involves measurement of the magnetic fields generated in the cerebral cortex, rather than changes in electrical potential, which are measured in electroencephalography. Brain tissue and the bony skull severely attenuate electric, but not magnetic fields, and MEG is, therefore, much better than EEG for functional imaging. The magnetic fields that it detects are strong enough that a three-dimensional image of field sources can be computed from them, including sources deep in the brain. Functional imaging of the brain with MEG can be performed with high temporal resolution but relatively low spatial resolution (as compared to fMRI).

Positron emission tomography, a scanning procedure involving radionuclides, is used to investigate metabolic processes in the brain. Oxygen and glucose consumption in the brain can be directly measured after the injection of the corresponding radioactively labeled substances into the body. Radioactively labeled drugs can also be used to visualize intracerebral synaptic activity and receptor distribution. The disadvantages of PET include the radiation dose to the patient, which is not always insignificant, and the technical difficulty and expense of the procedure. Some of the radioactive isotopes used in PET have very short half-lives and must be generated directly adjacent to the scanner, in an on-site cyclotron. Furthermore, the spatial resolution and temporal resolution of PET are relatively low.

Functional magnetic resonance imaging. Most of the problems associated with MEG and PET, as just described, do not affect fMRI. This technique is based on the different magnetic properties of oxyhemoglobin and deoxyhemoglobin. Regional cerebral activation is immediately followed not just by a change in blood flow but also by a change in the relative concentrations of the two forms of hemoglobin, which can be detected as a very small change in the MRI signal. fMRI is not known to have any harmful effect on the body, so that subjects can be examined at length or repeatedly. fMRI has now largely replaced PET for studies of cerebral activation, but it cannot yet be used reliably to visualize metabolic processes.

We will now describe some aspects of the new conception of functional localization in the cerebral cortex that has been obtained through the application of these new techniques.

Primary Cortical Fields

From the functional point of view, the cortex can be divided into primary cortical fields and unimodal (p. 384) and multimodal association areas (p. 385).

Most of the primary cortical fields have a receptive function: they are the final targets of the somatosensory and special sensory pathways (visual, auditory, etc.) in the CNS, and they receive their afferent input by way of a thalamic relay. The primary cortical fields serve to bring the respective sensory qualities to consciousness in raw form, i.e., *without interpretation.* The individual primary cortical fields have no distinctive gross anatomical features and do not correspond precisely to the pattern of convolutions on the brain surface. Rather, the extent of a primary cortical field is defined as the area of cortex in which the corresponding thalamic projection terminates.

In addition to the various primary receptive fields, there is also a primary motor area, which sends motor impulses through the pyramidal pathway to the spinal cord and, ultimately, to the muscles.

Primary Somatosensory and Motor Cortical Areas

Localization and function. The **primary somatosensory cortex** (**areas 3, 2, and 1**, Fig. 9.**18**) roughly corresponds to the postcentral gyrus of the parietal lobe and a portion of the precentral gyrus. It extends upward onto the medial surface of the hemisphere, where it occupies the posterior portion of the paracentral lobule. The primary somatosensory cortex is responsible for *the conscious perception of pain and temperature as well as somatic sensation and proprioception, mainly from the contralateral half of the body and face.* Its afferent input is derived from the ventral posterolateral and posteromedial nuclei of the thalamus (Fig. 6.**4**, p. 266). Even though some sensory stimuli, particularly painful stimuli, may already be vaguely perceived at the thalamic level, more precise differentiation in terms of localization, intensity, and type of stimulus cannot occur until impulses reach the somatosensory cortex. The conscious perception of vibration and position is not possible without the participation of the cortex.

The **primary motor cortex** (**area 4**) roughly corresponds to the precentral gyrus of the frontal lobe, including the anterior wall of the central sulcus, and extends upward into the anterior portion of the paracentral lobule on the medial surface of the hemisphere. The fifth cortical layer in area 4 contains the characteristic Betz pyramidal cells, which give off the rapidly conducting, thickly myelinated fibers of the pyramidal tract. Area 4 is thus considered the *site of origin of voluntary movement*, sending motor impulses to the muscles by way of the pyramidal tract and anterior horn cells of the spinal cord. It receives afferent input from other areas of the brain that participate in the planning and initiation of voluntary movement, particularly the ventro-oral posterior nucleus of the thalamus (cf. p. 265 f.), the premotor areas 6 and 8, and the somatosensory areas.

Somatotopy and plasticity. The primary somatosensory and motor fields of the neocortex contain somatotopic, i.e., point-to-point, representations of the periphery of the body, taking the form of a **homunculus** (a "little man," as it were, drawn on the surface of the brain; the Latin term is the diminutive of *homo*, man, in the sense of human being; cf. Fig. 9.**19**). The configuration of these

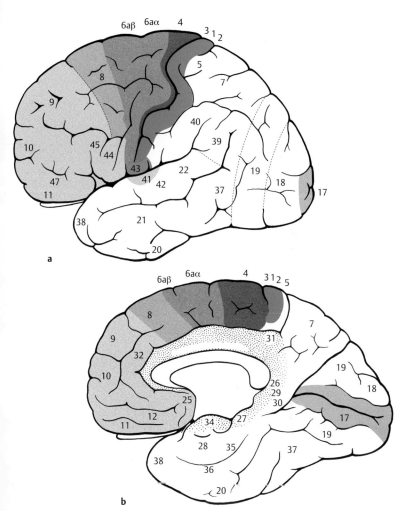

Fig. 9.**18 Primary cortical fields** and **premotor and prefrontal cortical areas** (diagram). **a** Lateral view. **b** Medial view.

maps of the body on the cortical surface was originally determined by pathoanatomical study (Fig. 9.20). The findings were confirmed and refined by the intraoperative electrical stimulation studies of Penfield (Fig. 9.21), by the somatosensory evoked potential mapping studies of Marshall, and, more re-

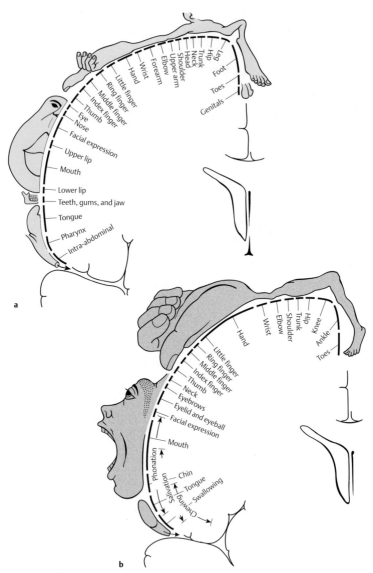

Fig. 9.19 Relative sizes of the cortical representations of different parts of the body in the human primary somatosensory (**a**) and motor (**b**) cortical fields. (From: Penfield W and Rasmussen T: The Cerebral Cortex of Man, Macmillan, New York, 1950.)

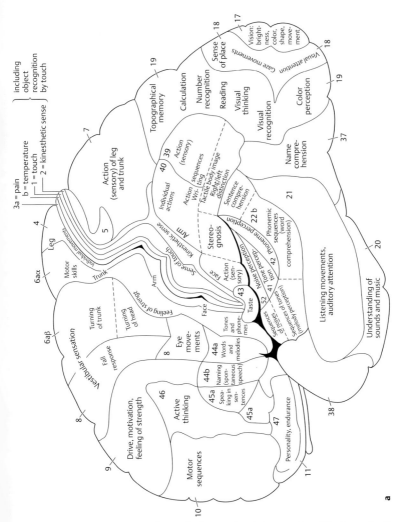

Fig. 9.20 Functional localization in the cerebral cortex in relation to cytoarchitecture, after K. Kleist. **a** Lateral view of left hemisphere.

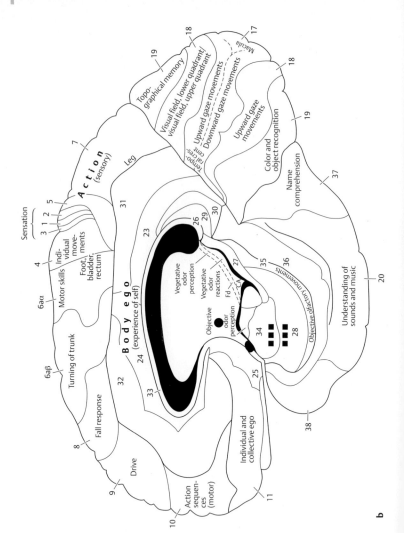

Fig. 9.**20** (continued) **Functional localization in the cerebral cortex in relation to cytoarchitecture,** after K. Kleist. **b** Medial view of right hemisphere. (Figs. 9.**20a** and **b** from: Kleist K: Gehirnpathologie. In: Handbuch der ärztlichen Erfahrungen im Weltkrieg 1914/18, vol. IV, Barth, Leipzig, 1922–1934.)

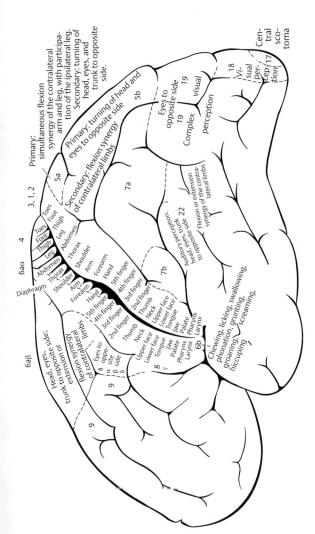

Fig. 9.21 Motor effects induced by electrical stimulation of individual cortical fields: overview. (From: Foerster O: Grosshirn. In: Handbuch der Neurologie, vol. VI. Ed. by O. Bumke and O. Foerster, Springer, Berlin, 1936.)

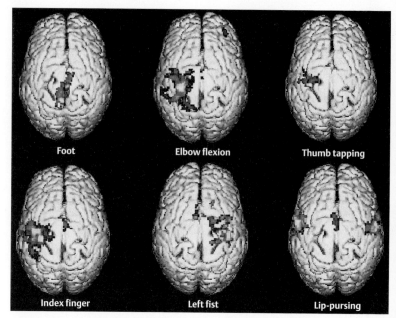

Foot   Elbow flexion   Thumb tapping

Index finger   Left fist   Lip-pursing

Fig. 9.**22 The cortical representation of regions of the body as revealed by functional MRI (fMRI) in normal persons.** fMRI data are shown projected onto a model of the brain surface. The data were obtained from 30 subjects who performed repetitive movements of the indicated body parts. Bright colors correspond to high levels of activation: i.e., brightly colored brain areas are activated during the respective movements. Localization, as determined by this technique, is in perfect accordance with the earlier findings of Penfield and Foerster (Fig. 9.**21**). fMRI is thus a noninvasive means of mapping the "homunculus" very reliably, either in normal persons or in patients. The images are reproduced with the kind permission of Professor Grodd. (From: Lotze M, Erb M, Flor H, et al.: Neuroimage 11 (2000) 473–481.)

cently, by PET, fMRI, and MEG studies (Fig. 9.**22**). fMRI enables visualization of the regions of the brain that are activated when *normal, healthy* subjects perform motor tasks.

These cortical maps are **not metrically proportional representations** of the body. In the cortical representation of superficial sensation, for example, parts of the body that are densely innervated by sensory fibers (such as the tongue, mouth, and face) are mapped to disproportionately large areas of cortex, and less densely innervated parts (arm, thigh, back) are mapped to smaller areas (Fig. 9.**19**).

Furthermore, and despite earlier assumptions, these maps are **not static**: rather, the cortical representation of a given body part can enlarge or shrink, depending on the degree to which that body part is put to use. Thus, if a tactile discrimination task involving the thumb and index finger (such as the palpation of a die to explore its surface) is carried out repetitively for a long enough time, the representation of these two fingers in the primary somatosensory cortex will enlarge. Similar, or even more extensive, changes of cortical representation are found after the injury or amputation of a limb. In such cases, the somatotopic map of the body in the cerebral cortex can be shifted by as much as several centimeters. When an arm is amputated, for example, the cortical area previously responsible for sensory impulses from the (now missing) hand can change its function and instead process sensory impulses from the face. This change is brought about by neuronal reorganization in the brain.

Much current research concerns the potential connection between shifting cortical representations and the generation of painful conditions such as phantom pain. If a connection exists, then some type of therapeutic alteration or suppression of this form of cortical "plasticity" might be used to treat, or even prevent, these conditions.

Cortical columns. In addition to the somatotopic cortical representation of superficial sensation (touch and pressure), which involves impulses that are generated in cutaneous mechanoreceptors and then transmitted to the cortex along the pathways that have been described, there are also other cortical maps for the remaining somatosensory modalities (proprioception, temperature, pain), which lie deeper within the cortex but have a generally similar configuration. Thus, somatic sensation as a whole is represented by *cortical columns:* each column deals with a particular, small region of the body surface, and cells at different depths within the column respond to different somatosensory modalities. This structural property enables the brain to process impulses from all somatosensory modalities simultaneously and in parallel, even though they have reached the cortex through distinct neuroanatomical pathways.

A lesion of the primary somatosensory cortex impairs or abolishes the sensations of touch, pressure, pain, and temperature, as well as two-point discrimination and position sense, in a corresponding area on the opposite side of the body (**contralateral hemihypesthesia** or **hemianesthesia)**.

A lesion in area 4 produces **contralateral flaccid hemiparesis**. Additional damage of the adjacent premotor area and the underlying fiber tracts is necessary to produce **spastic hemiparesis**, which reflects the interruption of nonpyramidal as well as pyramidal pathways. Focal epileptic seizures restricted to the somatosensory cortex are characterized by repetitive motor phenomena, such as twitching, or by paresthesia/dysesthesia on the opposite side of the body or face (motor or sensory **jacksonian** seizures).

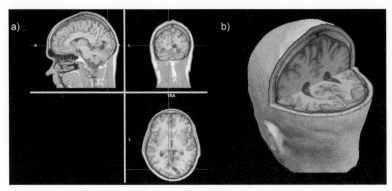

Fig. 9.**23 Functional localization in the primary visual cortex as revealed by fMRI.** Normal subjects viewed visual stimuli in the form of expanding rings, and the associated cortical activity is depicted, projected onto a model of the brain surface. There is activation of the primary visual cortex at the calcarine sulcus, as well as of the secondary visual areas. Images obtained by Professor Grodd. (From: Kammer T, Erb M, Beck S, and Grodd W: Zur Topographie von Phosphenen: Eine Studie mit fMRI und TMS. 3. Tübinger Wahrnehmungskonferenz (3rd Tübingen Conference on Perception), 2000).)

Primary Visual Cortex

Localization and retinotopy. The primary visual cortex corresponds to **area 17** of the occipital lobe (Figs. 9.**17**, 9.**18**). It is located in the depths of the calcarine sulcus, and in the gyri immediately above and below this sulcus on the medial surface of the hemisphere, and it extends only slightly beyond the occipital pole (Fig. 9.**23**). It is also called the *striate* ("striped") cortex because of the white stripe of Gennari, which is grossly visible within it in a perpendicular anatomical section. The visual cortex receives input by way of the optic radiation from the lateral geniculate body, in orderly, retinotopic fashion: the visual cortex of one side receives visual information from the temporal half of the ipsilateral retina and the nasal half of the contralateral retina. Thus, the right visual cortex subserves the left half of the visual field, and vice versa (p. 134). Visual information from the macula lutea is conveyed to the posterior part of area 17, i.e., the area around the occipital pole.

Columnar structure. The neurons of the primary visual cortex respond to stimuli having a particular position and orientation in the contralateral visual field. Neurons responding to similarly oriented stimuli are organized in vertical columns. Each column is 30-100 microns wide. Neighboring columns are organized in "pinwheels" (Fig. 9.**24**), in which every direction of the compass is represented once. The orientation columns are interrupted at regular distances by the "**blobs**" (Fig. 9.**24**), which contain neurons primarily responding to color. Finally, the **ocular dominance columns** are the third major structural component of the primary visual cortex. Each ocular dominance column responds to visual stimulation of a single eye; the adjacent column responds to visual stimulation of the other eye.

These three major components of the primary visual cortex together form a hypercolumn occupying an area of about 1 mm². The **hypercolumns**, in turn, make up a regularly repeating pattern on the surface of the primary visual cortex. They are interconnected through horizontal cells. The structural and functional organization of the visual cortex enables it to carry out an elementary analysis of visual stimuli for their shape and color. Direct electrical stimulation of the primary visual cortex (e. g., in awake patients undergoing brain surgery) induces the perception of flashes of light, bright lines, and colors.

A unilateral lesion of area 17 produces contralateral **hemianopsia**; a partial lesion produces **quadrantanopsia** in the part of the visual field that corresponds to the site of the lesion. Central vision is unimpaired as long as the lesion spares the posterior end of the calcarine fissure at the occipital pole.

Primary Auditory Cortex

Localization. The primary auditory cortex is located in the transverse gyri of Heschl (area 41), which form part of the upper surface of the superior temporal gyrus (see Figs. 9.**10**, 9.**17**, 9.**18**, and 9.**25**). It receives its afferent input from the medial geniculate body, which, in turn, receives auditory impulses from both organs of Corti by way of the lateral lemnisci. Thus, the primary auditory cortex of each side processes impulses arising in both ears (bilateral projection).

Tonotopy. The structure of the primary auditory cortex resembles that of the primary visual cortex in many respects. Its neurons are finely tuned for the detection and processing of tones of a particular frequency. The entire spectrum of audible sound is tonotopically represented: the cells for lower frequencies are found rostrolaterally, and those for higher frequencies caudomedially, along the sylvian fissure. The primary auditory cortex thus contains **iso-frequency bands** running in a medial-to-lateral direction. Area 41 neurons preferentially respond not only to a particular frequency but also to a particular intensity of sound.

Columnar structure. The primary auditory cortex also appears to possess a columnar organization for the processing of stimuli from the two ears. Two types of neurons respond in different ways to binaural stimuli. One responds

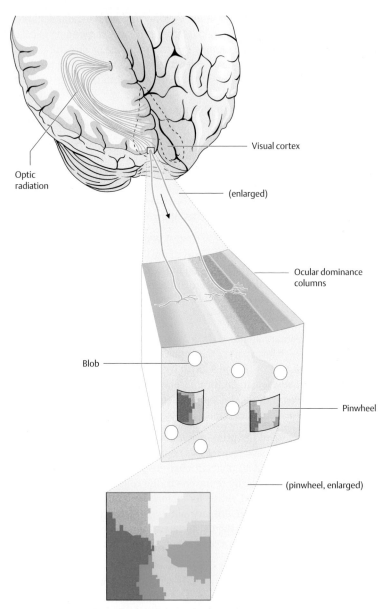

Optic radiation

Visual cortex

(enlarged)

Ocular dominance columns

Blob

Pinwheel

(pinwheel, enlarged)

Fig. 9.**24 Structure of the visual cortex: pinwheels and blobs** (diagram)

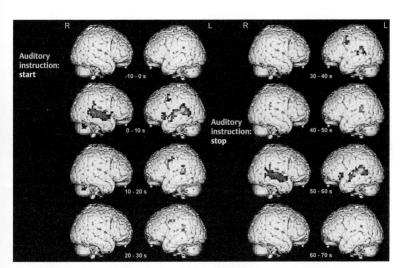

Fig. 9.**25 Functional localization of the auditory cortex and language centers by fMRI.** Eighteen subjects were asked to listen to and repeat spoken words (names of months). Listening is associated with activation of the primary auditory cortex bilaterally in the area of the transverse gyri of Heschl. Repetition, on the other hand, is associated with activity in the left hemisphere only; specifically, in the angular gyrus of the parietal lobe (Wernicke's area) and in the inferior frontal gyrus (Broca's area). Images obtained by Professor Grodd. (From: Wildgruber D, Kischka U, Ackermann H, et al.: Cognitive Brain Research 7 (1999) 285–294.)

more strongly to stimuli delivered to both ears than to stimuli in a single ear (*EE neurons*), while the other is inhibited by simultaneous binaural stimulation (*EI neurons*). Columns of cells of these two types are found in alternation on the surface of the primary auditory cortex, like the ocular dominance columns of the primary visual cortex (Fig. 9.**24**). These columns lie tangential to the isofrequency bands. A further special property of neurons of the primary auditory cortex is that different neurons are excited by auditory stimuli of the same frequency but different duration.

Direct electrical stimulation of the auditory cortex induces the perception of simple sounds of higher or lower frequency and greater or lesser volume, but never of words.

Unilateral lesions of the primary auditory cortex cause only subtle hearing loss because of the bilateral projections in the auditory pathway. The impairment mainly concerns **directed hearing**, and the ability to distinguish simple from complex sounds of the same frequency and intensity.

Primary Gustatory Cortex

Taste-related impulses are processed first in the rostral nucleus of the tractus solitarius in the brainstem and then conducted, by way of the central tegmental tract, to a relay station in the ventral posteromedial nucleus of the thalamus (parvocellular part). They then travel onward through the posterior limb of the internal capsule to the primary gustatory cortex, which is located in the *pars opercularis* of the inferior frontal gyrus, ventral to the somatosensory cortex and above the lateral sulcus (area 43, Fig. 9.**18**).

Primary Vestibular Cortex

Neurons of the vestibular nuclei in the brainstem project bilaterally to the ventral posterolateral and posteroinferior nuclei of the thalamus, as well as to its posterior nuclear group near the lateral geniculate body. Vestibular impulses are conducted from these sites to **area 2v** in the parietal lobe, which lies at the base of the intraparietal sulcus, directly posterior to the hand and mouth areas of the postcentral gyrus. Electrical stimulation of area 2v in humans induces a sensation of movement and vertigo. Area 2v neurons are excited by head movement. They receive visual and proprioceptive as well as vestibular input. Another cortical area receiving vestibular input is **area 3a**, at the base of the central sulcus adjacent to the motor cortex. The function of area 3a neurons is probably to integrate somatosensory, special sensory, and motor information for the control of head and body position.

Large lesions of area 2v in humans can impair spatial orientation.

Association Areas

Unimodal Association Areas

The unimodal association areas of the cortex are located next to the primary cortical areas. Their function, in very general terms, is to provide an initial *interpretation* of the sensory impulses that are processed in relatively raw form in the primary cortical areas. Sensory information transmitted to the association areas is compared with previously stored information, so that a meaning can be assigned to it. The visual association areas are **areas 18 and 19** (Fig. 9.**18**), which are adjacent to the primary visual cortex (area 17). These areas receive relatively basic visual information from area 17 and use it to perform a higher-level analysis of the visual world. The somatosensory association cortex lies just behind the primary somatosensory cortex in **area 5**, and the auditory association cortex is part of the superior temporal gyrus (**area 22**

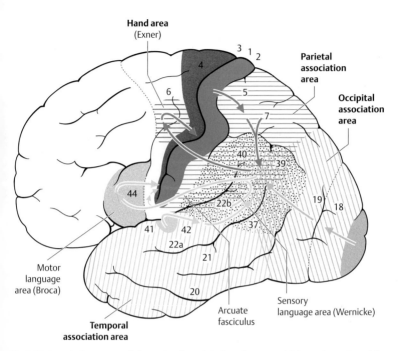

Fig. 9.26 Association areas of the parietal, occipital, and temporal lobes. These three lobes come together in the region of the angular gyrus. Broca's and Wernicke's areas are indicated, along with the association pathways from the secondary association areas to the tertiary association area, and from the latter to the premotor cortical fields for language and for the face and hand.

(Fig. 9.**18**). The unimodal association areas receive their neural input through association fibers from the corresponding primary cortical fields. They receive no direct input from the thalamus.

Multimodal Association Areas

Unlike the unimodal association areas, the multimodal association areas are not tightly linked to any single primary cortical field. They make afferent and efferent connections with many different areas of the brain and process information from multiple somatosensory and special sensory modalities (Fig. 9.**26**). They are the areas in which motor and linguistic concepts are first drafted, and in which neural representations are formed that do not directly depend on sensory input. The largest multimodal association area is the **multi-**

modal portion of the frontal lobe (to be described further below), accounting for 20% of the entire neocortex. Another important multimodal association area is found in the **posterior portion of the parietal lobe**. While the anterior portion of the parietal lobe processes somatosensory information (areas 1, 2, 3, and 5), its posterior portion integrates somatosensory with visual information to enable the performance of complex movements.

Frontal Lobe

The frontal lobe can be divided into three major components: the primary motor cortex (*area 4*, p. 372), which has already been described, the premotor cortex (*area 6*, see below), and the *prefrontal region*, a large expanse of cortex consisting of multimodal association areas (Fig. 9.**18**).

The primary motor cortex and the premotor cortex form a functional system for the planning and control of movement. The prefrontal cortex is primarily concerned with cognitive tasks and the control of behavior (p. 397).

Premotor cortex. The premotor cortex (**area 6**) is a *higher-order center for the planning and selection of motor programs*, which are then executed by the primary motor cortex. Just as the unimodal association areas adjacent to the primary somatosensory, visual, and auditory cortices are thought to store sensory impressions, so too the premotor cortex is thought to store learned motor processes, acting in cooperation with the cerebellum and basal ganglia. The stored "motor engrams" can be called up again for use as needed. Even tasks performed with a single hand activate the premotor cortex of both hemispheres. Another important function of the premotor cortex is the planning and initiation of eye movements by the frontal eye fields (**area 8**; Figs. 9.**17**, 9.**18**, and 9.**21**). Unilateral stimulation of area 8 induces conjugate movement of both eyes to the opposite side.

Lesions of area 8 that diminish its activity produce conjugate gaze deviation to the side of the lesion through the preponderant activity of the contralateral area 8 (**déviation conjuguée**, e. g., in stroke—"the patient looks toward the lesion").

Higher Cortical Functions and Their Impairment by Cortical Lesions

This section concerns the more important higher cortical functions and the typical clinical findings associated with their impairment. An adequate understanding of these very complex functions requires knowledge of certain basic concepts of neuropsychology and neuropsychological testing, which will be briefly explained where necessary. We will discuss *language, aspects of perception, the planning of complex patterns of movement and motor activities*, and *the control of social behavior*. These functions are mostly subserved by the multimodal association cortices, which make up more than half of the brain surface and which receive afferent input from the primary somatosensory, special sensory, and motor cortices, the mediodorsal and lateroposterior pulvinar portions of the thalamus, and other association areas in both hemispheres (Fig. 9.**26**).

Language and Lateralization—Aphasia

Language is one of the more important and complex activities of the human brain. In most individuals (ca. 95 %), language-related areas are located in the frontal and temporoparietal association cortices of the left hemisphere, which is usually contralateral to the dominant (right) hand. Some important aspects of language, however, including its emotional (affective) component, are subserved by the right hemisphere. The major speech centers are in the basal region of the left frontal lobe (**Broca's area**, **area 44**) and in the posterior portion of the temporal lobe at its junction with the parietal lobe (**Wernicke's area**, **area 22**) (Fig. 9.**26**).

These areas are spatially distinct from the primary sensory and motor cortical areas responsible for purely auditory perception (auditory cortex, transverse gyri of Heschl), purely visual perception (visual cortex), and the motor performance of the act of speaking (primary motor cortex). Experimental studies involving the measurement of regional cerebral blood flow (rCBF) with PET and fMRI have revealed that letter sequences that do not make up intelligible words mainly activate the visual cortex, and pure tones mainly activate the primary auditory cortex (cf. Fig. 9.**25**), while intelligible words or sentences presented to the eyes or ears activate Wernicke's area. The brain can thus distinguish words from nonwords after either visual or auditory presentation, and processes these two categories of stimuli in different cortical areas.

Broca's area is activated when an individual speaks, and even during "silent speech," i.e., when words and sentences are formulated without actually being spoken. Pure word repetition, on the other hand, is associated with activation in the insula. This suggests that two pathways are available for the generation of language. In "**automatic language**," an incoming stimulus is followed by activation of the primary visual or auditory cortex, then the insular cortex, and finally the primary motor cortex. In "**nonautomatic language**," activation of the primary cortices is immediately followed by activation of Broca's area. Wernicke's area is primarily concerned with the analysis of heard sounds that are classified as words.

Aphasia. A disturbance of language function is called *aphasia* (different subtypes of aphasia are sometimes collectively termed "the aphasias"). Some types of aphasia exclusively affect speech, writing (**dysgraphia** or **agraphia**), or reading (**dyslexia** or **alexia**). Aphasia is distinct from impairment of the physical act of speaking, which is called *dysarthria* or *anarthria* (caused, for example, by lesions of the pyramidal tract, cerebellar fiber pathways, the brainstem motor neurons innervating the muscles of speech, e. g., in bulbar paralysis, or the muscles themselves).

Dysarthria and anarthria affect articulation and phonation, i.e., *speech*, rather than language production *per se* (grammar, morphology, syntax, etc.). Aphasia is called *fluent* or *nonfluent*, depending on whether the patient speaks easily and rapidly, or only hesitantly and with abnormal effort. The more important types of aphasia, their distinguishing features, and their cortical localization are summarized in Table 9.**1**.

Broca aphasia. The most important clinical finding in Broca aphasia (Case Presentation 1, p. 390) is *markedly reduced or absent language production*. The patient can still understand words and name (simple) objects, but produces faulty sentences (*paragrammatism* or *agrammatism*) and makes *phonemic paraphasic errors* (substitution or exchange of sounds within words, such as "ackle" for "apple," "parket" for "carpet").

Wernicke aphasia. In classic Wernicke aphasia (Case Presentation 2, p. 392), *the understanding of language is severely impaired*. The patient's speech is fluent and of normal prosody (melody and rhythm) but marred by frequent *semantic paraphasic errors* (substitutions or exchanges of words within clauses or sentences) and by the use of neologisms (nonwords) instead of words. The patient's speech may be so severely disturbed as to be entirely unintelligible (*jargon aphasia* or *word salad*).

Disconnection Syndromes

Disconnection syndromes are produced by the **interruption of fiber pathways connecting different cortical areas**, while the cortical areas themselves remain intact. The responsible lesion may affect association, projection, and/or commissural fibers (p. 365 ff.).

Major insight into the function of the commissural fibers, in particular, has been gained from studies of so-called "*split-brain*" patients after surgical transection of the corpus callosum (callosotomy) for the treatment of medically in-

Tabelle 9.1 Types of Aphasia

Aphasia	Spontaneous Speech	Repetition	Articulation	Comprehension	Sentence Structure, Choice of Words	Naming	Commonly Associated Neurological Deficits
Broca aphasia	Markedly diminished	Severely impaired	Dysarthric	Normal	Agrammatism, phonemic paraphasic errors	Mildly impaired	Right hemiparesis and left apraxia
Wernicke aphasia	Normal	Severely impaired	Normal	Severely impaired	Paragrammatism, semantic paraphasic errors, neologisms	Severely impaired	Right homonymous hemianopsia
Conduction aphasia	Normal	Mildly impaired	Normal	Normal	Phonemic paraphasic errors	Mildly impaired	Right hemihypesthesia and apraxia
Global aphasia	Severely impaired	Severely impaired	Dysarthric	Severely impaired	Single words, empty phrases, semantic paraphasic errors	Severely impaired	Right hemiparesis and hemihypesthesia, right homonymous hemianopsia
Amnestic aphasia	Normal	Normal	Normal	Normal	Word substitutions, phonemic paraphasic errors	Severely impaired	None
Transcortical motor aphasia	Impaired	Normal	Mildly impaired	Normal	Semantic paraphasic errors	Impaired	Right hemiparesis

tractable epilepsy, as well as of persons whose corpus callosum failed to develop normally (*agenesis of the corpus callosum*).

For ease of presentation, we will discuss the disconnection systems here in relation to the various functional systems of the brain that they affect.

Case Presentation 1: *Broca Aphasia*

This previously healthy 48-year-old bank employee was dancing and chatting happily at his son's high school graduation when his dance partner suddenly noticed that he could no longer lead properly and had become unusually taciturn. From that moment onward, his speech seemed increasingly labored, even though he had been telling one joke after another only minutes before. He could barely produce even fragmentary sentences. He left the dance floor to take a break and, shortly afterward, dropped a glass from of his hand and began to complain of a "dim feeling." His wife took him to the hospital. Examining him, the neurologist on duty found a mild, predominantly motor right hemisyndrome. The patient's right limbs felt heavy to him, his right arm sank when he extended both arms in front of his chest, and the deep tendon reflexes were slightly brisker on the right. He also had motor aphasia: he barely spoke at all except in response to questions, to which he gave telegraphic, monosyllabic answers. He had difficulty finding words and naming objects, and his sentence construction was faulty.

For the further diagnostic work-up, the neurologist ordered Doppler ultrasonography of the great vessels of the neck and an MRI scan of the head. The former revealed near-occlusion of the left internal carotid artery, in which a dissection had apparently taken place, in the absence of any vascular risk factors. The cause was thought most likely to be the patient's suddenly turning his head while dancing (Fig. 9.**27d**, **e**, **f**). As a result of the carotid dissection, ischemia had developed in Broca's area in the left, language-dominant hemisphere, as seen in the MRI scan (Fig. 9.**27a**, **b**, **c**). The scan also showed a small area of ischemia in the precentral gyrus, which accounted for the patient's hemiparesis (Fig. 9.**27g**, **h**).

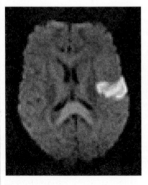
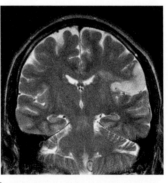

a   b

Fig. 9.**27 Cerebral infarct in Broca's area due to dissection of the left internal carotid artery** (MRI).
(a, b) a The axial diffusion-weighted image reveals the infarcted brain tissue, which appears brighter than the surrounding normal tissue. It lies in the central portion of the territory of the middle cerebral artery, mainly in the inferior frontal gyrus (Broca's area, area 44). This area is supplied by the prerolandic artery. **b** The coronal T2-weighted image reveals hyperintense signal, corresponding to infarction, in Broca's area. The infarct focally involves this portion of the inferior frontal gyrus on the upper bank of the sylvian fissure.

He was fully heparinized at once, and an overlapping treatment with warfarin was initiated. In cases of carotid dissection, therapeutic anticoagulation serves to prevent further microembolism from the dissection site. The blood clot within the vessel wall is usually resorbed over time, and the defect is covered with new endothelium, so that the internal carotid artery often regains its normal patency within 4–6 months.

During his stay in the hospital, the patient underwent a course of regular speech therapy and physical therapy. By the time he was discharged, the hemiparesis had fully resolved and his speech had become entirely clear and error-free. Six weeks later, he was asymptomatic. Warfarin was discontinued when normal patency of the internal carotid artery was demonstrated radiologically after five months of treatment.

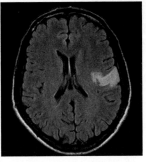
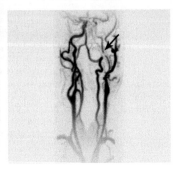

c   d

(Continued) Fig. 9.**27 (c, d) c** Axial T2-weighted FLAIR sequence. The infarct is hyperintense in comparison to the surrounding tissue. **d** Contrast-enhanced MR angiography. Flow is markedly reduced in the left internal carotid artery (arrow).

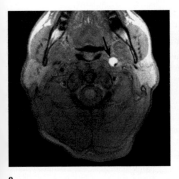
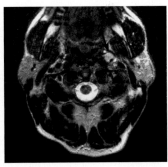

e   f

(Continued) Fig. 9.**27 (e, f)** Axial images at the C2 level, T1-weighted (**e**) and T2-weighted (**f**). Both images reveal a hyperintense mural hematoma in the left internal carotid artery, indicating arterial dissection (arrow).

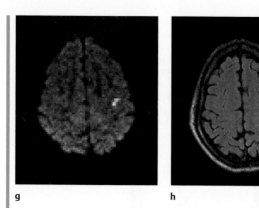

g   h

(Continued) Fig. 9.**27 (g, h) g** The axial diffusion-weighted image reveals a second area of infarction in the left precentral gyrus, accounting for the patient's right arm paresis. This area is supplied by the prerolandic artery. **h** The axial T2-weighted FLAIR sequence reveals this second infarcted area as a small zone of hyperintensity.

Case Presentation 2: *Wernicke Aphasia*

This 54-year-old housewife had been seeing her family doctor regularly because of a persistent cardiac arrhythmia in the aftermath of a bout of myocarditis. On one of these routine visits, the doctor's assistant, while performing an ECG, noticed that the patient was not following her instructions. Instead, she was talking nonstop in an unintelligible jargon, and she seemed increasingly anxious and helpless. The assistant summoned the doctor, whose neurological examination revealed a mild right hemiparesis in addition to the evident language disturbance. He arranged the patient's urgent admission to the hospital.

The admitting physician repeated the neurological examination and performed a battery of neuropsychological tests. The patient could easily imitate the examiner's movements and shake hands with him when asked to do so by pantomime, but linguistic communication was practically impossible, because of her severe jargon aphasia. When asked how she was, she replied, "More were marning"; when asked her name, she replied, "Be give with them dannifer." She could not name objects such as a

ball-point pen ("dadathig"), book ("oughta thissum higher"), or lamp ("here that sheller"). She answered open-ended questions ("How are you?") with long-drawn-out replies ("That from a fleddra, where is that here, are here, what's that doing down though, he says, is too where long"). Requests made with gestures, rather than with spoken language, such as to write her name on the hospital's admission sheet, copy written sentences and drawings, or perform written calculations, were complied with immediately and correctly. Interestingly, she could copy sentences of any length correctly, even longer ones, but she could not read them afterward, either silently or out loud. *[Readers please note: the jargon given here in quotation marks is an approximate English rendition of the patient's original German jargon.]*

An MRI scan showed the cause of the aphasia and mild hemiparesis to be a left parietal infarct involving Wernicke's area (Fig. 9.**28a–d**). This, in turn, was thought most likely to be due to embolism from the heart, in view of the patient's known, long-standing cardiac arrhythmia. Transesophageal echocardiography indeed revealed thrombotic vegetations in the left atrium. The patient was anticoagulated with heparin and an overlapping treatment with warfarin was initiated to prevent further embolization. Her spontaneous speech gradually became more intelligible with intensive speech therapy, though some aspects of her language deficit persisted until the day of her discharge from the hospital (semantic paraphasia and impaired comprehension).

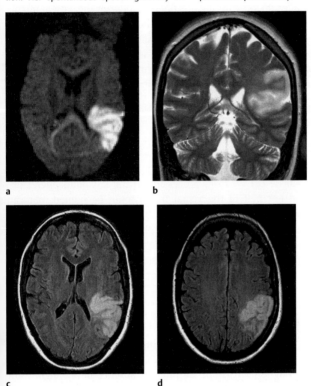

a   b

c   d

Fig. 9.28 **Infarct in Wernicke's area** (MRI).

(a, b) a The axial diffusion-weighted image reveals the infarct as a zone of hyperintensity in the posterior (i.e., parieto-occipital) portion of the territory of the middle cerebral artery, mainly involving the angular and supramarginal gyri. This area is supplied by the angular and posterior parietal arteries. **b** The coronal T2-weighted image reveals the infarct as a zone of hyperintensity above the sylvian fissure. The focal involvement of Wernicke's area is evident.

(c, d) Axial T2-weighted FLAIR sequences. The infarct, which is hyperintense in these images as well, is mainly in the cortex rather than the underlying white matter. It lies mainly in the parietal lobe, involving the parietal operculum and the angular and supramarginal gyri. The apical portion of the infarct likewise lies mainly in the parietal, postcentral region, but one can see that it also involves a small portion of the precentral gyrus, accounting for the patient's hemiparesis. **c** shows the infarct extending to the wall of the lateral ventricle; it thus presumably involves the optic radiation. This would be expected to cause a right visual field defect.

Disconnection in the olfactory system. The olfactory pathway is unique among sensory pathways in being uncrossed: the right and left olfactory nerves send their impulses to the olfactory cortex of the right and left hemispheres, respectively (cf. p. 128). The two primary olfactory centers are connected by the anterior commissure. A lesion interrupting this fiber tract makes the patient unable to identify smells presented via the right nostril, because no pathway exists for transmission of the olfactory information to the speech center in the left hemisphere. The patient cannot name the source of the smell (e. g., "cinnamon") spontaneously or pick the appropriate name out of a list. Smells presented via the left nostril, however, are identified immediately.

Disconnection in the visual system. The decussation of the fibers from the nasal half of each retina in the optic chiasm (cf. p. 132) ensures that the right and left halves of the visual field are separately represented in the left and right visual cortices, respectively. Therefore, if the connection between the two hemispheres is interrupted, visual stimuli presented in the left half of the visual field will be cut off from processing in the left hemisphere: objects shown in the left half of the visual field cannot be named, nor can words be read (**selective aphasia and alexia**). Object naming and word reading are unimpaired, however, in the right half of the visual field. Conversely, complex spatial constructions presented in the right half of the visual field are cut off from processing in the right hemisphere, and so cannot be correctly analyzed. Complex geometric figures, for example, cannot be copied (**acopia**).

Complex Movements—Apraxia

The term "apraxia" was coined in the 1870s by Hughlings Jackson to denote the complete inability of some of his aphasic patients to perform certain voluntary movements (e. g., tongue protrusion), despite the absence of any significant weakness and retention of the ability to move the same part of the body automatically or involuntarily (e. g., when licking the lips). Later, in the early years of the twentieth century, Liepmann classified the different types of apraxia (the "apraxias") systematically. In his classification, which remains in use, *ideational* and *ideomotor* apraxias mainly affecting the motor system are distinguished from *construction apraxia*s mainly affecting the visuospatial system. Apraxia, in general, is a complex disturbance of voluntary movement that does not result from weakness or other dysfunction of the primary motor areas, or from the patient's lack of motivation or failure to comprehend the task. It manifests itself as an inability to combine individual, elementary movements into complex movement sequences, or to assemble these sequences themselves into still higher-order motor behaviors. The individual movements themselves, however, can still be carried out.

Motor apraxia. A patient with severe motor apraxia cannot execute basic sequences of movements, such as reaching out and grasping an object, even though isolated testing of the individual muscle groups involved reveals no weakness in the arm or hand.

Ideomotor apraxia results from lesions of the language-dominant (left) hemisphere, either in the motor association areas or in the association and commissural fibers by which they are innervated and interconnected. A typical clinical finding is the omission, or premature termination, of individual components of a sequence of movements. Individual components can also be unnecessarily repeated (motor perseveration), so that they start at inappropriate times and thereby impede or interrupt the course of the next movement.

Patients with motor apraxia whose lesions lie in the parietal lobe cannot correctly imitate the examiner's movements (e. g., a military salute). These patients can often still copy facial expressions, while patients with left frontal lobe lesions can copy complex arm movements, but not facial expressions.

Ideational apraxia. In this rarer type of apraxia, a temporoparietal lesion in the language-dominant (left) hemisphere impairs the planning and initiation of complex motor activities. The patient remains able, in principle, to carry out a complex sequence of movements, but seems not to comprehend its meaning or purpose. The patient either fails to initiate the movement or terminates it prematurely.

Construction apraxia. Patients with construction apraxia have difficulty drawing spatial constructions such as geometrical figures or objects. This disturbance usually results from a lesion in the parietal lobe of the non-language-dominant (right) hemisphere.

Most apraxic patients are also aphasic. Patients can suffer from ideomotor, ideational, and constructive apraxia simultaneously, depending on the site and extent of the lesion.

Perceptual Integration—Agnosia and Neglect

The anterior portion of the parietal lobe, as we have seen, processes somatosensory signals, while its posterior portion and the visual association cortices are concerned with the integration of somatosensory, visual, and motor information. Complex activities, such as pouring a drink while carrying on a conversation, require the simultaneous integration of many different perceptual and motor processes: the objects handled (glass, bottle) must be recognized, which requires conjugate eye movements and visual processing; reaching, grasping, and pouring movements must be smoothly executed; and, at the same time, language must be heard, understood, formulated, and spoken.

In order to perform these tasks, the brain needs internal representations of the body, information about the positions of the limbs, and a conception of the outside world. These representations must, in turn, be linked to incoming visual and auditory signals, and to the brain's plans for intended movement. The association cortices and the posterior portion of the parietal lobe play an essential role in these complex integrative processes. As an illustration of this role, the posterior portion of the parietal lobe is activated not only by intended grasping movements induced by visual stimuli, but also by palpation of an unseen object.

Lesions of the visual association cortices and the parietal lobe can produce many different types of *agnosia*, i.e., complex disturbances of perception. A patient with agnosia cannot recognize objects or spatiotemporal contexts despite intact primary perception (normal vision, hearing, and somatic sensation) and motor function (absence of weakness). Agnosia can be visual, auditory, somatosensory, or spatial.

Visual object agnosia. If the visual association areas are damaged, the patient can still comprehend the spatial structure of familiar objects, but can no longer identify them. A bottle, for example, can be correctly drawn, but cannot be identified as a bottle. Other, more complex types of visual agnosia include **prosopagnosia** (the inability to recognize faces) and **alexia** (the inability to read).

Somatosensory agnosias. **Astereognosia** is the inability to recognize an object by touch alone, even though sensation is intact and objects can otherwise be named without difficulty. **Asomatognosia** is a generally diminished, or even absent, ability to perceive one's own body. **Gerstmann syndrome** consists of the inability to name one's own fingers (finger agnosia) along with an impairment of writing (dysgraphia or agraphia), calculation (dyscalculia or acalculia), and the ability to distinguish right from left. Gerstmann first described these findings in 1924 in a patient with an ischemic stroke in the territory of the middle cerebral artery affecting the left parietal lobe.

Balint syndrome. This complex type of agnosia is caused by bilateral parieto-occipital lesions. The patient originally described by Balint could not voluntarily fix his gaze on a given point in space. When his attention was directed to a particular object, he could not perceive any other visual stimuli. He also could not follow a moving object with his eyes (visual ataxia).

Neglect. Patients sometimes pay less attention to the side of the body or visual field opposite a cortical lesion, or ignore it altogether; this is called *neglect*. There is often an accompanying unawareness of the deficit (**anosognosia**). Neglect usually involves vision, hearing, somatic sensation, spatial perception, and movement simultaneously. The causative lesion is usually in the parietal lobe of the non-language-dominant (right) hemisphere. A patient with motor neglect moves one side of the body very little, or not at all, even though it is not paralyzed. Sensory neglect is revealed by the so-called **extinction phenomenon**: when the examiner simultaneously taps the same spot on both arms with equal strength, the patient reports having been touched only on one side, even though all modalities of touch are intact bilaterally. The patient can still perceive a single tap on the arm on the abnormal side, but may report it to have been felt on the other side (**allesthesia**). Similarly, simultaneous bilateral visual or auditory stimuli will only be perceived on one side.

Normal and Impaired Control of Behavior, Including Social Behavior

Prefrontal cortex. Cognition and the control of behavior are the main functions of the multimodal association areas in the frontal lobe that constitute the prefrontal cortex (Fig. 9.**18**). Experimental electrical stimulation of the prefrontal cortex does not induce any motor response. This portion of the frontal lobe is extraordinarily enlarged in primates, and particularly in humans; thus, it has long been presumed to be the seat of higher mental functioning. The frontal cortical fields make reciprocal connections with the medial nucleus of the thalamus (cf. p. 268), through which they receive input from the hypothalamus. They also make very extensive connections with all other areas of the cerebral cortex.

The task of the prefrontal cortex is the rapid storage and analysis of objective and temporal information. The dorsolateral prefrontal cortex plays an essential role in the planning and control of behavior, and the orbital prefrontal cortex does the same in the planning and control of sexual behavior.

Lesions of the prefrontal convexity. Patients with bilateral prefrontal lesions can barely concentrate on a task and are extremely easy to distract with any new stimulus. They can carry out complex tasks only in part, or not at all. They have no sense of advance planning and take no account of future events or of possible problems in the execution of a task. They often stick rigidly to an idea and fail to adapt to changing circumstances. In extreme cases, they manifest **perseveration**, i.e., they perform the same task again and again, always with the same mistakes. This deficit is strikingly brought out by the Wisconsin Card Sorting Test, in which the patient sorts cards bearing various symbols and

Case Presentation 3: *Neglect*

This 69-year-old retiree, living alone, had had poorly controlled arterial hypertension for a number of years and two brief episodes of left arm weakness in recent months. On another occasion, he had been unable to see anything with his right eye for a few minutes. He had paid no further attention to these transient disturbances, because he otherwise felt well. Getting up from bed one night, he suddenly fell to the ground and could not stand up again. He shouted for help, waking a neighbor who had a spare key to his apartment. She notified the emergency physician on call, who took him to the hospital.

The admitting house officer performed a thorough neurological examination and found a mild left hemiparesis, with sinking of the left arm and leg and impaired fine motor control of the left hand. The patient failed to notice a light tap on the left side of his body when simultaneously tapped at a mirror-image location on the right side (tactile extinction). He did not react when spoken to from his left side. When the doctor asked him to draw a house and a tree, he drew only the right sides of these objects. He generally tended to look to the right and appeared to be conscious only of the right side of space. The cause of these acute neurological deficits was an approximately 80% stenosis of the right internal carotid artery, which had led to a right hemispheric infarct in the distribution of the middle cerebral artery (Fig. 9.29).

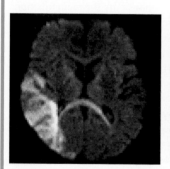

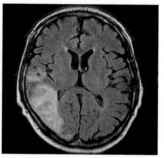

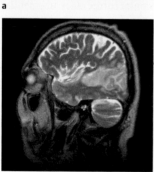

Fig. 9.**29 Infarct in the territory of the right middle cerebral artery, causing neglect** (MRI). **a** Axial EPI sequence. **b** Axial T2-weighted FLAIR sequence. The axial images reveal an infarct affecting the posterior portion of the middle cerebral artery territory on the right, reaching far back into the occipital lobe and to the wall of the lateral ventricle. Involved areas include the temporal lobe, the angular and supramarginal gyri of the parietal lobe, and the occipital lobe. The patient's hemianopsia is due to involvement of the optic radiation and occipital lobe. **c** Sagittal T2-weighted image. The hyperintense zone of infarction is seen behind and under the sylvian fissure.

a

b

c

colors according to some criterion (e. g., shape), after seeing the examiner do so. Performance in the first round is usually relatively normal. The examiner confirms the patient's success, then changes the sorting criterion (e. g., to color) without explicitly saying so. A patient with a prefrontal lesion realizes about as rapidly as a normal individual that the task has changed, yet keeps sorting according to the old criterion, despite being immediately informed of each mistake.

Markedly reduced drive and **lack of spontaneity** are also characteristic clinical signs of prefrontal dysfunction. These deficits are revealed by very poor performance on the Word Fluency Test, in which the patient is given a short period of time to say as many words as possible that begin with a particular letter of the alphabet. Patients with prefrontal lesions do badly despite relatively normal verbal memory. They do badly on nonverbal tests as well: normal subjects can draw about 35 pictures in five minutes, patients with left frontal lesions 24, patients with right frontal lesions 15. Because they lack spontaneity in all forms of communication, these patients seem lazy, lethargic, and unmotivated. They neglect many activities of daily life, spend the morning in bed, fail to wash or groom themselves or to get dressed without help, and do no regular work. Nonetheless, their formal IQ and long-term memory are largely intact!

Fronto-orbital lesions. Social and sexual behavior are controlled and regulated by highly complex processes. Behavior of these types, too, is abnormal in patients with frontal lobe lesions. Fronto-orbital lesions, in particular, produce two characteristic types of personality disturbance. **Pseudo-depressive** patients are apathetic and indifferent and display markedly reduced drive, diminished sexual desire, and little or no variation in their emotional state. **Pseudo-psychopathic** patients, on the other hand, are hypomanic and restless in their movements, fail to keep an appropriate distance from others, and lack normal kinds of inhibition. They display markedly increased drive and sexual desire. They are unwilling or unable to hold to the same normal conventions of behavior that they followed unquestioningly before becoming ill.

Case Presentation 4: *Frontal Lobe Disturbance*

This case illustrating the typical course of one type of frontal lobe disturbance comes from an earlier era—not so long ago—when today's powerful neuroimaging techniques were not yet available. The diagnostic work-up does not meet the current standards. The neurological findings, however, are just as relevant now as they were then.

A 57-year-old Norwegian clergyman recovered from a cold and noticed that he could no longer smell. Over the next three years, his sense of smell never returned, his vision gradually worsened, and he became less and less interested in his job. He failed to keep up with the administrative paperwork with which the church had entrusted him. His superiors rebuked him many times for leaving their letters unanswered. He raised eyebrows among his parishioners by making an unduly jocular speech at a friend's funeral. Six months before his admission to the hospital (see below), he was given an assistant, because he was increasingly neglecting his work. Shortly thereafter, he was relieved of his duties entirely and admitted to a psychiatric institution.

His vision deteriorated further, and he began to experience episodic headaches. Visual hallucinations arose in which he saw snakes and the like. He did not consider himself ill, saying instead that he was entirely well but had been hospitalized at his superiors' request. His judgment and drive were severely impaired. His mood was highly euphoric, and he constantly made jokes, sometimes quite indecent ones. He viewed his physicians with distrust.

As time went on, his headaches grew worse, and he vomited in the morning on several occasions. A neurologist, called to examine him, found that he had anosmia and an absolute central scotoma on the right, along with an upper temporal visual field defect on the right. The nasal aspect of both optic disks was somewhat blurred. Suspecting an intracranial mass, the neurologist had him transferred to a specialized clinic in Oslo.

There, a craniotomy revealed a large, typical (i.e., histologically benign) meningioma, arising from the olfactory groove and compressing the frontal lobes from below, without invading or adhering to them. The tumor was removed in its entirety, and the postoperative course was uneventful. The patient's mental state recovered with remarkable speed. A few days after the operation, he clearly understood that he had been ill. He was deeply ashamed of his previous conduct, vaguely sensing its impropriety. From being garrulous, distrustful, ill-mannered, and unkempt, he was transformed within a few days back into a kind, peaceful man, not without a certain sacerdotal dignity. He was discharged from the hospital, resumed his ministerial duties two months later, and exercised them without the slightest difficulty.

10 Coverings of the Brain and Spinal Cord; Cerebrospinal Fluid and Ventricular System

10 Coverings of the Brain and Spinal Cord; Cerebrospinal Fluid and Ventricular System

The brain and spinal cord are covered by three layers (meninges) of mesodermal origin: the tough **dura mater** is outermost, followed by the **arachnoid** and, lastly, the **pia mater**. The pia matter lies directly on the surface of the brain and spinal cord. Between the dura mater and the arachnoid is the (normally only virtual) *subdural space;* between the arachnoid and the pia mater is the *subarachnoid space*. The subarachnoid space contains the cerebrospinal fluid (CSF).

The **cerebrospinal fluid** is formed in the choroid plexuses of the four cerebral ventricles (right and left lateral ventricles, third ventricle, and fourth ventricle). It flows through the ventricular system (internal CSF space) and then enters the subarachnoid space surrounding the brain and spinal cord (external CSF space). It is resorbed in the arachnoid granulations of the superior sagittal sinus and in the perineural sheaths of the spinal cord. An **increased volume of cerebrospinal fluid** (because of either diminished resorption or—less commonly—increased production) manifests itself in increased CSF pressure and enlargement of the ventricles (**hydrocephalus**).

Coverings of the Brain and Spinal Cord

The three meninges (*dura mater, arachnoid, pia mater*) are depicted in Figs. 10.**1** and 10.**2**. The dura mater is also called the *pachymeninx* ("tough membrane"), while the arachnoid and pia mater are collectively called the *leptomeninges* ("delicate membranes").

Dura Mater

The dura mater consists of two layers of tough, fibrous connective tissue.

Outer and inner layers. The outer layer of the cranial dura mater is the periosteum of the inside of the skull. The inner layer is the actual meningeal layer; it forms the outer limit of the very narrow subdural space. The two dural layers separate from each other at the sites of the dural sinuses. Between the superior and inferior sagittal sinuses, a double fold of the inner dural layer forms the *falx*

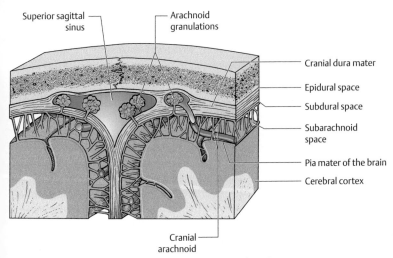

Superior sagittal sinus
Arachnoid granulations
Cranial dura mater
Epidural space
Subdural space
Subarachnoid space
Pia mater of the brain
Cerebral cortex
Cranial arachnoid

Fig. 10.**1 Meninges of the brain** (schematic drawing, coronal view)

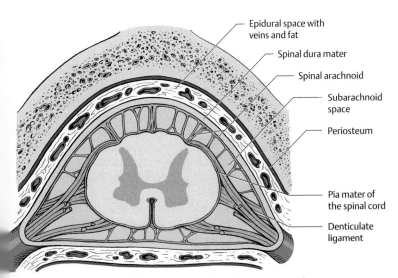

Epidural space with veins and fat
Spinal dura mater
Spinal arachnoid
Subarachnoid space
Periosteum
Pia mater of the spinal cord
Denticulate ligament

Fig. 10.**2 Meninges of the spinal cord** (schematic drawing, transverse view)

cerebri, which lies in the midsagittal plane between the two cerebral hemispheres; the falx cerebri is continuous with the *tentorium*, which separates the cerebellum from the cerebrum. Other structures formed by a double fold of inner dura mater are the *falx cerebelli* separating the two cerebellar hemispheres, the *diaphragma sellae* and the *wall of Meckel's cave*, which contains the gasserian (trigeminal) ganglion.

Blood supply of the dura mater. The dural arteries are relatively large in caliber because they supply the bony skull as well as the dura mater. The largest is the **middle meningeal artery**, whose branches are distributed over the entire lateral convexity of the skull. This artery is a branch of the maxillary artery, which is, in turn, derived from the external carotid artery; it enters the skull through the foramen spinosum. The **anterior meningeal artery** is relatively small and supplies the midportion of the frontal dura mater and the anterior portion of the falx cerebri. It enters the skull through the anterior portion of the cribriform plate. It is a branch of the anterior ethmoidal artery, which is, in turn, a branch of the ophthalmic artery; it therefore carries blood from the internal carotid artery. The **posterior meningeal artery** enters the skull through the jugular foramen to supply the dura mater of the posterior cranial fossa.

The middle meningeal artery makes an anastomotic connection in the orbit to the lacrimal artery, a branch of the ophthalmic artery. The ophthalmic artery branches off of the internal carotid artery near the internal aperture of the optic canal. Thus, in some cases, the central retinal artery can obtain blood by way of the middle meningeal artery, even if the ophthalmic artery is proximally occluded.

Spinal dura mater. The two layers of the dura mater adhere tightly to each other within the cranial cavity but separate from each other at the outer rim of the foramen magnum. The outer dural layer continues as the periosteum of the spinal canal, while the inner layer forms the dural sac enclosing the spinal cord. The space between the two layers is called the epidural or extradural space, even though it is, strictly speaking, inside the dura mater. It contains loose connective tissue, fat, and the internal venous plexus (Fig. 10.**2**, Fig. 11.**20**, p. 442). The two layers of the spinal dura matter join where the spinal nerve roots exit from the spinal canal through the intervertebral foramina. The lower end of the dural sac encloses the cauda equina and terminates at the S2 level (Fig. 3.**22**, p. 86 f.). Its continuation below this level is the filum of the dura mater, which is anchored to the sacral periosteum by the fibrous coccygeal ligament.

Orbital dura mater. A similar division of the two layers of the dura mater is found in the orbit, which the dura mater reaches from the cranial cavity by extension along the optic canal. The outer dural layer is the periosteal lining of the bony orbit. The inner dural layer surrounds the optic nerve, together with its pia mater and arachnoid, as well as the perioptic subarachnoid space in between. This space communicates with the subarachnoid space of the cranial cavity. The inner dural layer is continuous with the sclera as the optic nerve enters the globe.

Papilledema. The dural sheath of the optic nerve can be stretched if elevated intracranial pressure is transmitted to the perioptic subarachnoid space. Retrobulbar stretching of the dural sheath is a major factor in the development of papilledema. Another cause of papilledema is acute intracranial subarachnoid hemorrhage (due to a ruptured aneurysm or vascular malformation) with blood extending into the perioptic subarachnoid space.

Innervation. The dura mater above the tentorium is innervated by branches of the trigeminal nerve, its infratentorial portion by branches of the upper cervical segmental nerves and the vagus nerve. Some of the dural nerves are myelinated, while others are unmyelinated. Their endings evidently respond to stretch, because mechanical stimulation of the dura can be consciously felt, and is often painful. The afferent fibers accompanying the meningeal arteries are particularly sensitive to pain.

Arachnoid

The arachnoid of both the brain and the spinal cord is a thin, delicate, avascular membrane closely applied to the inner surface of the dura matter. The space between the arachnoid and the pia mater (the subarachnoid space) contains the cerebrospinal fluid. The arachnoid and the pia mater are connected to each other across this space by delicate strands of connective tissue. The pia mater adheres to the surface of the brain along all of its foldings; thus, the subarachnoid space is narrower in some places, and wider in others. Enlargements of the subarachnoid space are called *cisterns*. The cranial and spinal subarachnoid spaces communicate directly with each other across the foramen magnum. Most of the arterial trunks supplying the brain, and most of the cranial nerves, run in the subarachnoid space.

Cisterns. The subarachnoid cisterns of the head have individual names, e. g., the cerebellomedullary cistern, also called the *cisterna magna*. The more important named cisterns are depicted in Fig. 10.**4**, p. 408.

Pia Mater

The pia mater consists of thin layers of mesodermal cells resembling endothelium. Unlike the arachnoid, it covers not just the entire externally visible surface of the brain and spinal cord but also all of the hidden surfaces in the depths of the sulci (Figs. 10.**1** and 10.**2**). It is fixed to the central nervous tissue beneath it by an ectodermal membrane consisting of marginal astrocytes (pial-glial membrane). Blood vessels that enter or leave the brain and spinal cord by way of the subarachnoid space are surrounded by a funnel-like sheath of pia mater. The space between a blood vessel and the pia mater around it is called the *Virchow-Robin space.*

The sensory nerves of the pia mater, unlike those of the dura mater, do not respond to mechanical or thermal stimuli, but they are thought to respond to vascular stretch and changes in vascular wall tone.

Cerebrospinal Fluid and Ventricular System

Structure of the Ventricular System

The ventricular system (Fig. 10.**3**) consists of the **two lateral ventricles** (each of which has a frontal horn, central portion = *cella media*, posterior horn, and inferior horn); the narrow **third ventricle**, which lies between the two halves of the diencephalon; and the **fourth ventricle**, which extends from pontine to medullary levels. The lateral ventricles communicate with the third ventricle through the interventricular foramina (of Monro); the third ventricle, in turn, communicates with the fourth ventricle through the cerebral aqueduct. The fourth ventricle empties into the subarachnoid space through three openings: the single median aperture (foramen of Magendie) and the paired lateral apertures (foramina of Luschka).

Cerebrospinal Fluid Circulation and Resorption

Properties of the cerebrospinal fluid. The normal cerebrospinal fluid is *clear and colorless*, containing *only a few cells* (up to 4/μl) and *relatively little protein* (ratio of CSF albumin to serum albumin = $6.5 \pm 1.9 \times 10^{-3}$). Its composition differs from that of blood in other respects as well. The cerebrospinal fluid is not an ultrafiltrate of blood; rather, it is actively secreted by the choroid plexus, mainly within the lateral ventricles. The blood within the capillaries of the choroid plexus is separated from the subarachnoid space by the so-called *blood-CSF barrier*, which consists of vascular endothelium, basal membrane, and plexus epithe-

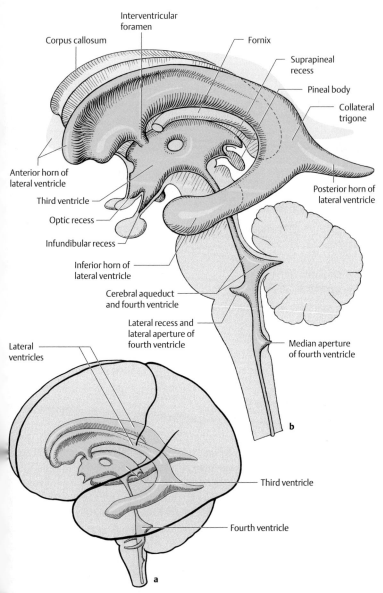

Fig. 10.**3 Ventricular system. a** Position of the ventricular system in the brain. **b** Anatomical structure.

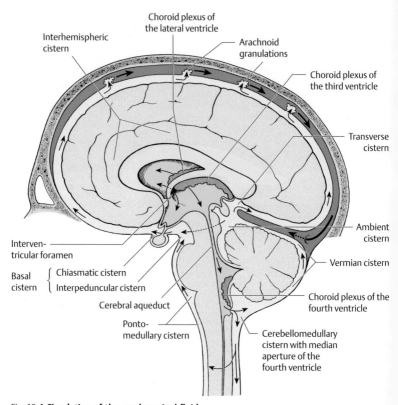

Fig. 10.**4 Circulation of the cerebrospinal fluid**

lium. This barrier is permeable to water, oxygen, and carbon dioxide, but relatively impermeable to electrolytes and completely impermeable to cells.

The **circulating CSF volume** is generally between 130 and 150 ml. Every 24 hours 400-500 ml of CSF are produced; thus, the entire CSF volume is exchanged three or four times daily. The **CSF pressure** (note that the CSF pressure is not the same as the intracranial pressure) in the supine position is normally 70-120 mmH$_2$O.

Infectious or neoplastic processes affecting the CNS alter the composition of the cerebrospinal fluid in characteristic ways, as summarized in Table 10.1.

Circulation. The CSF is produced by the choroid plexus of the lateral ventricles, third ventricle, and fourth ventricle (Fig. 10.**4**). It flows through the foramina of

Tabelle 10.1 CSF Findings in Diseases of the Central Nervous System

Diagnosis	Appearance	Pandy Reaction	Cell Count, Cytology	Biochemistry	Other Findings
Normal lumbar CSF	Clear, colorless	—	Up to 4 cells/μl, mainly lymphocytes (85%)	Lactate <2.1 mmol/l. Albumin quotient: Adults over 40 years, <8; under 40 years, <7; children under 15 years, <5	Glucose 50–60% of blood level
Purulent (bacterial) meningitis	Turbid	+++	Several thousand/μl, mainly neutrophils	Lactate >3.5 mmol/l; albumin quotient >20 × 10⁻³	Demonstration of bacteria
Brain abscess	Clear, occasionally turbid	+/-	A few hundred/μl, mononuclear cells and/or neutrophils	Albumin quotient normal or mildly elevated	Low glucose, bacteria sometimes demonstrable, local IgA synthesis
Encephalitis (herpes simplex)	Clear, colorless	+/-	Normal or mononuclear pleocytosis (lymphocytes)	Albumin quotient >10 × 10⁻³	IgG, IgM, IgA elevated; demonstration of specific Ab, PCR positive for HSV
Viral meningitis	Clear	+	Up to several hundred mononuclear cells, including activated B lymphocytes	Albumin quotient up to 20 × 10⁻³; lactate <3.5 mmol/l	
Tuberculous meningitis	Yellow-tinged	+++	Up to 1500/μl, mixed cellular picture, mostly mononuclear cells	Albumin quotient >20 × 10⁻³; glucose <50% of serum glucose	IgG and IgA elevated; mycobacteria demonstrated by culture and PCR
Neurosyphilis	Clear or turbid	+/-	Mononuclear pleocytosis		Immunoglobulins elevated, TPHA positive

Tabelle 10.1 (Continued) **CSF Findings in Diseases of the Central Nervous System**

Diagnosis	Appearance	Pandy Reaction	Cell Count, Cytology	Biochemistry	Other Findings
Diagnosis	Appearance	Pandy Reaction	Cell Count, Cytology	Biochemistry	Other Findings
Multiple sclerosis	Clear, colorless	+/-	Up to 40 mononuclear cells/μl	Albumin quotient $< 20 \times 10^{-3}$	Oligoclonal bands revealed by isoelectric focusing
Acute neuroborreliosis (Lyme disease)	Clear		Up to a few hundred mononuclear cells/μl	Albumin quotient $< 50 \times 10^{-3}$	Immunoglobulins elevated, demonstration of antibody
Fungal meningitis	Clear		Up to a few hundred mononuclear cells/μl		Immunoglobulins elevated, demonstration of fungi by culture and special stains
Polyradiculitis (Guillain-Barré syndrome)	Clear		No more than mild pleocytosis	Albumin quotient up to 50×10^{-3} ("albumino-cytological dissociation")	

Luschka and Magendie (Figs. 10.**3b** and 10.**4**) into the subarachnoid space, circulates around the brain, and flows down into the spinal subarachnoid space surrounding the spinal cord. Some of the CSF is resorbed at spinal levels (see below). The composition of the CSF is the same at all points; it is not more dilute or more concentrated at either end of the pathway.

Resorption. CSF is resorbed (i.e., removed from the subarachnoid space) intracranially and along the spinal cord. Some of the CSF leaves the subarachnoid space and enters the bloodstream through the many villous **arachnoid granulations** located in the superior sagittal sinus and in the diploic veins of the skull. The remainder is resorbed in the perineural sheaths of the cranial and spinal nerves, where these nerves exit the brainstem and spinal cord, respectively, and across the ependyma and capillaries of the leptomeninges.

Thus, CSF is constantly being produced in the choroid plexuses of the ventricles and resorbed again from the subarachnoid space at various locations.

Bottlenecks of the CSF circulation. As it flows through the ventricular system, the CSF must traverse a number of narrow passageways: the *interventricular foramina*, the slender *third ventricle*, the *cerebral aqueduct* (narrowest point!), and the *exit foramina of the fourth ventricle* and the tentorial aperture.

Disturbances of Cerebrospinal Fluid Circulation—Hydrocephalus

General aspects of pathogenesis. Many different diseases cause an imbalance of CSF production and resorption. If too much CSF is produced or too little is resorbed, the ventricular system becomes enlarged (hydrocephalus). Elevated CSF pressure in the ventricles leads to displacement, and eventually atrophy, of the periventricular white matter, while the gray matter is not affected, at least at first. As animal experiments have shown, hydrocephalus causes seepage (diaedesis) of CSF through the ventricular ependyma into the periventricular white matter. The elevated hydrostatic pressure in the white matter impairs tissue perfusion, causing local tissue hypoxia, damage to myelinated nerve pathways, and, ultimately, irreversible gliosis. The histological and clinical abnormalities caused by hydrocephalus can regress only if the intraventricular pressure is brought back to normal in timely fashion.

Types of Hydrocephalus

Different clinical varieties of hydrocephalus can be conveniently classified by etiology, by the site where CSF flow is blocked, and by the dynamic status of the pathological process (e. g., active hydrocephalus due to congenital aqueductal stenosis).

Classification by etiology and pathogenesis. Hydrocephalus due to obstruction of the CSF pathways is called **occlusive hydrocephalus**, while that due to inadequate CSF resorption is called **malresorptive hydrocephalus** (see Fig. 10.**6**). Occlusive hydrocephalus is typically due to an intracranial space-occupying lesion (e. g., tumor, infarct, or hemorrhage, particularly in the posterior fossa) or malformation (e. g., aqueductal stenosis, colloid cyst of the third ventricle). Malresorptive hydrocephalus often arises in the aftermath of subarachnoid hemorrhage and meningitis, both of which can produce occlusive adhesions of the arachnoid granulations. Hydrocephalus can also result from traumatic brain injury and intraventricular hemorrhage. **Hypersecretory hydrocephalus**, due to overproduction of CSF, is much rarer; it is usually caused by a tumor (papilloma) of the choroid plexus.

Older, alternative, and essentially synonymous terms for malresorptive and occlusive hydrocephalus are "communicating" and "noncommunicating" hydrocephalus, respectively. In **communicating hydrocephalus**, the CSF circulates freely from the ventricular system to the subarachnoid cisterns. In **noncommunicating hydrocephalus**, there is an obstruction to CSF flow within the ventricular system, so that the connection from the ventricles to the CSF-resorbing structures is no longer patent, or can only be kept open under abnormally high pressure.

Classification by dynamics. Hydrocephalus is called **active** if the intraventricular pressure is continuously elevated. There are two types of active hydrocephalus. In *compensated active hydrocephalus*, the ventricular size and the patient's symptoms and signs remain constant over time; in *uncontrolled hydrocephalus*, the patient's condition worsens while the ventricles continue to enlarge. Active hydrocephalus is not the same as normal pressure hydrocephalus (see below), in which the CSF pressure is only intermittently elevated.

Normal pressure hydrocephalus (NPH). NPH is a special case among types of hydrocephalus, generally involving communicating hydrocephalus with abnormal CSF flow dynamics and only intermittently elevated intraventricular pressure. The characteristic clinical triad of NPH consists of *apraxic gait disturbance*, *dementia*, and *urinary incontinence* (Case Presentation 1). Its cause is unclear; it may be the common clinical expression of a number of different disease processes (aqueductal stenosis, malresorptive hydrocephalus, etc.).

Differential diagnosis: "hydrocephalus ex vacuo." Degenerative diseases of the brain, such as Alzheimer disease and Pick disease, cause brain atrophy, with secondary enlargement of the internal and external CSF spaces. This may create the impression of hydrocephalus. Strictly speaking, however, hydrocephalus is present only when the internal CSF spaces (i.e., the ventricular system) are enlarged out of proportion to the external spaces, and not when both are enlarged by atrophy. The older term "hydrocephalus ex vacuo" for the latter condition is, therefore, not recommended. Unlike NPH, in which the ventricles are enlarged but the sulci are of relatively normal width, neurodegenerative diseases cause enlargement of the internal and external CSF spaces to a roughly comparable extent.

Case Presentation 1: *Normal Pressure Hydrocephalus*

This retired 80-year-old man suffered for several months from urge incontinence, which was initially attributed to his benign prostatic hypertrophy. Over time, however, other symptoms developed: he felt unsteady while walking, walked with his feet wide apart, and fell multiple times. He sometimes complained that he could barely lift his feet off the ground. His family physician ordered an MRI scan of the head (Fig. 10.**5**) and, after viewing the images, referred him for admission to the hospital. The patient's wife, in response to the specific questions of the admitting neurologist, reported that he had become increasingly forgetful and inattentive in recent months. Neurological examination revealed an unsteady, apraxic gait.

The clinical and radiological diagnosis was normal pressure hydrocephalus (NPH).

Transient improvement of gait after removal of a large quantity of cerebrospinal fluid is considered to confirm the diagnosis of NPH. Even in this 80-year-old patient, a lumbar puncture and removal of 40 ml of cerebrospinal fluid resulted in marked improvement of gait, as well as complete resolution of urinary incontinence. His cognitive difficulties were unchanged, however. He was transferred to the neurosurgical service for the insertion of a shunt. In the ensuing months, his gait became normal and his urinary incontinence resolved completely. His cognitive difficulties remained, but did not progress.

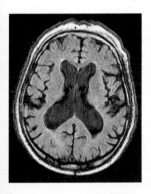
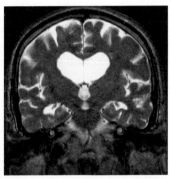

a   b

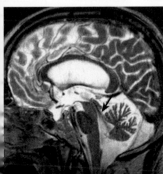

c

Fig. 10.**5 Normal pressure hydrocephalus (NPH)** (communicating hydrocephalus), as seen on MRI. Axial T2-weighted FLAIR image (**a**), coronal image (**b**), and sagittal T2-weighted spin-echo image (**c**). The ventricles are disproportionately enlarged in relation to the subarachnoid space. The sagittal image (**c**) reveals low signal intensity in the aqueduct and neighboring portions of the third and fourth ventricles (arrow) because of rapid CSF flow ("flow void"). Recent studies have shown that CSF pulsatility is greater than normal, as a rule, in patients with NPH. The images are mildly blurred because of patient movement; persons with NPH and other dementing illnesses are often unable to cooperate fully with MRI studies.

General Aspects of the Clinical Presentation, Diagnostic Evaluation, and Treatment of Hydrocephalus

Epidemiology. Many types of hydrocephalus begin in childhood, usually accompanying other abnormalities of development, such as the Chiari malformation, spina bifida, or meningo(myelo)cele. The prevalence of hydrocephalus in the first three months of postnatal life is 0.1-0.4%.

Manifestations in children. The cranial sutures do not close until one year after birth; throughout the first year of life, the skull bones can respond to elevated intracranial pressure by spreading wider apart. Thus, the most obvious clinical sign of childhood hydrocephalus is *abnormal growth of the head*, with disproportionate enlargement of the skull in relation to the face. Further signs include gaping cranial sutures, stasis of the scalp veins, frontal bossing, and tightly bulging fontanelles. Percussion of the head produces a rattling sound (MacEwen sign). The affected children appear well at first, because the intracranial pressure is only mildly raised as long as the sutures are open and the head is still able to expand. Decompensation occurs later, giving rise to *signs of intracranial hypertension*, including vomiting (including projectile vomiting and dry heaves). These children may also present with the *sunset phenomenon* (upward gaze paresis) and general *failure to thrive*.

Diagnostic evaluation in children. At present, hydrocephalus can be diagnosed before birth by routine prenatal ultrasonography. Hydrocephalus arising after birth is detected by routine serial measurement and documentation of the child's head circumference: if the head grows faster than normal (according to the reference curves on the chart), then hydrocephalus should be suspected, and further diagnostic studies should be done to guide potential treatment. After birth, children with hydrocephalus are evaluated not just with ultrasound but also with CT and MRI. This enables the identification of potential treatable causes of hydrocephalus, as well as other potential causes of disproportionate growth of the head, such as subdural hematomas and hygromas, and familial macrocephaly.

Manifestations in adults. In children with closed sutures, and in adults, hydrocephalus presents with manifestations of *intracranial hypertension*, including headache, nausea, and vomiting (particularly morning dry heaves and projectile vomiting), and signs of *meningeal irritation*, including nuchal rigidity, head tilt, opisthotonus, and photophobia. As the condition progresses, further manifestations may include fatigue, cognitive decline, unsteady gait, cranial nerve deficits (particularly abducens palsy), Parinaud syndrome, papilledema, and impairment of consciousness.

Diagnostic evaluation in adults. CT and MRI readily demonstrate ventricular enlargement and often reveal the cause of hydrocephalus.

Treatment. If no underlying, treatable cause of hydrocephalus can be identified, the elevated intraventricular pressure can be relieved by the insertion of a *cerebrospinal fluid shunt*. Many different types of shunts are available; for further information, the reader is directed to textbooks of neurosurgery.

Case Presentation 2: **Malresorptive Hydrocephalus after Subarachnoid Hemorrhage (SAH)**

This 52-year-old man was admitted to the hospital because of an acute, severe headache—the worst headache of his life—and mild somnolence. A CT scan of the head revealed the cause: acute subarachnoid hemorrhage (SAH). Cerebral angiography showed the source of bleeding to be a ruptured aneurysm of the left middle cerebral artery. The blood in the subarachnoid space blocked the outflow and resorption of CSF, leading to widening of the ventricles (hydrocephalus, Fig. 10.**6**). A temporary external ventricular drain was inserted to treat the hydrocephalus, and the aneurysm was then clipped in an open neurosurgical procedure.

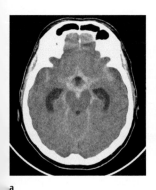 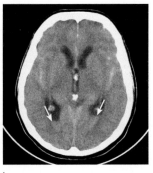

a   b

Fig. 10.6 Malresorptive hydrocephalus after aneurysmal subarachnoid hemorrhage (SAH); CT of head. The subarachnoid space is filled with hyperdense (bright) blood (**a**), which impairs CSF circulation and resorption. The ventricles are dilated, particularly the temporal horns (**b**). The ventricles are black in the CT scan because they contain very little blood. A small amount of blood has entered the ventricular system by reflux and can be seen in the posterior horns of the lateral ventricles (blood–CSF levels, arrows, **b**).

11 Blood Supply and Vascular Disorders of the Central Nervous System

11 Blood Supply and Vascular Disorders of the Central Nervous System

The cerebral blood supply is derived from the **internal carotid** and **vertebral arteries** The internal carotid artery on either side delivers blood to the brain through its major branches, the middle and anterior cerebral arteries and the anterior choroidal artery (**anterior circulation**). The two vertebral arteries unite in the midline at the caudal border of the pons to form the basilar artery, which delivers blood to the brainstem and cerebellum, as well as to part of the cerebral hemispheres through its terminal branches, the posterior cerebral arteries (**posterior circulation**). The anterior and posterior circulations communicate with each other through the arterial circle of Willis. There are also many other anastomotic connections among the arteries supplying the brain, and between the intracranial and extracranial circulations; thus, occlusion of a major vessel does not necessarily lead to stroke, because the brain tissue distal to the occlusion may be adequately perfused by collateral vessels.

The **venous blood** of the brain flows from the deep and superficial cerebral veins into the venous sinuses of the dura mater, and thence into the internal jugular veins on both sides.

Protracted interruption of blood flow to a part of the brain causes loss of function and, finally, ischemic necrosis of brain tissue (**cerebral infarction**). Cerebral ischemia generally presents with the sudden onset of a neurological deficit (hence the term "stroke"), due to loss of function of the affected part of the brain. Sometimes, however, the deficit appears gradually rather than suddenly. The most common causes of ischemia on the arterial side of the cerebral circulation are **emboli** (usually arising from the heart or from an atheromatous plaque, e. g., in the aorta or carotid bifurcation) and direct occlusion of small or middle-sized vessels by arteriolosclerosis (**cerebral microangiopathy**, usually due to hypertension). Cerebral ischemia can also be due to impairment of venous drainage (cerebral venous or venous sinus thrombosis).

Another cause of the stroke syndrome is **intracranial hemorrhage**, which may be either into the brain parenchyma itself (intracerebral hemorrhage) or into the neighboring meningeal compartments (subarachnoid, subdural, and epidural hemorrhage and hematoma).

The **blood supply of the spinal cord** is mainly supplied by the unpaired anterior spinal artery and the paired posterolateral spinal arteries The anterior spinal artery receives contributions from many segmental arteries. Like the brain, the spinal cord can be damaged by hemorrhage or by ischemia of arterial or venous origin.

Arteries of the Brain

Extradural Course of the Arteries of the Brain

Four great vessels supply the brain with blood: the right and left **internal carotid arteries** and the right and left **vertebral arteries**. The internal carotid arteries are of the same caliber on both sides, but the two vertebral arteries are often of very different sizes in a single individual. All of the arteries supplying the brain are anastomotically interconnected at the base of the brain through the arterial circle of Willis. They are also interconnected extracranially through small branches in the muscles and connective tissue, which may become important in certain pathological processes affecting the vasculature, but which are normally too small to be demonstrated.

The structures of the anterior and middle cranial fossae are mainly supplied by the internal carotid arteries (the so-called **anterior circulation**), while the structures of the posterior fossa and the posterior portion of the cerebral hemispheres are mainly supplied by the vertebral arteries (the so-called **posterior circulation**).

Common carotid artery. The internal carotid artery is one of the two terminal branches of the common carotid artery, which, on the right side, arises from the aortic arch in a common (brachiocephalic) trunk that it shares with the right subclavian artery (Fig. 11.**1**). The left common carotid artery usually arises directly from the aortic arch, but there are frequent anatomical variants. In 20% of individuals, the left common carotid artery arises from a left brachiocephalic trunk.

The *internal carotid artery* originates at the bifurcation of the common carotid artery at the level of the thyroid cartilage and ascends to the skull base without giving off any major branches. It passes through the *carotid canal* of the petrous bone, where it is separated from the middle ear only by a thin, bony wall, and then enters the *cavernous sinus* (Fig. 11.**1**). For its further intracranial course, see p. 421.

Anastomotic connections of the arteries of the brain with the external carotid artery. The second branch of the common carotid artery, the external carotid artery, supplies the *soft tissues of the neck and face*. It makes numerous anastomotic connections with the opposite external carotid artery, as well as with the vertebral arteries (see Fig. 11.**11**, p. 433) and the intracranial territory of the internal carotid artery (e. g., through the ophthalmic artery [Fig. 11.**11**] or the inferolateral trunk, see p. 432). These connections can dilate in the setting of slowly progressive stenosis or occlusion of the internal carotid artery, thereby assuring continued delivery of blood to the brain.

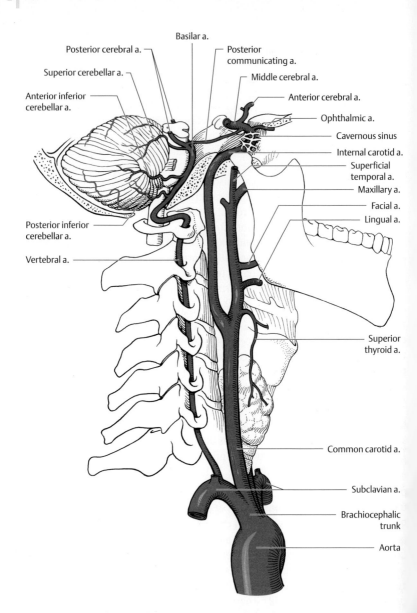

Fig. 11.1 Extracranial course of the major arteries supplying the brain (common carotid artery, vertebral artery)

Vertebral artery. The vertebral arteries arise from the subclavian arteries on either side and are often of different caliber on the two sides. The left vertebral artery rarely arises directly from the aortic arch. The vertebral artery travels up the neck in the bony canal formed by the transverse foramina of the cervical vertebrae, which it enters at the C6 level (i.e., it does not pass through the transverse foramen of C7). At the level of the atlas (C1), it leaves this bony canal and curves around the lateral mass of the atlas dorsally and medially, sitting in the *sulcus of the vertebral artery* on the upper surface of the posterior arch of C1. It then runs ventrally between the occiput and the atlas and passes through the atlanto-occipital membrane. It usually penetrates the dura mater at the level of the foramen magnum.

In the subarachnoid space, the vertebral artery curves ventrally and cranially around the brainstem, then joins the contralateral vertebral artery in front of the caudal portion of the pons to form the **basilar artery**. The vertebral artery gives off many branches to the muscles and soft tissues of the neck; its major intracranial branches are the **posterior inferior cerebellar artery** (PICA) and the **anterior spinal artery** (Fig. 11.**2**). The origin of the PICA (cf. also p. 427) is just distal to the point where the vertebral artery enters the subarachnoid space; a ruptured aneurysm at the origin of the PICA may, therefore, be extracranial and nonetheless produce a subarachnoid hemorrhage. The **branches of the vertebral artery to the spinal cord** have a variable anatomy. They supply blood to the upper cervical spinal cord and form anastomoses with segmental spinal arteries arising from the proximal portion of the vertebral artery, and with the nuchal arteries.

Arteries of the Anterior and Middle Cranial Fossae

Internal Carotid Artery (ICA)

After it exits the carotid canal, the internal carotid artery courses rostrally, next to the clivus and beneath the dura mater, to the cavernous sinus. It curves upward and backward within the cavernous sinus, forming a loop that is open posteriorly (the carotid siphon, Fig. 11.**1**). Fine extradural branches of the internal carotid artery supply the floor of the tympanic cavity, the dura mater of the clivus, the semilunar ganglion, and the pituitary gland.

Injury or rupture of the internal carotid artery within the cavernous sinus produces a "short-circuit" connection between its arterial blood and the venous blood of the sinus (carotid-cavernous fistula). If an *intracavernous aneurysm of the internal carotid artery* ruptures, exophthalmos develops but there is no subarachnoid hemorrhage, because the aneurysm is extradural. The patient's vision in the ipsilateral eye deteriorates thereafter because of outflow obstruction and congestion of the retinal veins.

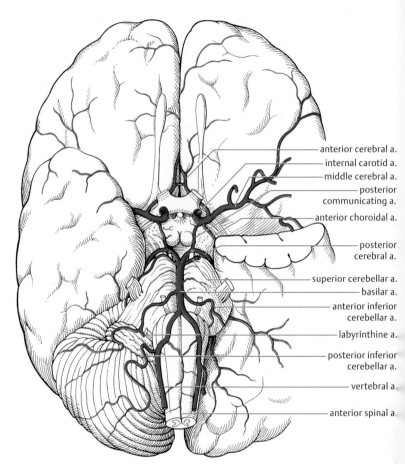

anterior cerebral a.
internal carotid a.
middle cerebral a.
posterior communicating a.
anterior choroidal a.
posterior cerebral a.
superior cerebellar a.
basilar a.
anterior inferior cerebellar a.
labyrinthine a.
posterior inferior cerebellar a.
vertebral a.
anterior spinal a.

Fig. 11.**2 Arteries of the base of the skull**

Ophthalmic artery. The internal carotid artery enters the subarachnoid space medial to the anterior clinoid process. The ophthalmic artery arises at this point from the internal carotid artery; it is thus already intradural at its site of origin (Fig. 11.**1**). It enters the orbit together with the optic nerve and supplies not only the *contents of the orbit*, but also the *sphenoid sinus*, the *ethmoid air cells*, the *nasal mucosa*, the *dura mater of the anterior cranial fossa*, and the *skin of the forehead, root of the nose, and eyelids*. The cutaneous branches of the ophthalmic artery form anastomoses with branches of the external carotid artery which can be an important path for collateral circulation around a stenosis or occlusion of the internal carotid artery (ophthalmic collaterals). Ruptured aneurysms or injuries of the ICA distal to the origin of the ophthalmic artery cause subarachnoid hemorrhage.

Posterior communicating artery. The next angiographically visible artery arising from the internal carotid artery along its intradural course is the posterior communicating artery (Figs. 11.**1** and 11.**2**). In the early stages of embryonic development, this artery is the proximal segment of the posterior cerebral artery, which is at first a branch of the internal carotid artery and only later comes to be supplied by the basilar artery. In some 20 % of cases, the posterior communicating artery remains the main source of blood for the posterior cerebral artery; this is equivalent to a direct origin of the posterior cerebral artery from the ICA, or *fetal origin of the posterior cerebral artery*, as it is traditionally called. The fetal pattern, if present, is usually seen only on one side, while the contralateral posterior cerebral artery arises from an asymmetric basilar tip. Sometimes, however, both posterior cerebral arteries arise directly from the ICA through unusually large posterior communicating arteries. In such cases, the basilar tip is smaller than usual, and the basilar artery appears to terminate where it gives off the two superior cerebellar arteries.

The posterior communicating artery ends where it joins the proximal segment of the posterior cerebral artery some 10 mm lateral to the basilar tip. It is a component of the circle of Willis and *the most important anastomotic connection between the anterior and posterior circulations.*

The posterior communicating artery gives off fine perforating branches to the *tuber cinereum, mamillary body, rostral thalamic nuclei, subthalamus,* and *part of the internal capsule.*

The origin of the posterior communicating artery from the ICA is a preferred site for the formation of aneurysms (so-called PComm aneurysms; see p. 481). Such aneurysms usually arise from the side wall of the internal carotid artery, and only rarely from the posterior communicating artery itself.

Anterior choroidal artery. This artery arises from the internal carotid artery immediately distal to the posterior communicating artery (Fig. 11.**2**), runs toward the occiput parallel to the optic tract, and then enters the choroidal fissure to supply the *choroid plexus of the temporal horn of the lateral ventricle.* Along its course, it gives off branches to the *optic tract, uncus, hippocampus, amygdala, part of the basal ganglia,* and *part of the internal capsule.* It is clinically significant that the anterior choroidal artery also supplies part of the *pyramidal tract.* It has anastomotic connections with the lateral posterior choroidal artery (see Fig. 11.**10**, p. 431).

Terminal branches. The internal carotid artery bifurcates above the clinoid process, giving rise to the **anterior cerebral artery** medially and the **middle cerebral artery** laterally.

Middle Cerebral Artery

The middle cerebral artery (MCA) is the largest branch of the internal carotid artery (Fig. 11.**2**). After its origin from the ICA above the anterior clinoid process, it travels laterally in the sylvian fissure (lateral sulcus). The main trunk of the middle cerebral artery gives off numerous *perforating branches to the basal ganglia* and to the *anterior limb and genu of the internal capsule*, as well as to the *external capsule and claustrum* (Fig. 11.**3**).

The middle cerebral artery divides into its major cortical branches within the insular cistern. These branches supply *large areas of the frontal parietal, and temporal lobes.*

The **major branches of the middle cerebral artery** (Fig. 11.**4**) are the orbitofrontal (I), prerolandic (II), rolandic (III), anterior parietal (IV), and posterior parietal (V) arteries, the artery of the angular gyrus (VI), and the temporo-occipital, posterior temporal (VII), and anterior temporal (VIII) arteries. The cortical areas supplied by the middle cerebral artery include, among others, the primary sensory and motor cortices (except for their parasagittal and medial portions), the language areas of Broca and Wernicke, the primary auditory cortex, and the primary gustatory cortex.

The middle cerebral artery has cortical anastomotic connections with the anterior and posterior cerebral arteries.

Anterior Cerebral Artery

The anterior cerebral artery (ACA) originates from the bifurcation of the internal carotid artery and then courses medially and rostrally. The anterior cerebral arteries of the two sides come to lie adjacent to each other across the midline in front of the lamina terminalis; from this location, the two arteries course in parallel upward and posteriorly. This is also the site of the anastomotic connection between the two anterior cerebral arteries through the *anterior communicating artery*, a further important component of the circle of Willis (see Fig. 11.**12**, p. 434). The anterior communicating artery and the neighboring segments of the anterior cerebral arteries are preferred sites for the formation of aneurysms (so-called AComm aneurysms, p. 481).

Branches of the anterior cerebral artery. The proximal (basal) segment of the anterior cerebral artery gives off numerous small perforating branches that

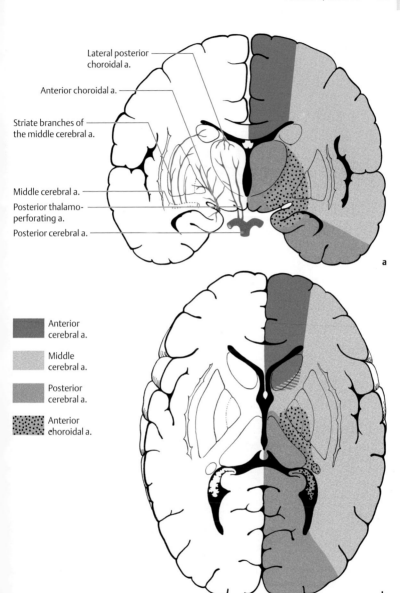

Lateral posterior choroidal a.

Anterior choroidal a.

Striate branches of the middle cerebral a.

Middle cerebral a.

Posterior thalamo-perforating a.

Posterior cerebral a.

Anterior cerebral a.

Middle cerebral a.

Posterior cerebral a.

Anterior choroidal a.

a

b

Fig. 11.**3 Arterial supply of the interior of the brain. a** Coronal section. **b** Horizontal section.

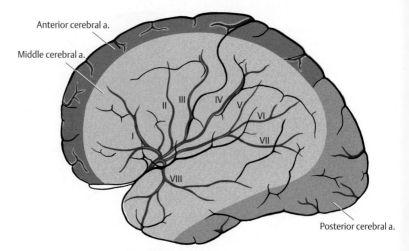

Fig. 11.4 Territory and branches of the middle cerebral artery on the convexity of the brain. See text, p. 424.

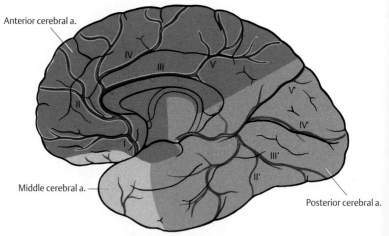

Fig. 11.5 Territories and branches of the anterior cerebral, posterior cerebral, and middle cerebral arteries on the medial surface of the brain. I′, anterior temporal artery; II′, posterior temporal artery; III′, posterior occipital artery; IV′, calcarine artery; V′, parieto-occipital artery. For labels I–V, see text, p. 427.

supply the *paraseptal region, rostral portion of the basal ganglia* and *diencephalon*, and the *anterior limb of the internal capsule* (Fig. 11.**3**). The *recurrent artery of Heubner* is a large branch of the proximal segment of the anterior cerebral artery that supplies the basal ganglia; it is sometimes visible on an angiogram (see Fig. 11.**12**, p. 434).

In their further course, the anterior cerebral arteries wind around the genu of the corpus callosum and then course posteriorly until they reach the central region, where they make anastomotic connections with the posterior cerebral arteries Along the way, they give off branches to the *corpus callosum*, the *medial surfaces of the cerebral hemispheres*, and the *parasagittal region*. Areas of the brain receiving their blood supply from the anterior cerebral artery include the *leg areas of the primary sensory and motor cortices* and the *cingulate gyrus*. The anterior cerebral artery makes anastomotic connections with the middle cerebral artery as well as the posterior cerebral artery.

The major cortical branches of the anterior cerebral artery (Fig. 11.**5**) are the orbital (I), frontopolar (II), frontal, pericallosal (III), callosomarginal (IV), and internal parietal (V) arteries.

Arteries of the Posterior Fossa

Vertebral Artery

Just after it enters the dura mater, the vertebral artery gives off branches to the cervical spinal cord. The vascular anatomy in this area is variable, but the **ante-**

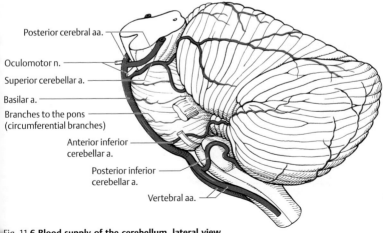

Posterior cerebral aa.

Oculomotor n.

Superior cerebellar a.

Basilar a.

Branches to the pons
(circumferential branches)

Anterior inferior
cerebellar a.

Posterior inferior
cerebellar a.

Vertebral aa.

Fig. 11.**6 Blood supply of the cerebellum, lateral view**

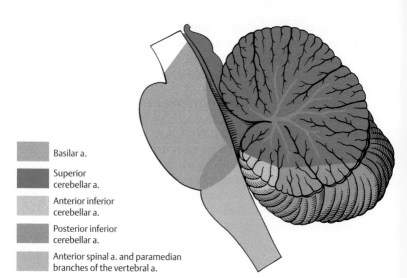

Basilar a.

Superior
cerebellar a.

Anterior inferior
cerebellar a.

Posterior inferior
cerebellar a.

Anterior spinal a. and paramedian
branches of the vertebral a.

Fig. 11.**7 Territories of the cerebellar and brainstem arteries in midline sagittal section**

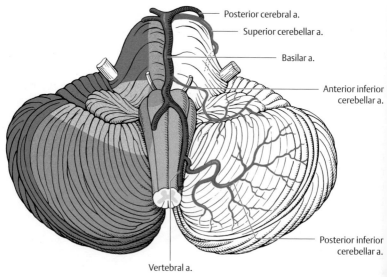

Posterior cerebral a.

Superior cerebellar a.

Basilar a.

Anterior inferior
cerebellar a.

Posterior inferior
cerebellar a.

Vertebral a.

Fig. 11.**8 Blood supply of the cerebellum and territories of the cerebellar arteries, inferior view**

rior spinal artery almost always arises from the intradural portion of the vertebral artery.

Posterior inferior cerebellar artery (PICA). The PICA is the largest branch of the vertebral artery (Figs. 11.**1**, 11.**2**, and 11.**6**-11.**8**) and likewise arises from its intradural portion, just before the vertebral artery joins its counterpart from the opposite side to form the basilar artery. The PICA supplies the *basal portion of the cerebellar hemispheres*, the *lower portion of the vermis*, part of the *cerebellar nuclei*, and the *choroid plexus of the fourth ventricle*, as well as the *dorsolateral portion of the medulla*. It makes numerous anastomotic connections with the remaining cerebellar arteries.

The size of the PICA territory is inversely related to that of the anterior inferior cerebellar artery (AICA) territory; furthermore, the PICA and its territory may be of very different sizes on the two sides. If one PICA is particularly small, the basal portion of the cerebellum will be supplied by the AICA ipsilaterally and the larger PICA contralaterally. A congenitally small ("*hypoplastic*") vertebral artery may terminate as the PICA and give off no contribution to the basilar artery, which, in such cases, is simply a continuation of the contralateral vertebral artery. This is a fairly common normal variant.

Basilar Artery

The basilar artery arises from the union of the right and left vertebral arteries in front of the brainstem at a lower pontine level (Fig. 11.**2**). Its major branches are the two pairs of cerebellar arteries and the posterior cerebral arteries. The basilar artery also gives off numerous small perforating branches to the brainstem—the *paramedian branches* as well as the *short* and *long circumferential branches* (Fig. 4.**58**, p. 225). Occlusions of these branches produce the brainstem syndromes described in Chapter 4 (p. 223 ff.).

Anterior inferior cerebellar artery (AICA). The first major branch of the basilar artery is the AICA (Figs. 11.**1**, 11.**2**, and 11.**6**-11.**8**), which supplies the *flocculus* and the *anterior portion of the cerebellar hemisphere*. Its territory is inversely related in size to the ipsilateral PICA territory: in some individuals, part of the cerebellar hemisphere that is usually supplied by the PICA is actually supplied by the AICA (as discussed above). The AICA also gives off the *labyrinthine artery* to the inner ear.

Superior cerebellar artery (SCA). The superior cerebellar artery (Figs. 11.**1**, 11.**2**, and 11.**6**-11.**8**) arises from the basilar artery below its tip and supplies the *rostral portion of the cerebellar hemisphere* and the *upper portion of the vermis*. As it curves around the midbrain, it gives off *branches to the tegmentum*.

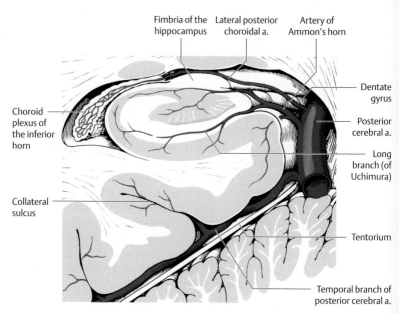

Fig. 11.**9 Anatomical relation of the posterior cerebral artery to the tentorial edge**; blood supply of Ammon's horn

The **basilar tip** (end of the basilar artery) is the site where the artery divides into the two posterior cerebral arteries (Fig. 11.**2**).

Posterior Cerebral Artery

The posterior cerebral artery (PCA) has connections to both the anterior and posterior circulation. Most of the blood flowing within it is usually derived from the basilar tip, but there is also a smaller contribution from the internal carotid artery by way of the posterior communicating artery (Fig. 11.**1**). At an earlier stage in ontogenetic development, the posterior cerebral artery is a branch of the internal carotid artery (as discussed above, p. 423). The posterior communicating artery joins the posterior cerebral artery some 10 mm distal to the basilar tip. The segment of the posterior cerebral artery proximal to this point is called the precommunicating segment, or, in Fischer's terminology, the P1 segment, while the segment distal to this point is the postcommunicating or P2 segment. Both the posterior cerebral artery and the posterior communicating artery give off *perforating branches to the midbrain and thalamus* (Fig. 11.**3**).

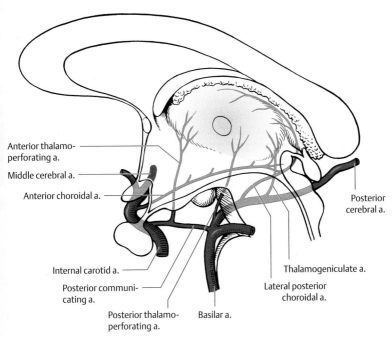

Fig. 11.**10 Arterial blood supply of the thalamus**

The posterior cerebral artery originates at the basilar bifurcation and then curves around the midbrain and enters the ambient cistern, where it has a close spatial relation to the tentorial edge (Fig. 11.**9**). Within the ambient cistern, the posterior cerebral artery divides into its major cortical branches, including the *calcarine* and *occipitotemporal arteries* and the *temporal branches* (Fig. 11.**5**).

The anterior and posterior thalamoperforating arteries (Fig. 11.**10**). The anterior thalamoperforating artery is a branch of the posterior communicating artery that mainly supplies the *rostral portion of the thalamus.* The posterior thalamoperforating artery arises from the posterior cerebral artery proximal to the insertion of the posterior communicating artery and supplies the *basal and medial portions of the thalamus*, as well as the *pulvinar*. The posterior thalamoperforating arteries of the two sides may share a common trunk, called the *artery of Percheron;* this is often seen in association with unilateral hypo-plasia of the P1 segment and fetal origin of the posterior cerebral artery (cf. p. 423). An alternative nomenclature is sometimes used for the anterior and posterior thalamoperforating arteries, in which the former is called the thalamotuberal artery, and the latter is called the thalamoperforating artery.

The thalamogeniculate artery arises from the posterior cerebral artery distal to the origin of the posterior communicating artery (Fig. 11.**10**). It supplies the *lateral portion of the thalamus.*

The medial and lateral posterior choroidal arteries also arise distal to the origin of the posterior communicating artery (Figs. 11.**9**-11.**10**). They supply the *geniculate bodies, medial* and *posteromedial thalamic nuclei,* and *pulvinar.* The medial posterior choroidal artery gives off *branches to the midbrain* and supplies the choroid plexus of the third ventricle. The lateral posterior choroidal artery supplies the choroid plexus of the lateral ventricle and has an anastomotic connection with the anterior choroidal artery.

Cortical branches of the posterior cerebral artery. The territories of the posterior cerebral artery and middle cerebral artery vary widely in extent. In some cases, the posterior cerebral artery territory is delimited by the sylvian fissure; in others, the middle cerebral artery supplies the entire convexity of the brain all the way back to the occipital pole. The *visual cortex of the calcarine sulcus* is always supplied by the posterior cerebral artery. The optic radiation, however, is often supplied by the middle cerebral artery, so that homonymous hemianopsia does not always imply an infarct in the territory of the posterior cerebral artery. The posterior cerebral artery supplies not only the occipital lobe but also the medial temporal lobe through its temporal branches.

Collateral Circulation in the Brain

External-to-Internal Collateralization

When the internal carotid artery is stenotic, blood is diverted from branches of the external carotid artery into the internal carotid artery distal to the stenosis, enabling continued perfusion of the brain. The facial or superficial temporal artery, for example, can form an anastomotic connection with the **ophthalmic artery** by way of the angular artery; retrograde flow in the ophthalmic artery then takes the blood back into the carotid siphon (Fig. 11.**11**). Collaterals to the ophthalmic artery can also be fed by the buccal artery. Further external-to-internal anastomotic connections exist between the ascending pharyngeal artery and meningeal branches of the ICA. These arteries, usually too small to be seen by angiography, are known collectively as the **inferolateral trunk.**

External-Carotid-to-Vertebral Collateralization

The branches of the external carotid artery and vertebral artery that supply the cervical and nuchal muscles are anastomotically connected at multiple points.

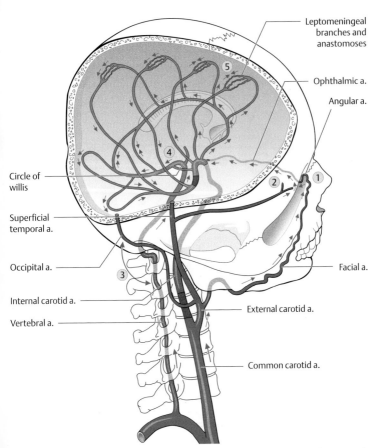

Fig. 11.**11 Anastomoses of the arteries of the brain.** The following collateral pathways are shown: **Collaterals from the external to the internal carotid circulation: 1**, external carotid artery–facial artery–angular artery–internal carotid artery; **2**, external carotid artery–superficial temporal artery–angular artery–internal carotid artery. **3, Collaterals from the external to the vertebral circulation:** external carotid artery–occipital artery–vertebral artery. **4, Circle of Willis. 5, Lepto-meningeal collaterals** between the anterior, middle, and posterior cerebral arteries. After Poeck K and Hacke W: Neurologie, 11th ed., Springer, Berlin/Heidelberg, 2001.

The most important branch of the external carotid artery in this respect is the **occipital artery**. Collaterals can form in either direction (Fig. 11.**11**): proximal occlusion of the vertebral artery can be compensated by blood from nuchal branches of the occipital artery, while occlusion of the common carotid artery

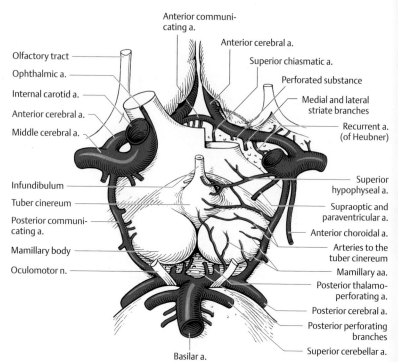

Fig. 11.**12 Circle of Willis**

or proximal occlusion of the internal carotid artery can be compensated by blood entering the anterior circulation from the muscular branches of the vertebral artery by way of the occipital artery. As another example, if a proximal occlusion of the common carotid artery has cut off both the internal and the external cerebral arteries from the circulation, then blood from the vertebral artery can flow in the external carotid artery in retrograde fashion down to the carotid bifurcation, and then up again in the internal carotid artery, restoring perfusion in the ICA territory.

Arterial Circle of Willis

The cerebral arteries are connected to each other through a wreathlike arrangement of blood vessels at the base of the brain known as the circle of Willis (after Thomas Willis, an English anatomist of the seventeenth century). This interconnection enables continued perfusion of brain tissue even if one of the great vessels is stenotic or occluded. The circle itself consists of **segments of the great vessels** and the so-called **communicating arteries** linking them to one another. Traveling around one side of the circle from anterior to posterior, we find the *anterior communicating artery*, the *proximal (A1) segment of the anterior cerebral artery*, the *distal segment of the internal carotid artery*, the *posterior communicating artery*, the *proximal (P1) segment of the posterior cerebral artery*, and the *basilar tip* (Fig. 11.**12**). Decreased blood flow in a great vessel due to slowly progressive stenosis below the circle of Willis can usually be compensated by increased collateral flow around the circle, so that hemodynamic infarction will not occur (see below). There are, however, frequent anatomical variants of the circle of Willis in which one or more of its constituent arterial segments may be hypoplastic or absent. The unlucky combination of a stenotic great vessel with an anatomical variant of the circle of Willis preventing adequate collateral flow can result in hemodynamic infarction (p. 445 and Fig. 11.**21**).

Callosal Anastomoses

The anterior and posterior cerebral circulations are anastomotically connected through the callosal arteries (Fig. 11.**1**). Thus, when the anterior cerebral artery is occluded, blood from the posterior cerebral artery may continue to supply the central region.

Leptomeningeal Anastomoses

Furthermore, the branches of the anterior, posterior, and middle cerebral arteries are anastomotically linked to each other through the arteries of the pia mater and arachnoid (Fig. 11.**11**). There are also leptomeningeal anastomoses linking the branches of the three main cerebellar arteries.

Veins of the Brain

Superficial and Deep Veins of the Brain

The veins of the brain, unlike those of the rest of the body, do not run together with its arteries. The territories of the cerebral arteries do not coincide with the drainage areas of the cerebral veins. Venous blood from the brain parenchyma crosses the subarachnoid and subdural spaces in short **cortical veins** whose anatomy is relatively invariable: these include the *superior anastomotic vein* (*of Trolard*), the *dorsal superior cerebral vein*, the *superficial middle cerebral vein*, and the *inferior anastomotic vein* (*of Labbé*) on the lateral surface of the temporal lobe (Fig. 11.**13**).

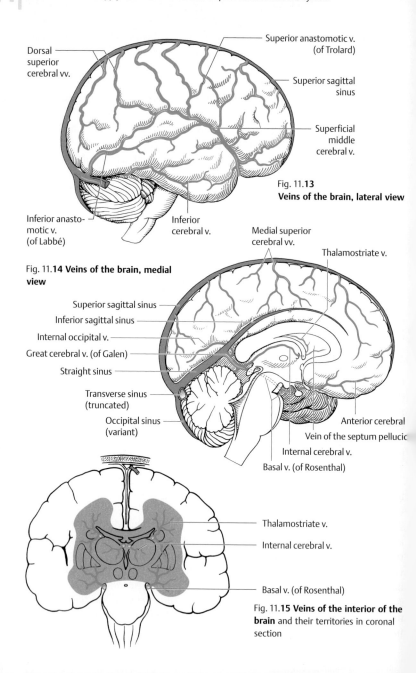

Dorsal superior cerebral vv.

Superior anastomotic v. (of Trolard)

Superior sagittal sinus

Superficial middle cerebral v.

Fig. 11.**13**
Veins of the brain, lateral view

Inferior anastomotic v. (of Labbé)

Inferior cerebral v.

Fig. 11.**14 Veins of the brain, medial view**

Medial superior cerebral vv.

Thalamostriate v.

Superior sagittal sinus

Inferior sagittal sinus

Internal occipital v.

Great cerebral v. (of Galen)

Straight sinus

Transverse sinus (truncated)

Occipital sinus (variant)

Anterior cerebral

Vein of the septum pellucid

Internal cerebral v.

Basal v. (of Rosenthal)

Thalamostriate v.

Internal cerebral v.

Basal v. (of Rosenthal)

Fig. 11.**15 Veins of the interior of the brain** and their territories in coronal section

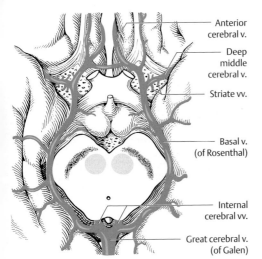

Fig. 11.**16 Veins of the base of the skull**

- Anterior cerebral v.
- Deep middle cerebral v.
- Striate vv.
- Basal v. (of Rosenthal)
- Internal cerebral vv.
- Great cerebral v. (of Galen)

Venous blood from deep regions of the brain, including the basal ganglia and thalamus, drains into the paired **internal cerebral veins** and the paired **basal veins of Rosenthal**. The internal cerebral veins are created by the confluence of the vein of the septum pellucidum (septal vein) with the thalamostriate vein. These four veins, coming from the two sides, join behind the splenium to form the **great vein of Galen**. From here, venous blood drains into the straight sinus (sinus rectus) and then into the confluence of the sinuses (confluens sinuum, torcular Herophili), which is the junction of the straight sinus, the superior sagittal sinus, and the transverse sinuses of the two sides (Figs. 11.**14-16**).

Dural Sinuses

The superficial and deep veins of the brain drain into the *cranial venous sinuses* formed by double folding of the inner dural membrane (Fig. 11.**17**). Most of the venous drainage from the cerebral convexities travels from front to back in the **superior sagittal sinus**, which runs in the midline along the attachment of the falx cerebri. At the point in the back of the head where the falx cerebri merges with the tentorium, the superior sagittal sinus is joined by the **straight sinus**, which runs in the midline along the attachment of the tentorium and carries blood from deep regions of the brain. Venous blood from the superior sagittal sinus and straight sinus is then distributed to the two **transverse sinuses** in the torcular Herophili ("winepress of Herophilus," after Herophilus of Alexandria); from each transverse sinus, blood drains into the **sigmoid sinus**, which then

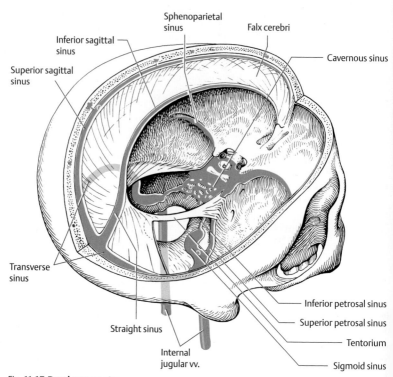

Fig. 11.17 Dural venous sinuses

continues below the jugular foramen as the internal jugular vein. The sinuses are often asymmetric, and there are a number of anatomical variants of the venous drainage pattern in the region of the torcular.

Blood from the brain drains not only into the internal jugular system, but also, by way of the pterygoid plexus, into the venous system of the viscerocranium. The **cavernous sinus**, formed by a double fold of dura mater at the base of the skull, also drains some of the venous blood from basal regions of the brain. It mainly receives blood from the temporal lobe and from the orbit (by way of the **superior** and **inferior ophthalmic veins**). It drains into a variety of venous channels. One of these is the sigmoid sinus, to which it is connected by the **superior** and **inferior petrosal sinuses**. Some of its blood also enters the pterygoid plexus.

Pathologically elevated venous pressure in the cavernous sinus, caused, for example, by the intracavernous rupture of an aneurysm of the internal carotid artery, causes reversal of flow in these veins, resulting in chemosis and exophthalmos.

Blood Supply of the Spinal Cord

Arterial Anastomotic Network

The spinal cord receives blood from an anastomotic network of arteries on its surface. There are three named longitudinal arteries, but these are multiply interconnected as they travel down the spinal cord, so that the vascular pattern resembles a chain of anastomoses rather than three distinct, independent vessels.

Anterior spinal artery. The unpaired (single) anterior spinal artery runs down the ventral surface of the spinal cord at the anterior edge of the anterior median fissure. It receives segmental contributions from a number of arteries (see below) and supplies the ventral part of the spinal gray matter through perforating vessels known as the *sulco-commissural arteries*. These arteries branch off segmentally from the anterior spinal artery and run transversely through the median fissure, from which they enter the parenchyma. Each sulco-commissural artery supplies one half of the spinal cord. Important structures supplied by the anterior spinal artery include the *anterior horns*, the *lateral spinothalamic tract*, and *part of the pyramidal tract* (Fig. 11.**18**).

Posterolateral spinal arteries. The posterolateral spinal arteries are the major longitudinal vessels on the dorsal side of the spinal cord; they run down the cord between the posterior roots and the lateral columns on either side. Like the anterior spinal artery, they arise from a confluence of segmental arteries; this confluence can be incomplete in places. The posterolateral spinal arteries supply the *posterior columns*, the *posterior roots*, and the *dorsal horns* (Fig. 11.**18**). The longitudinal axes are connected by radicular anastomoses. These supply the anterior and lateral columns through perforating branches.

The arteries of the spinal cord are interconnected by many anastomoses. Thus, proximal stenosis or occlusion of one of these arteries is usually asymptomatic. In the periphery, however, the arteries of the spinal cord are functional end arteries; intramedullary embolic occlusion of a sulco-commissural artery therefore causes *infarction of the spinal cord.*

Arteries Contributing to the Arterial Network of the Spinal Cord

The embryonic spinal cord receives its blood supply from segmental arteries, in accordance with the metameric segmentation of the spine. Over the course of development, many of these arteries regress, leaving only a few major ones to supply the cord. There is no way to know which of the original segmental arteries has persisted in the mature individual, except by angiography. Yet the blood

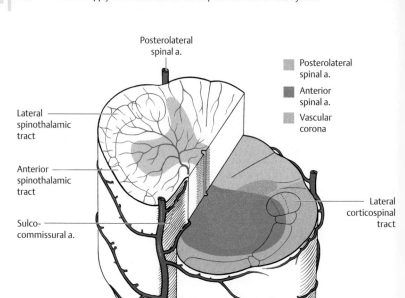

Fig. 11.**18 Arterial network of the spinal cord**

supply of the spinal cord does receive relatively constant contributions from a number of segmental levels (Fig. 11.**19**).

In the upper cervical region, the anterior spinal artery receives most of its blood from the **vertebral artery**. In principle, both vertebral arteries may supply blood to the anterior spinal artery, but the vertebral artery of one side is usually dominant. Further down the cord, the anterior and posterior longitudinal vessels receive most of their blood either from the vertebral artery or from cervical branches of the **subclavian artery** (or both). Spinal cord arteries preferentially arise from the *costocervical* or *thyrocervical trunk*. From T3 downward the anterior spinal artery is fed by aortic branches: the *thoracic and lumbar segmental arteries*, in addition to the branches that they give off to the musculature, connective tissue, and bones, also contribute a few branches to the anterior spinal artery or the posterolateral spinal artery. These spinal branches are the segmental spinal cord arteries that did not regress during embryonic development. Each one divides into an anterior and a posterior branch, which

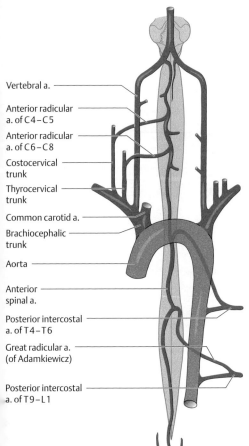

Fig. 11.19 Contributions of the segmental arteries to the arterial network of the spinal cord. After Thron A in Poeck K and Hacke W: Neurologie, 11th ed., Springer, Berlin/Heidelberg, 2001.

Vertebral a.

Anterior radicular a. of C4–C5

Anterior radicular a. of C6–C8

Costocervical trunk

Thyrocervical trunk

Common carotid a.

Brachiocephalic trunk

Aorta

Anterior spinal a.

Posterior intercostal a. of T4–T6

Great radicular a. (of Adamkiewicz)

Posterior intercostal a. of T9–L1

enter the spinal canal with the anterior and posterior root, respectively. Because the spinal cord elongates to a lesser extent than the vertebral column during development, each radicular artery enters the spinal cord some distance above its level of origin. There is usually one particularly large segmental artery supplying the lower spinal cord, which is called the **great radicular artery** or, more commonly, the *artery of Adamkiewicz*. The developmental "ascent" of the spinal cord makes this artery join the anterior spinal artery at an acute angle (hairpin configuration).

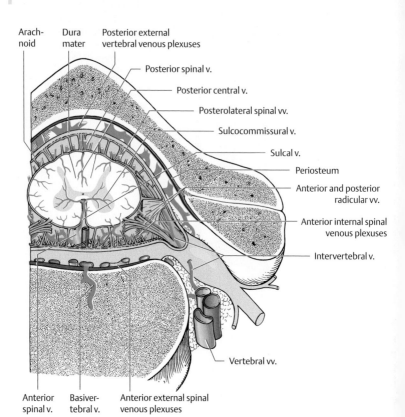

Fig. 11.**20 Venous drainage of the spinal cord**

Venous Drainage

The venous blood of the spinal cord drains into epimedullary veins that form a venous network in the subarachnoid space, called the internal spinal venous plexus or the e**pimedullary venous network**. These vessels communicate via radicular veins with the epidural venous plexus (external venous plexus, anterior and posterior external vertebral venous plexus). The venous blood then drains from the **epidural venous plexus** into the large veins of the body. The venous drainage of the spinal cord is shown in detail in Figure 11.**20**.

The finite ability of the radicular veins to drain blood from the epimedullary veins may be exceeded in the presence of arteriovenous malformations, even when the shunt volume is relatively low. The result is a rapid increase of venous pressure. Even small pressure increases can damage spinal cord tissue (see the section on impaired venous drainage, p. 473).

Cerebral Ischemia

Ischemic lesions of the brain parenchyma are caused by persistent disruption of the brain's blood supply, usually either by **blockage of the supplying (arterial) vessels** or, more rarely, **by an impediment to venous outflow** leading to stasis of blood in the brain, with secondary impairment of the delivery of oxygen and nutrients.

Arterial Hypoperfusion

General Pathophysiology of Cerebral Ischemia

The central nervous system has a **very high demand for energy** that can only be met by the continuous, uninterrupted delivery of metabolic substrates. Under normal conditions, this energy is derived exclusively from the aerobic metabolism of glucose. The brain has no way of storing energy to tide itself over potential interruptions of substrate delivery. If its neurons are not given enough glucose and oxygen, they can cease functioning within seconds.

Very different amounts of energy are needed to keep brain tissue alive (structurally intact) and to keep it functioning. The minimal blood flow requirement for **maintenance of structure** is about 5-8 ml per 100 g per minute (in the first hour of ischemia). In contrast, the minimal blood flow requirement for **continued function** is 20 ml per 100 g per minute. It follows that there may be a functional deficit in the absence of death of tissue (infarction). If the endangered blood supply is rapidly restored, as by spontaneous or therapeutic thrombolysis, the brain tissue remains undamaged and recovers its function as before, i.e., the neurological deficit regresses completely. This is the sequence of events in a **transient ischemic attack** (**TIA**), which is clinically defined as a transient neurological deficit of no more than 24 hours' duration. Eighty percent of all TIAs last less than 30 minutes. Their clinical manifestations depend on the particular vascular territory of the brain that is affected. TIAs in the territory of the middle cerebral artery are common; patients report transient contralateral paresthesiae and sensory deficits, as well as transient contralateral weakness. Such attacks are sometimes hard to distinguish from focal epileptic seizures. Ischemia in the vertebrobasilar territory, on the other hand, causes transient brainstem symptoms and signs, including vertigo.

Neurological deficits due to ischemia can sometimes regress even though they have lasted for more than 24 hours; in such cases, one speaks, not of a TIA, but of a **PRIND** (**prolonged reversible ischemic neurological deficit**).

If hypoperfusion persists longer than the brain tissue can tolerate, cell death ensues. **Ischemic stroke** is not reversible. Cell death with collapse of the blood-brain-barrier results in an influx of water into the infarcted brain tissue (accompanying **cerebral edema**). The infarct thus begins to swell within hours of the ischemic event, is maximally swollen a few days later, and then gradually contracts again.

In patients with large infarcts with extensive accompanying edema, **clinical signs of life-threatening intracranial hypertension such as headache, vomiting, and disturbances of consciousness must be noted and treated appropriately** (see below). The critical infarct volume needed for this situation to arise varies depending on the patient's age and brain volume. Younger patients with normal-sized brains are at risk after extensive infarction in the territory of the middle cerebral artery alone. In contrast, older patients with brain atrophy may not be in danger unless the infarct involves the territories of two or more cerebral vessels. Often, in such situations, the patient's life can be saved only by timely medical treatment to lower the intracranial pressure, or by surgical removal of a large piece of the skull (hemicraniectomy) in order to decompress the swollen brain.

In the aftermath of infarction, the dead brain tissue liquefies and is resorbed. What remains is a **cystic cavity filled with cerebrospinal fluid**, perhaps containing a few blood vessels and strands of connective tissue, along with reactive glial changes (astrogliosis) in the surrounding parenchyma. No scar is formed in the proper sense of the term (proliferation of collagenous tissue).

The importance of collateral circulation. The temporal course and extent of cerebral parenchymal edema depend not only on the patency of the blood vessel(s) that normally supply the brain region at risk, but also on the availability of collateral circulation through other pathways. In general, the arteries of the brain are functional end arteries: collateral pathways normally cannot provide enough blood to sustain brain tissue distal to a suddenly occluded artery. If an artery becomes narrow very slowly and progressively, however, the capacity of the collateral circulation can increase. Collaterals can often be "trained" by chronic, mild tissue hypoxia to the extent that they can meet the energetic needs of tissue even if the main arterial supply is blocked for relatively long periods of time. The infarct is then much smaller, and far fewer neurons are lost than one would otherwise see if the same artery were suddenly occluded from a state of normal patency.

Collateral blood supply may arrive from the basal anastomotic ring of vessels (circle of Willis) or from superficial leptomeningeal anastomoses of the cerebral arteries. As a rule, collateral circulation is better at the periphery of an infarct than at its center. The ischemic brain tissue at the periphery that is at risk of dying (infarction) but, because of collateral circulation, has not yet been irreversibly damaged is called the **penumbra** (half-shadow) of the infarct. Rescuing this area is the goal of all forms of acute stroke therapy, including thrombolytic therapy (cf. Case Presentations 4 and 5, p. 456 ff.).

Causes of Cerebral Ischemia: Types of Infarction

Embolic Infarction

Eighty percent of ischemic strokes are caused by emboli. Blood clots, or pieces of debris that have broken away from an atheromatous plaque in the wall of one of the extracranial great vessels, are carried by the bloodstream into the brain, where they become lodged in the lumen of a functional end artery. Proximal embolic occlusion of the main trunk of a cerebral artery causes extensive infarction in its entire territory (**territorial infarction**).

Most emboli arise either from **atheromatous lesions of the carotid bifurcation** or from the **heart**. Rarely, emboli arising in the peripheral venous circulation are carried by the bloodstream into the brain (*so-called paradoxical emboli*). A precondition for this occurrence is a patent foramen ovale, which furnishes the necessary connection between the venous and arterial circulations at the level of the atria. In the normal case, the foramen ovale is closed and venous thrombi are filtered out of the circulation in the lungs, so that they cannot pass through to the arterial side.

Embolic thrombi are sometimes spontaneously dissolved by the fibrinolytic activity of the blood. If this happens rapidly, the patient's neurological deficit may regress, with full recovery and no lasting damage. If the thrombus is not dissolved for hours or days, however, cell death ensues and the neurological deficit is usually irreversible.

Hemodynamic Infarction

Hemodynamic infarction is caused by a **critical drop in perfusion pressure** in a distal arterial segment as the result of a more proximal stenosis. Such events usually occur in the territories of long, perforating arteries deep within the cerebral white matter. The resulting infarcts are seen to lie like chains in the white matter of the centrum semiovale.

Hemodynamic infarction is much rarer than embolic infarction. This fact may, at first, seem incompatible with the observation that the risk of stroke increases in proportion to the degree of carotid stenosis; in fact, however, only very few patients with slowly progressive carotid stenosis ever develop hemodynamic infarcts. This is because the area of brain at risk often receives an adequate collateral blood supply from the contralateral internal carotid artery and the vertebral arteries, and, in addition, anastomotic channels open up to convey blood from the external carotid artery to intracranial branches of the internal carotid artery (cf. p. 432). The real reason that patients with tighter stenoses are at greater risk of stroke is that, in such patients, an embolus is more likely to form or break away from the atheromatous plaque in the carotid wall.

Hemodynamic infarcts are usually found in the **hemispheric white matter** (see Fig. 11.**21**). They are aligned in chains running from anterior to posterior. Cortical ischemia, in contrast, is almost always of embolic origin. Incompleteness of the circle of Willis due to hypoplasia or absence of some of its component arterial segments has been shown to be a precondition for the occurrence of hemodynamic stroke. If the circle of Willis is intact, a single great vessel of the neck can suffice to supply blood to the entire brain!

Hemodynamic infarction differs from embolic infarction in a number of characteristic ways that facilitate its diagnosis. It often causes a **fluctuating neurological deficit**, corresponding to fluctuations of blood flow in the poststenotic arterial segment. Because the overall perfusion drops slowly in such situations, there may be a protracted period of time in which the brain tissue at risk lacks the blood it needs to function properly but is still receiving enough to sustain its structural metabolism. In embolic infarction, on the other hand, the regional blood flow immediately sinks below the level needed to maintain tissue structure—at least at the center of the infarct. This explains why neurological deficits due to hemodynamic ischemia are often reversible for a longer period of time than those due to embolic stroke.

Case Presentation 1: *Hemodynamic Infarction*

This retired 72-year-old man had suffered from arterial hypertension and diabetes mellitus for many years, but felt generally well. His last routine medical check-up had revealed a high serum cholesterol concentration. One afternoon, while taking a walk with his family, he noticed that his left arm felt heavy and that he could no longer walk steadily. His daughter took him to the hospital, where the admitting physician found a left hemiparesis, more severe in the arm than in the leg, with sinking of both left limbs in postural testing. He walked unsteadily because of the left leg weakness, but had no sensory abnormality.

A diffusion-weighted MRI scan of the head revealed multiple, neighboring zones of acute ischemia in the deep white matter of the right cerebral hemisphere, appearing to form a chain

(Fig. 11.**21a**, **b**). These lesions were interpreted as arterial end-zone infarcts due to hemodynamic insufficiency. MR angiography (Fig. 11.**21c**, **d**) and Doppler ultrasonography (Fig. 11.**21e**) revealed a hemodynamically significant 90–95% stenosis of the right internal carotid artery. As soon as the diagnostic evaluation was complete, the patient underwent thrombendarterectomy, without complication. He went on to recover fully from his hemiparesis and was discharged home one week after admission.

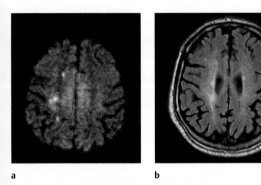

a   b

Fig. 11.21 Hemodynamic infarction due to high-grade stenosis of the right internal carotid artery

c MR angiography of the arteries of the base of the brain. In the flow-sensitive image, the right internal carotid artery is less well visualized than its counterpart on the left side. This finding suggests that there may be a hemodynamically significant stenosis proximal to the area of impaired flow.

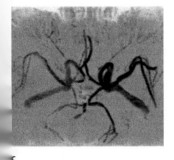

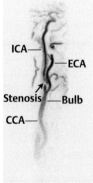

d Contrast-enhanced MR angiography.

c

d

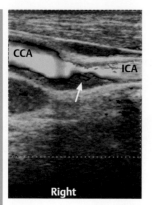

(Continued) Fig. 11.**21 Hemodynamic infarction due to high-grade stenosis of the right internal carotid artery e** Color duplex sonography reveals high-grade stenosis at the origin of the internal carotid artery, with ulceration. Blood is flowing from left to right, from the common carotid artery into the internal carotid artery. The color indicates the speed of flow. A plaque is evident as a dark structure behind the lumen, which contains flowing blood. The red-colored area in the craterlike pit (plaque) shows that there is flowing blood here, too: this finding implies ulceration (arrow). (Image kindly supplied by Dr. H. Krapf, Tübingen.)

Lacunar Infarction

Lacunar infarcts are caused by **microangiopathic changes of smaller arteries** with progressive narrowing of the lumen and subsequent occlusion. The most important risk factor is *arterial hypertension*, which leads to hyalinosis of the vascular wall of smaller arteries. The perforating, long, and thin lenticulostriate arteries are most commonly involved; thus, lacunar infarction commonly occurs in the *internal capsule*, the *basal ganglia*, the *hemispheric white matter*, and the *pons*. The **lesions are typically spherical or tubular**, appearing round on CT or MRI; they are usually less than 10 mm in diameter. Lacunar infarction also occurs in the territory of the perforating brainstem arteries. Because lacunar infarction usually occurs in the setting of arterial hypertension, it is often accompanied by microangiopathic abnormalities of the deep cerebral white matter ("*microangiopathic leukoencephalopathy*" or *leukoaraiosis*). Acute lacunar infarcts can be distinguished from older ones only by diffusion-weighted MRI, or by comparison with previously obtained radiological studies.

Case Presentation 2: *Lacunar Infarction*

This 58-year-old lawyer had had arterial hypertension for many years. This had initially been well controlled; in recent months, however, there had been multiple, prolonged, and dangerous elevations of blood pressure, despite medication. One night, he awoke with a feeling of weakness in the right leg, which lasted only a few minutes before returning to normal. He felt fully well the next day and went to work as usual. A short time later, while talking and drinking coffee with a client, he suddenly noticed that the coffee was dribbling out of the right corner of his mouth, and he had difficulty articulating words properly. At the same time, his right arm felt very weak. He no longer had the strength to get up and walk. His secretary called an ambulance, and he was taken to the hospital.

The admitting neurologist found a mainly brachiofacial right hemiparesis, without any accompanying sensory deficit. MRI revealed the cause, a small infarct in the left internal capsule. The diffusion-weighted image revealed an acute ischemic process (Fig. 11.**22a**), and the

better spatial resolution of the T2-weighted image enabled its precise anatomical localization (Fig. 11.**22b**).

Diagnostic studies of the heart revealed no abnormality. The patient remained in the hospital for two weeks, during which time his antihypertensive medication was readjusted for better blood pressure control. He was given an inhibitor of platelet aggregation to prevent recurrent infarction. His hemiparesis resolved to a marked, but incomplete, extent, and he was transferred from the hospital to an inpatient rehabilitation unit.

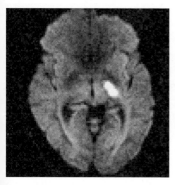 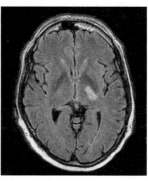

a   b

Fig. 11.**22 Lacunar infarct in the left internal capsule. a** Diffusion-weighted image. The infarct in the posterior limb of the internal capsule and the posterior portion of the thalamus is markedly hyperintense, implying acute infarction. This image was obtained 24 hours after the onset of symptoms. **b** The T2-weighted FLAIR image reveals the same hyperintense infarct in the internal capsule and thalamus. T2 hyperintensity persists long after the acute event; thus, a T2-weighted image alone is insufficient for estimation of the age of the lesion.

The Diagnostic Evaluation of Cerebral Ischemia

The goals of diagnostic evaluation are to determine **the site and extent of the ischemic lesion** and, most importantly, its **cause**. Only a precise etiological diagnosis will lead to the appropriate treatment that, in favorable cases, can halt the progression of an infarct and prevent future recurrences.

The diagnostic tools used in this evaluation are a precise case history and a clinical neurological and general physical examination, along with specifically chosen, complementary laboratory tests and imaging studies. **CT** and **MRI** are used to demonstrate the presence of ischemia and differentiate it from hemorrhage (see below). Furthermore, the site and visual "gestalt" of an infarct may provide initial clues regarding its type (embolic/territorial, hemodynamic, lacunar, cf. p. 445 ff.) and, therefore, its cause: for example, a territorial infarct in the middle cerebral artery territory is probably of embolic origin, and the embolus, in turn, probably came from the carotid bifurcation or the heart. The search for an etiology also includes cardiovascular studies: **ECG** and **cardiac ultrasonography** provide information about possible underlying heart disease predisposing to cerebral ischemia (e. g., insufficient cardiac pumping activity due to arrhythmia or any of the myriad causes of congestive heart failure; intracardiac thrombi as a source of embolism). Abnormalities of the cerebral blood vessels themselves can be detected with **extracranial and transcranial ultrasonography** and with **angiography**—for example, stenosis or atherosclerotic plaque as a source of arterioarterial embolism. MR angiography, in combination with ultrasonography, often suffices to establish the diagnosis of vascular pathology, but conventional angiography with digital subtraction (DSA) is still occasionally necessary.

We will now briefly discuss each of the major diagnostic methods individually.

Ancillary Diagnostic Studies in Cerebral Ischemia

Computerized tomography (CT) reveals ischemic areas no sooner than two hours after the onset of hypoperfusion. It does, however, show intracranial hemorrhage immediately and reliably. Any patient with the sudden or subacute onset of a neurological deficit should therefore receive a CT scan as soon as possible, so that a hemorrhage can be diagnosed or ruled out. A further advantage of CT, compared to MRI, is its rapid availability. Its inability to demonstrate the initial phase of acute ischemia is a major disadvantage: CT scans are generally normal precisely at the moment when causal treatment of cerebral ischemia is still possible. Furthermore, for technical reasons (artifact), infarcts in the posterior fossa and purely cortical ischemia are often not revealed by CT until late in their course, or may never be seen at all. If the initial CT scan reveals no lesion, it is reasonable to repeat the study ca. 24 hours later as an initially invisible infarct may be demonstrable the second time. Alternatively, an MRI scan can be obtained immediately after the initial, negative CT scan.

Recently, CT techniques have been developed that enable the detection of vascular occlusion in the acute phase (CT angiography), or an interruption of blood supply to an area of the brain that otherwise appears normal (perfusion CT). The clinical usefulness of these methods is currently being assessed.

There is no evidence to suggest that the administration of contrast medium increases the size of infarcts, despite earlier speculation to that effect. Nonetheless, intravenous contrast medium is only rarely needed in the subacute phase. Infarcts begin to take up contrast medium strongly on the fourth to sixth day after the acute ischemic event because of disruption of the blood-brain barrier. This phenomenon, when combined with an imprecise history, may lead to the misdiagnosis of an infarct as a neoplasm (e.g., lymphoma).

Magnetic resonance imaging (MRI) reveals ischemia within a few minutes of onset. Brain cells deprived of energy swell with water because their energy-dependent membrane pumps cease to function (cytotoxic edema). Edema, in turn, slows the water molecules in the blood vessels of the infarct zone, and this slowing can be demonstrated immediately after the onset of ischemia, and very rapidly, with diffusion-weighted MR sequences. Combined with conventional sequences for anatomical imaging, diffusion-weighted MRI detects ischemia highly reliably anywhere in the brain. MRI also reveals cerebral infarcts that are not seen by CT in patients with transient or only mild neurological deficits (e.g., purely cortical infarcts in the so-called noneloquent areas of the brain, such as the frontal association cortex or right insula). Brainstem infarcts, too, are readily seen. Furthermore, the blood vessels supplying the brain are well visualized both extracranially and intracranially. MR angiography is risk-free, which cannot be said of conventional angiography with intra-arterial contrast medium; its quality, however, still falls short of the standard set by DSA. Two disadvantages of MRI are its limited availability as an emergency study and the relatively long time needed to perform it, which makes it susceptible to movement artifacts.

Of all neuroimaging methods, **digital subtraction angiography (DSA)** (i.e., visualization of the blood vessels of the brain with intra-arterially injected radiographic contrast medium) still provides the best morphological view of pathological changes in the extracranial and intracranial vessels. Each study, however, carries its own small risk of stroke or other complications, and its indications are therefore being progressively limited to a small number of specific clinical situations. Contemporary ultrasound and MRI techniques are available as risk-free alternatives. Because angiography does not visualize brain tissue, it can only reveal infarcts indirectly.

Ultrasonography is routinely used in the diagnostic evaluation of cerebral ischemia. Modern color-coded methods enable rapid, risk-free, and reliable assessment of the great vessels of the neck, with quantification of any stenoses that might be present (Fig. 11.**21**). Some of the intracranial vessels can even be studied by Doppler ultrasonography through the bony skull (i.e., trans-cranially), but this technique is of limited reliability.

Radionuclide studies. In addition to the techniques discussed above for the morphological study of the brain and the cerebral vasculature, modern nuclear medicine provides other techniques for the study of functional parameters such as regional cerebral blood flow (rCBF). The two most important types of functional study are **positron emission tomography** (**PET**) and **single-photon emission computerized tomography** (**SPECT**). Very recently, sophisticated MRI and CT techniques for the measurement of rCBF have also been introduced. As a comment on all of these types of studies, it should be noted that, because most strokes are due to emboli rather than preexisting deficiencies of regional perfusion, measuring blood flow is generally useless as a means of predicting stroke. Thus, the assessment of rCBF by any of these techniques is only indicated in certain specific situations.

Case Presentation 3: **The Use of Imaging Studies for Definitive Diagnosis in Neurology**

This case illustrates how clinical problems in neurology can be solved by precise correlation of the findings of clinical history-taking, physical examination, and ancillary studies. The history and physical examination often enable fairly precise localization of the lesion, but further laboratory tests and neuroimaging are usually needed to pinpoint its etiology.

This previously healthy 59-year-old school-teacher suddenly became weak on the entire right side of his body, most severely in the leg, and was well again a short time later. During the episode, he also had transient sensory abnormalities in *both* legs. An MRI scan of the brain with diffusion-weighted (Fig. 11.**23a**) and T2-weighted sequences (not shown) revealed a small, acute infarct in the left parietal lobe. MR angiography (Fig. 11.**23b**, **c**) and intra-arterial digital subtraction angiography (Fig. 11.**23d**, **e**)

revealed a high-grade, calcific stenosis of the left internal carotid artery. The infarct had apparently been caused by transient hemodynamic insufficiency on the basis of this stenotic lesion. The infarct sufficed to explain the patient's transient right hemiparesis, but not the transient sensory abnormality in his *left* leg, which could only be attributed to hypoperfusion in the territory of the *right* anterior cerebral artery. Because this vessel is ordinarily not a branch of the left internal cerebral artery, a possible second cause of cerebral ischemia had to be sought.

The left carotid lesion described above had no counterpart in the right internal carotid artery, which was normal. The MR angiogram, however, showed *both* anterior cerebral arteries receiving blood from the left internal carotid artery; a normal anatomical variant was pre sent, in which the initial, or "precommunicating," segment of the left anterior cerebral artery (the left A1 segment) was hypoplastic. The left carotid stenosis thus sufficed to explain all of the patient's symptoms, including weak-ness in the left leg, due to hypoperfusion in the territory of the left anterior cerebral artery. In this case, definitive diagnosis would have been impossible without imaging studies of the cerebral vasculature.

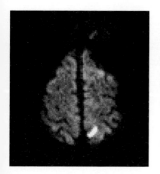

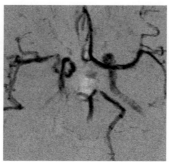

a

b

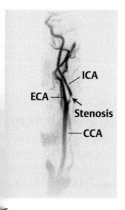

c

Fig. 11.**23 Infarct in the territory of the left anterior cerebral artery and transient ischemia in the right anterior circulation due to high-grade stenosis of the left internal carotid artery. a** Diffusion-weighted MRI. Abnormally bright signal is seen in the parasagittal portion of the left postcentral gyrus, indicating acute ischemia in the territory of the left anterior cerebral artery. **b** MR angiography of the arteries of the base of the brain. Both anterior cerebral arteries are supplied by the left internal carotid artery. **c** Contrast-enhanced MR angiography of the arteries of the neck. High-grade stenosis at the origin of the left internal carotid artery is the probable cause of the embolic infarction in the left anterior circulation, clinically manifest as right hemiparesis mainly affecting the leg. The patient had also reported a transient sensory disturbance in the left leg, which was most likely due to a transient impairment of flow in the right anterior cerebral artery. Because both anterior cerebral arteries are supplied by the left internal carotid artery in this patient, the bi-hemispheric symptoms can be traced back to a *single* common cause (left ICA stenosis).

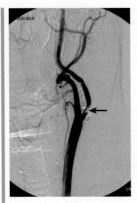 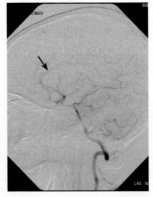

d   **e**

(Continued) **Fig. 11.23 Infarct in the territory of the left anterior cerebral artery and transient ischemia in the right anterior circulation due to high-grade stenosis of the left internal carotid artery. d** This intra-arterial digital subtraction angiogram demonstrates the high-grade stenosis of the left ICA very well (arrow). **e** This angiographic image, obtained after injection of contrast medium into one of the vertebral arteries, reveals a further sign of carotid stenosis: there is intracranial reversal of flow in the posterior communicating artery, which is supplied with blood in retrograde fashion from the basilar artery. The pericallosal artery (arrow) obtains blood from the posterior communicating artery and can thus be seen after vertebral injection. Normal flow in the posterior communicating artery is from the anterior to the posterior circulation (internal carotid to posterior cerebral artery).

The Treatment of Ischemic Stroke

Acute Treatment

In the acute phase of ischemic stroke, the physician's efforts are mainly directed at limiting irreversible neuronal loss in the ischemic area, to whatever extent this is possible. Treatment is aimed at rescuing brain tissue that has become dysfunctional because of ischemia, but is still structurally intact (the ischemic penumbra, p. 445). The rescue strategy is to **restore "normal" circulation in the ischemic area as rapidly as possible**.

In consideration of this overall strategy, the most obvious therapeutic approach—at least in theory—is the **rapid recanalization of the blocked vessel**. If the vessel is obstructed by an embolus, for example, the embolus can be dissolved by accelerating the body's fibrinolytic system (**thrombolytic therapy**). The thrombolytic agent, either *recombinant tissue plasminogen activator* (*rtPA*) or *urokinase*, can be given either intravenously (i.e., systemically) or intra-arterially. The possible indications for thrombolytic therapy must be considered in all patients with acute stroke. Only 5-7% of patients will turn out to be candidates for it, however, because it is effective only when performed according to the study criteria, i.e., very soon after the onset of neurological signs and symptoms—within three hours for systemic thrombolysis, and within six hours for local thrombolysis. Intracranial hemorrhage must be ruled out by CT or MRI before thrombolysis is performed.

In all patients suffering from acute stroke, whether or not they can be treated with thrombolysis, a number of clinical factors must be carefully controlled to assure the best possible outcome. In general, an **adequate perfusion pressure must be maintained** in the area of brain at risk. Thus, the *arterial blood pressure is closely monitored*, and no antihypertensive therapy is given unless the systolic pressure exceeds 180 mmHg. The *cardiovascular parameters are optimally stabilized* (adequate hydration, treatment of hemodynamically significant arrhythmia or heart failure). Furthermore, **pathological energy-consuming and oxygen-consuming metabolic processes must be counteracted**: hyperglycemia and fever, for example, markedly worsen the patient's prognosis. The vital signs and the serum electrolyte concentrations should be monitored. Dysphagic patients should be treated early with parenteral nutrition to reduce the risk of aspiration pneumonia and consequent hypoxia. Over the last decade, it has been found to be very useful to care for acute stroke patients in specialized *stroke units* in which the necessary diagnostic testing can be accomplished rapidly and all of the therapeutic measures just discussed can be efficiently implemented.

In patients with large infarcts, the **clinical signs of elevated intracranial pressure must be watched for and treated** (headache, nausea, vomiting; finally, loss of consciousness and perhaps anisocoria). Nonsurgical measures may suffice to bring the intracranial pressure back down to safe levels, as long as the infarct and surrounding edema are not too large: such measures include *elevating the head of the bed to 30°*, *hyperventilation* (if the patient is attached to a ventilator), and *mannitol infusion*. In younger patients with very large infarcts, hemicraniectomy should be considered at an early stage before the increasing intracranial pressure further impairs cerebral perfusion.

The administration of so-called neuroprotective drugs has been found to affect infarct size favorably in animal models of stroke, but the hope that these drugs would bring similar results in acute stroke patients has, so far, not been borne out statistically in clinical trials. One reason for the apparent failure of neuroprotection may be that the trial inclusion criteria to date have not been strict enough; future studies will screen potential patients with MRI and select only those considered most likely to benefit from the treatment. Likewise, full heparinization and hemodilution have not been shown to have any beneficial effect in acute ischemic stroke, except in special situations.

Case Presentation 4: Thrombolysis in the Middle Cerebral Artery

This 69-year-old man was admitted to the oph-thalmology service of a teaching hospital for an elective retinal procedure. While undergoing preoperative evaluation, he suddenly developed left hemiplegia. A CT scan of the head, ordered as an emergency, was normal and was followed within 15 minutes by an MRI scan, in-cluding visualization of the blood vessels and diffusion-weighted sequences. The cause of the acute left hemiplegia was found to be a distal

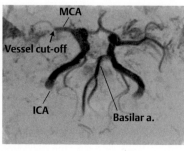
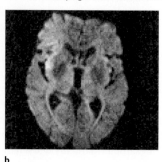

a   b

Fig. 11.**24 Thrombolysis in the right middle cerebral artery after acute thrombotic occlusion of its main stem. a** MR angiography of the arteries of the base of the brain. "Cut-off" of the right middle cerebral artery (MCA) indicates occlusion. **b** Diffusion-weighted MRI. Only a mild abnormal-ity of diffusion is visible as an area of hyperintensity in the right insular cortex. There is thus no definitive evidence of irreversible ischemic injury (i.e., infarction).

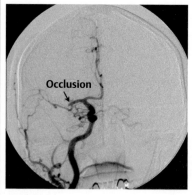
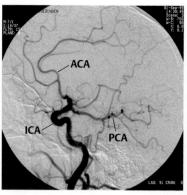

c   d

(Continued) Fig. 11.**24 Thrombolysis in the right middle cerebral artery after acute thrombotic occlusion of its main stem. c and d** Intra-arterial digital subtraction angiography in A-P (**c**) and lateral (**d**) projections after injection of contrast medium into the right common carotid artery The main stem of the middle cerebral artery is occluded distal to the origin of a large temporal branch. The anterior and posterior cerebral arteries (ACA, PCA) can be seen more easily than usual on the lateral projection because the normally overshadowing branches of the MCA are absent.

occlusion of the main trunk of the right middle cerebral artery (Fig. 11.**24a**). The diffusion-weighted image showed no evidence of irreversible infarction (Fig. 11.**24b**).

The patient was transferred to the neurology service. Intra-arterial thrombolysis was considered to be indicated, because less than three hours had elapsed from the onset of the neurological deficit, and because it did not appear that major, irreversible parenchymal injury had already occurred. He was taken to the angiography suite. First, the vascular occlusion was de-

monstrated angiographically (Fig. 11.**24c**, **d**). Then, a microcatheter was introduced into the middle cerebral artery just proximal to the thrombus, and 1 million units of urokinase were infused through it (Fig. 11.**24e**). This resulted in the complete dissolution of the thrombus (Fig. 11.**24f**, **g**). The patient's hemiplegia resolved completely, though a cortical infarct in the insular region remained visible by MRI (Fig. 11.**24h**). He was discharged eight days after the acute event and received further care as an outpatient.

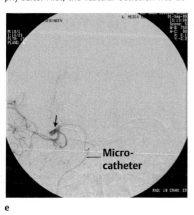

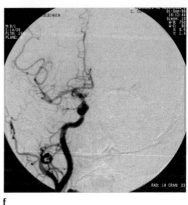

e f

(Continued) Fig. 11.**24 Thrombolysis in the right middle cerebral artery after acute thrombotic occlusion of its main stem. e** A microcatheter has been introduced by way of the internal carotid artery into the middle cerebral artery; its tip lies just proximal to the thrombus (arrow). Urokinase was infused through this catheter. **f** A follow-up angiogram obtained ca. 90 minutes after intra-arterial thrombolysis demonstrates restoration of flow in the middle cerebral artery.

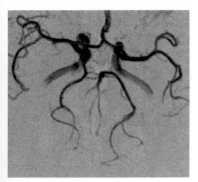

g Follow-up MR angiography also demonstrates recanalization of the middle cerebral artery (compare to **b**).

g

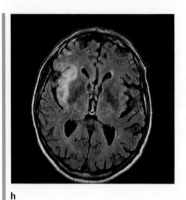

(Continued) Fig. 11.**24 Thrombolysis in the right middle cerebral artery after acute thrombotic occlusion of its main stem.**

h T2-weighted FLAIR image. Despite rapid recanalization of the right middle cerebral artery, infarction has occurred in part of the insular cortex. The underlying white matter does not appear to be involved to any significant extent. The prompt treatment of this patient with thrombolysis probably prevented much more extensive infarction.

h

Case Presentation 5: *Thrombolysis in a Case of Basilar Artery Thrombosis*

This 27-year-old student was riding a bicycle when she noticed a "fuzzy feeling." Because she could no longer ride straight, she got off her bicycle and sat down by the side of the road. A short time later, she became nauseated and vomited several times. The driver of a passing car stopped and got out to help. She could not respond adequately to his questions, but merely mumbled unintelligibly and lost consciousness shortly afterward. The driver notified the emergency medical service and the patient was taken to the hospital.

On admission, she was unconscious and withdrew her limbs from noxious stimuli on the right side only; therefore, a left hemiparesis was suspected. Her pupils were equal in size. The physician on duty in the emergency room ordered a CT scan to rule out an intracranial hemorrhage. The CT scan was normal, and was therefore immediately followed by an MRI scan including visualization of the cerebral vessels (Fig. 11.**25a**) and a diffusion-weighted image (Fig. 11.**25b**). The cause of the neurological deficits was found to be thrombosis of the basilar artery (Fig. 11.**25a**). No irreversible parenchymal injury was found to have occurred up to this point (Fig. 11.**25b**). Conventional transfemoral catheter angiography confirmed distal occlusion of the basilar artery (Fig. 11.**25c, d**); the tip of the basilar artery and the two posterior cerebral arteries were still patent and were supplied by the carotid artery by way of the posterior communicating artery (Fig. 11.**25e, f**). A microcatheter was introduced to the level of the thrombus (Fig. 11.**25g**) and 100 mg of rtPA were infused, resulting in disappearance of most of the thrombus (Fig. 11.**25h**). The patient's deficits resolved fully within two days, though a follow-up MRI scan revealed small infarcts in the pons and cerebellum (Fig. 11.**25i, j**). An exhaustive diagnostic evaluation failed to reveal the cause of the basilar artery thrombosis. The patient was asymptomatic on her discharge from the hospital 15 days after admission.

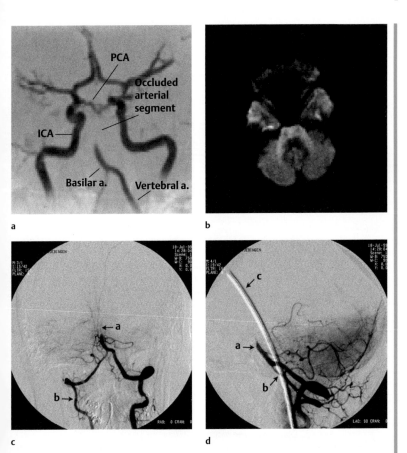

Fig. 11.**25 Thrombolysis in basilar artery thrombosis. a** The initial MR angiogram reveals lack of flow in the distal portion of the basilar artery (the course of the occluded arterial segment is sketched in dotted lines). The basilar tip receives blood from the anterior circulation through the circle of Willis. **b** The diffusion-weighted image of the brain is normal. Despite occlusion of the basilar artery, no infarction has occurred. The relatively intense signal in the pons is normal and is due to the middle cerebellar peduncles. The bright areas in the temporal lobes are due to artefact. **c and d** Digital subtraction angiography after injection of contrast medium into the left vertebral artery; A-P (**c**) and lateral (**d**) projections. The basilar artery is occluded distally (arrow a). Resistance to forward flow in the basilar artery causes reflux of the injected contrast medium into the opposite (right) vertebral artery (arrow b). Because the anterior and posterior inferior cerebellar arteries remain open, a vascular flush is seen in the inferior portion of the cerebellum. The superior cerebellar arteries, however, lie distal to the obstruction, and there is therefore no flush in the superior portion of the cerebellum. In **d** an artefact caused by an ECG cable lying in the path of the x-ray beam is seen (arrow c).

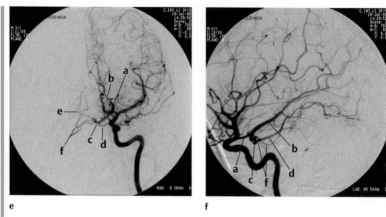

e   f

(Continued) Fig. 11.**25 Thrombolysis in basilar artery thrombosis. e and f** Digital subtraction an-giography after injection of contrast medium into the left internal carotid artery. A large posterior communicating artery (a) supplies the left posterior cerebral artery (b) with blood from the anterior circulation. The basilar tip (c), too, fills with contrast medium derived in retrograde fashion from the initial segment of the posterior cerebral artery (the P1 segment). Vessels filling with contrast from the basilar artery include the left superior cerebellar artery (d), the right posterior cerebral artery (e), and the doubled right superior cerebellar artery (f). The apparently weak filling of the right posterior cerebral artery is caused by "washout" of contrast medium by contrast-free blood that enters this vessel from the anterior circulation via the right posterior communicating artery, as was independ-ently confirmed by injection of the right internal carotid artery (study not shown).

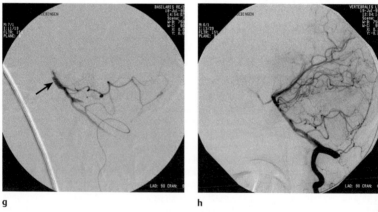

g   h

(Continued) Fig. 11.**25 Thrombolysis in basilar artery thrombosis. g** Superselective microcathe-terization of the basilar artery. The tip of the microcatheter lies just proximal to the thrombus (arrow). 100 mg of rtPA (recombinant tissue plasminogen activator) were injected through it. **h** Fol-low-up study 90 minutes after rtPA injection: the basilar artery is fully recanalized (cf. **d**).

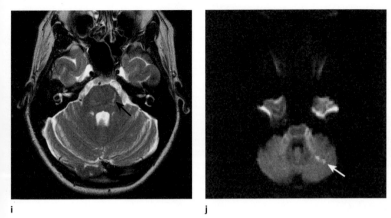

i   j

(Continued) Fig. 11.**25 Thrombolysis in basilar artery thrombosis. i and j** Follow-up MRI two days later. The patient was asymptomatic at this time. **i** The T2-weighted image reveals a small left pontine lesion (arrow) but no more extensive infarct. **j** The diffusion-weighted image additionally reveals a small lesion in the left cerebellar hemisphere (arrow).

Primary and Secondary Prophylaxis

In addition to the treatment of acute cerebral ischemia, a number of therapeutic measures are directed at the prevention of a first or second stroke in patients at risk for these events.

Primary prophylaxis. The goal of primary prophylaxis is to prevent a first stroke by treating the predisposing risk factors (Table 11.**1**). Its most important component is the effective **treatment of arterial hypertension**, which, besides age, is the single most important risk factor for stroke. High blood pressure also increases the patient's risk of intracerebral or subarachnoid hemorrhage. Normalization of blood pressure can reduce the risk of ischemic stroke by 40%. Other controllable risk factors include *cigarette smoking, diabetes mellitus*, and *atrial fibrillation*. The administration of aspirin and other inhibitors of platelet aggregation is not a component of primary prophylaxis.

The surgical treatment of asymptomatic stenosis of the internal carotid artery is also performed for primary prophylaxis, despite the absence of clear statistical evidence of benefit. Commonly used indications for this procedure at present include rapidly progressive, hemodynamically significant carotid stenosis, or occlusion of one internal carotid artery and simultaneous high-grade stenosis of the contralateral internal carotid artery.

Table 11.1 Risk Factors for Ischemic Stroke

Risk Factor	Relative Risk*
Age 65–74	6
Age 75–80	12
Hypertension	7
Smoking	2
Diabetes mellitus	2
Obesity	2
Hyperlipidemia	2
Atrial fibrillation	10

* I.e., the ratio of the probability of stroke in persons with the risk factor to the probability of stroke in persons without the risk factor.

Secondary prophylaxis. The goal of secondary prophylaxis is to prevent stroke after at least one episode of cerebral ischemia has already occurred. Both medical and surgical methods are used for secondary prophylaxis. The administration of **low-dose aspirin** (100 mg/day) lowers the risk of recurrent stroke by about 25%. There is no evidence that higher doses are better. Other inhibitors of platelet aggregation, such as *ticlopidine* and *clopidogrel*, have a more pronounced protective effect than aspirin, but this advantage is offset by their greater expense and some serious side effects. Therapeutic anticoagulation with warfarin is extremely effective in reducing the risk of stroke in patients with atrial fibrillation and an irregular heartbeat (patients with this type of arrhythmia are at increased risk of intracardiac thrombus formation with subsequent embolization into the brain); the relative risk reduction in this setting is 60-80%.

Large-scale studies have shown that the **surgical treatment of symptomatic, high-grade (i.e., at least 70–80%) stenosis of the internal carotid artery** lowers the relative risk of stroke in the follow-up period by ca. 50%, and is therefore worthwhile, as long as the operation can be performed with acceptably low perioperative morbidity and mortality. A newer method of treating carotid stenosis is **endoluminal dilation and stenting**. This method has already been in use for some time in other blood vessels, including the renal and coronary arteries. Studies comparing it to carotid endarterectomy for the treatment of carotid stenosis are currently underway.

The usefulness of a medication or operation used for secondary prophylaxis can only be expressed in terms of *statistical reduction of the risk of stroke*.

Stroke cannot be predicted with certainty in any individual case. As we have already pointed out several times, stroke is usually caused by emboli, rather than by slowly progressive arterial stenosis and occlusion leading to progressive hypoperfusion of an area of the brain. It follows that the surgical construction of a collateral circulation to improve cerebral perfusion (e. g., extracranial-intracranial bypass operations) only makes sense in very rare, exceptional cases.

Particular Cerebrovascular Syndromes

The dynamics of clinical ischemia, i.e., the manner in which the clinical picture unfolds over time, depends mainly on the type of infarct (embolic, hemodynamic, or lacunar; see above), but the particular neurological deficits that are present are a function of the site of the lesion. In the following sections, we will discuss the most important cerebrovascular syndromes caused by the occlusion of individual arteries supplying the brain.

Vascular Syndromes of the Cerebral Hemispheres

Ischemic Syndromes in the Anterior Circulation

Cerebral ischemia most commonly arises in the territory of the internal carotid artery. It is usually caused either by cardiogenic emboli or by arterioarterial emboli arising in atherosclerotic plaques at the bifurcation of the common carotid artery. Other, rarer causes include primary diseases of the vascular wall of the ICA (such as fibromuscular dysplasia) and traumatic or spontaneous dissection of the ICA, leading to occlusion. Dissection, usually spontaneous, is a common cause of carotid occlusion in younger patients.

Ischemic lesions can develop in the territory of any of the branches of the ICA, or in all of these territories combined. The neurological deficits resulting from ischemia in each vascular territory will be briefly described.

Ophthalmic artery. Small emboli can pass through the ophthalmic artery and lodge in the central retinal artery, causing retinal ischemia and thus monocular blindness. This is usually transient (*amaurosis fugax*), because the embolus usually undergoes spontaneous lysis. Permanent blindness is exceptional. Proximal obstruction of the ophthalmic artery does not cause transient monocular blindness, because the central retinal artery also obtains blood through collaterals from the external carotid artery.

Posterior communicating artery. The next two branches of the internal carotid artery are the posterior communicating artery and the anterior choroidal artery. Emboli entering the posterior communicating artery cause ischemia either in the territory of the posterior cerebral artery (see below) or in the thalamus. The clinical manifestations are thus *contralateral homonymous hemianopsia* and/or a *thalamic deficit* (cf. p. 468).

Anterior choroidal artery. The territory of the anterior choroidal artery includes the medial portion of the temporal lobe with the hippocampal formation, the genu of the internal capsule, and parts of the optic tract and radiation. The manifestations of ischemia in this territory are *contralateral hemiparesis and hemihypesthesia* as well as *contralateral homonymous hemianopsia*. It is often to difficult to distinguish an infarct in the territory of the anterior choroidal artery from a lenticulostriate infarct on clinical grounds alone. Ischemia of the medial portion of the temporal lobe is a sure sign that the anterior choroidal artery is involved; though this is not readily seen in a CT scan, MRI can demonstrate it with high sensitivity.

Bifurcation ("T") of the internal carotid artery. Embolic occlusion of the internal carotid artery at its bifurcation, cutting off blood flow from the internal carotid artery into the middle cerebral artery and the anterior cerebral artery, is a life-threatening situation. When this happens, the circle of Willis provides no collateral pathway for blood to flow into the middle cerebral artery. The usual result is *extensive infarction in the territory of the middle cerebral artery*, with the corresponding neurological deficits (see below). The anterior cerebral artery, on the other hand, can often be filled with blood from the contralateral anterior cerebral artery by way of the anterior communicating artery. If it cannot be filled in this way because the anterior communicating artery is hypoplastic, or because embolic material has occluded it distal to the insertion of the anterior communicating artery, there is additional *infarction in the territory of the anterior cerebral artery* (see below). Furthermore, the infarct in the territory of the middle cerebral artery is larger, because this territory cannot be supplied by collateral circulation into through the superficial leptomeningeal anastomoses.

In addition to the extensive and severe neurological deficits (see below), the infarcted territories swell rapidly (cytotoxic edema), causing a rapid *rise in intracranial pressure*. Therefore, permanent occlusion of the internal carotid artery at its bifurcation is usually fatal. It should be remembered, however, that embolic stroke is a dynamic event. The embolus undergoes spontaneous lysis by endogenous plasmin, even as it continues to form because of the absence of blood flow. The net result of these two competing processes may be in either direction: if thrombolysis prevails, the artery is spontaneously recanalized, perhaps with distal propagation of smaller fragments of clot; if clot formation prevails, the artery is permanently occluded.

Middle cerebral artery. Emboli in the territory of the middle cerebral artery are the most common cause of cerebral ischemia. The clinical manifestations depend on the site of arterial occlusion.

Main stem occlusion. The main stem (trunk) of the middle cerebral artery gives off the small lenticulostriate arteries at a right angle; these arteries supply the basal ganglia and internal capsule. Within the sylvian fissure, the middle cerebral artery divides into its main branches, which supply large portions of the frontal, parietal, and temporal lobes (cf. Fig. 11.**4**).

Occlusion of the main stem of the middle cerebral artery leads to loss of neurons in the basal ganglia, and, a short time later, to necrosis in the internal capsule as well. The basal ganglia, which lack a collateral circulation, tolerate ischemia poorly. Regional differences in ischemic tolerance depend not only on circulatory factors, however, but also on the intrinsic properties of neurons in different parts of the brain.

Because the middle cerebral artery supplies an extensive area of the cerebral hemisphere, occlusion of its main stem causes a large assortment of neurological deficits: *contralateral, mainly brachiofacial hemiparesis and hemihypesthesia*, occasionally *contralateral homonymous hemianopsia*, and *neuropsychological deficits* including motor/sensory aphasia, acalculia, agraphia, and motor apraxia if the lesion is in the dominant hemisphere, or constructive apraxia and, possibly, anosognosia if it is in the nondominant hemisphere. In the acute phase of infarction, there may also be *turning of the head to the opposite side*, as well as *fixed gaze deviation to the opposite side* (*déviation conjuguée*).

Large infarcts in the territory of the middle cerebral artery and the extensive accompanying cerebral edema generally cause *intracranial hypertension*, which, if untreated, can lead to death.

Occlusion of peripheral branches of the middle cerebral artery causes infarction in the respective territories. The neurological manifestations vary accordingly; they are most pronounced when the infarct involves the central region (*contralateral focal motor and/or sensory deficits*). Ischemia in the peri-insular region on the left (dominant) side, particularly in the inferior frontal gyrus or the angular gyrus, causes *motor* or *sensory aphasia* (p. 387 ff.). The neuropsychological deficits caused by lesions in corresponding areas on the right side (*constructive apraxia, anosognosia*) are less obvious and may only become evident on close examination. Because the exact border between the territories of the middle cerebral artery and the posterior cerebral artery is variable, the former sometimes supplies part of the optic radiation; if this is the case, occlusion of a branch of the middle cerebral artery can cause *contralateral homonymous hemianopsia*. Prefrontal and rostral temporal infarcts are clinically silent.

Anterior cerebral artery. Infarcts in the territory of the anterior cerebral artery are relatively rare (10-20% of all brain infarcts). They may be unilateral or bilateral, depending on variations in vascular anatomy. Bilateral infarcts often occur when both anterior cerebral arteries are supplied by a single internal carotid artery. Emboli from an atherosclerotic plaque in the carotid bifurcation can then enter both anterior cerebral arteries within a short period of time (cf. Case Presentation 3, p. 452). Less commonly, there may be only one (azygous) anterior cerebral artery, as a normal anatomical variant. Further causes of infarction in the territory of the anterior cerebral artery include aneurysms of the anterior communicating artery and stenosis of inflammatory/infectious origin, which often occurs in the pericallosal segment of the anterior cerebral artery.

Unilateral infarcts in the territory of the anterior cerebral artery are often clinically silent. Infarction rarely occurs in the far rostral portion of this arterial territory, because of the many anastomotic connections between the vessels of the two hemispheres. Further toward the back of the head, however, the territories of the two anterior cerebral arteries are separated by the falx cerebri, so that neither side can obtain collateral circulation from the other. Possible manifestations of an infarct in this (central) area are *hemiparesis mainly affecting the leg, isolated leg paresis,* and *paraparesis* (in bilateral infarction). These deficits are usually only transient, however, because of restitution of blood flow through collateral circulation from the posterior cerebral artery. Unilateral damage of the medial aspect of the frontal lobe usually does not produce any severe deficit, but bilateral damage produces a *very severe disturbance of drive*: the patient no longer participates in any of the normal activities of life, becomes totally apathetic, and spends most of the day in bed. This problem is often accompanied by further *mental abnormalities, neuropsychological deficits* (apraxia), *bladder dysfunction* (incontinence), *and pathological, "primitive" reflexes* (grasp, suck, and palmomental reflexes).

Ischemic Syndromes in the Posterior Circulation

Ischemia in the posterior circulation, as in the anterior circulation, is usually of **embolic** origin. Most of the responsible emboli arise from atheromatous plaques in the wall of the vertebral artery. In contrast to the common carotid artery, in which atheroma tends to form at the carotid bifurcation, the vertebral artery contains no preferred sites of atheroma formation. Atheromatous plaques can be found anywhere along its length.

This fact makes it difficult to **localize the source of emboli** precisely. Furthermore, atheromatous plaques in the right or left vertebral artery may give rise to emboli that travel distally into the basilar artery or into the posterior cerebral artery on *either* side. An indication of the side of origin of emboli is present, however, when the posterior inferior cerebellar artery is involved, because this vessel is a direct branch of the terminal segment of the vertebral artery. The radiographic demonstration of acute occlusion of one vertebral artery is also helpful in this respect. Stenosis of the vertebral artery, like stenosis of the internal carotid artery, usually causes stroke not by diminished perfusion but rather by acting as a source of emboli. It is unclear to what extent cardiogenic emboli might be responsible for ischemia in the posterior circulation.

The vertebral and basilar arteries supply the brainstem, among other parts of the brain. Because the brainstem controls many essential functions, including respiration and cardiovascular function, **brainstem infarction** often has much more serious consequences than infarction in the territory of the internal carotid artery. Occlusion of the basilar artery including the basilar tip is uniformly fatal. Furthermore, because there is only limited room in the posterior fossa for swollen brain tissue to expand, even a relatively small cerebellar infarct can cause life-threatening intracranial hypertension. Compression of the aqueduct or fourth ventricle by infarcted tissue can cause occlusive hydrocephalus, raising the intracranial pressure even higher. Emergency external ventricular drainage with or without consecutive neurosurgical decompression of the posterior fossa is a life-saving procedure in such cases.

Basilar artery. The two vertebral arteries unite in front of the brainstem to form the basilar artery. This vessel gives off many small branches to the brainstem, the anterior inferior cerebellar artery (AICA), and the superior cerebellar artery (SCA, p. 429) before dividing, at the level of the midbrain, into the two posterior cerebral arteries (basilar tip). The vascular syndromes caused by occlusion of the perforating or circumferential branches of the basilar artery were described in Chapter 4 (p. 231 ff.); those caused by occlusion of the cerebellar arteries are described on p. 470.

Posterior cerebral artery. The arteries in the neighborhood of the basilar tip are of particular clinical significance, because their perforating branches supply the important structures of the midbrain and thalamus. Midbrain infarction due to basilar tip occlusion is always fatal.

Embolic occlusion of the basilar artery or of the proximal (P1) segment of the posterior cerebral artery does not always produce an ischemic lesion in the peripheral territory of the posterior cerebral artery, because collateral circulation from the internal carotid artery by way of the posterior communicating artery can often provide an adequate flow of blood distal to the occlusion. Thus, basilar artery occlusion (embolic or thrombotic) is by no means excluded by normal findings in head CT and Doppler ultrasonography!

Among the numerous perforating arteries in this area, a few of the larger ones will be singled out for discussion:

- *Medial and lateral posterior choroidal arteries.* Ischemia in these territories is usually accompanied by ischemia in the territory of the posterior cerebral artery; thus, relatively little is known about the neurological deficits caused by isolated occlusions of these two small arteries. Deficits that have been described in isolated occlusion of the lateral posterior choroidal artery include homonymous quadrantanopsia due to infarction of the lateral geniculate body, hemisensory deficits, and neuropsychological abnormalities (transcortical aphasia, amnesia). Isolated occlusion of the medial posterior choroidal artery, which is even rarer, has been reported to produce midbrain damage, with resulting oculomotor dysfunction.

- *Cortical branches of the posterior cerebral artery.* Occlusion of one or more cortical branches of the posterior cerebral artery can produce a wide variety of neurological deficits, not just because these vessels take a highly variable course but also because the territory of the posterior cerebral artery varies in extent. Its border with the territory of the middle cerebral artery runs differently in different individuals, and the sizes of these two territories are reciprocally related. In a case of focal cortical infarction, it is important to determine in which vascular territory the lesion lies, because this will, in turn, imply the probable source of emboli. If the lesion is in the territory of the middle cerebral artery, the embolus probably arose from the ipsilateral common carotid bifurcation; if it is in the territory of the posterior cerebral artery, the embolus probably arose from the ipsilateral or contralateral vertebral artery.

- *Calcarine artery.* This is clinically the most important branch of the posterior cerebral artery because it supplies the visual cortex. A unilateral infarct produces *contralateral homonymous hemianopsia*; bilateral lesions can produce *cortical blindness*. Often, however, an infarct in the territory of the calcarine artery produces no more than a partial visual field defect (a *quadrantanopsia* or a blind patch called a *scotoma*), because the visual cortex is also supplied by leptomeningeal collaterals from the middle cerebral artery.

Thalamic Vascular Syndromes

Anterior thalamoperforating artery (thalamotuberal artery). This artery originates from the posterior communicating artery and mainly supplies the rostral portion of the thalamus. Infarction in its territory causes a *rest or intention tremor* and *choreoathetotic motor restlessness with thalamic hand* (an abnormally contracted posture of the hand). Sensory disturbances and pain are typically absent.

Posterior thalamoperforating artery (thalamoperforating artery). The thalamoperforating arteries of the two sides sometimes arise from a common trunk (the *artery* of *Percheron*, cf. p. 431). Occlusion of this artery causes bilateral infarction of the intralaminar nuclei of the thalamus, resulting in a *severe impairment of consciousness*.

Thalamogeniculate artery. The lateral portion of the thalamus is mainly supplied by the thalamogeniculate artery, which arises from the P2 segment of the posterior cerebral artery, i.e., distal to the posterior communicating artery. Infarcts in the territory of the posterior cerebral artery often involve ischemia in

---

Case Presentation 6: *Thalamic Infarction*

Out of a clear blue sky, this 45-year-old office worker suddenly became nauseated, vomited, felt very dizzy, and saw double. Thinking he had caught an acute stomach virus, he went home to bed. When he got up a few hours later to call a friend, he found he was still very dizzy and had double vision. While talking on the phone, he could only produce words with the greatest difficulty; his friend expressed surprise at his atypically monosyllabic responses. He was now worried enough to take himself directly to the emergency room of a nearby hospital.

The admitting house officer found skew deviation of the eyes and an unsteady gait, but no weakness. There was also a conduction-type aphasia (cf. Table 9.1, p. 389). Suspecting a process involving the basilar artery, the physician ordered an MRI scan, which revealed a left thalamic infarct.

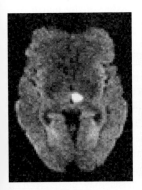 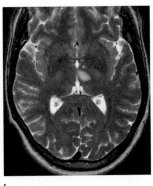

a   b

Fig. 11.**26 Thalamic infarct.** Diffusion-weighted (**a**) and T2-weighted (**b**) images. An acute infarct is seen in the territory of the left posterior thalamoperforating artery. Acute edema and a marked diffusion abnormality are present. Bilateral infarcts in this area can severely impair consciousness (cf. Case Presentation 3 in Chapter 7, p. 327).

A more rostrally lying lesion that additionally affects the subthalamic nucleus and the pallidothalamic fibers innervating the ventrolateral nuclei can cause (usually transient) hemiballism or, more commonly, chorea (cf. Case Presentation 3 in Chapter 8, p. 346). In such cases, the further clinical course is often marked by the development of a so-called "thalamic hand," with involuntary flexion of the wrist and hyperextension of the finger joints. The thumb is either abducted or pressed against the palm.

the distribution of the thalamogeniculate artery. The corresponding deficits were first described by Dejerine and Roussy: transient *contralateral hemiparesis*, persistent *contralateral hemianesthesia for touch and proprioception* (with lesser impairment of pain and temperature sensation), *spontaneous pain*, mild *hemiataxia* and *astereognosis*, and *contralateral choreoathetotic motor restlessness*.

The contralateral hemiparesis usually resolves rapidly. It is attributed to compression of the internal capsule by the neighboring, edematous thalamic tissue. The internal capsule itself is not ischemic, as it is not supplied by the thalamogeniculate artery.

Cerebellar Vascular Syndromes

The cerebellar arteries have numerous collaterals; thus, the occlusion of a single vessel often causes no more than a small infarct, which may be clinically silent. More extensive ischemia, which is less commonly seen, produces cerebellar neurological deficits, particularly in the acute phase. The accompanying brain edema may cause rapidly progressive compression of the fourth ventricle, resulting in occlusive hydrocephalus and impending brainstem herniation.

Posterior inferior cerebellar artery (PICA). Proximal occlusion of the PICA causes ischemia of the dorsolateral portion of the medulla, usually producing a partial or complete *Wallenberg syndrome* (p. 226 ff.). The PICA also supplies part of the cerebellum, but to a highly variable extent (p. 429); thus, there may be accompanying *cerebellar deficits* of variable severity, such as *hemiataxia*, *dysmetria*, *lateropulsion*, or *dysdiadochokinesia*. The cerebellar deficits are always found on the side of the infarct. They are also often accompanied by nausea and vomiting; if the latter are misinterpreted as being of gastrointestinal rather than neurological origin, the diagnosis may be delayed or missed, with potentially catastrophic results (see Case Presentation 7). Occasionally, if the PICA is occluded very near its origin, cerebellar signs may be entirely absent; conversely, brainstem signs may be absent in distal occlusions.

Case Presentation 7: *Cerebellar Infarction*

This 63-year-old master carpenter threw a big party for all of his employees to celebrate the 30th anniversary of his business. As usual at such events, the alcohol flowed plentifully.

Late that night, he awoke with severe dizziness, a headache, and nausea. When he tried to stand up, he fell to the ground at once and had a great deal of trouble pulling himself back into bed. About half an hour later, he began to vomit repeatedly, at brief intervals. His wife called the physician on night duty, despite the patient's repeated assurances that he had simply had too much to drink. The physician arrived a few minutes later, took the history, and performed a rapid general medical and neurological examination. The basic neurological tests were all normal: the patient's muscular strength, sensation, and reflexes were intact and symmetrical throughout. He was, however, completely unable to sit up from a lying position, remain upright in a seated position, or stand up and walk. The physician attributed these findings to hypovolemia because of vomiting induced by

an acute gastrointestinal infection. He gave the patient metoclopramide and advised him to drink plenty of fluids and to call his primary care physician the first thing in the morning.

The patient continued to vomit through the night and became increasingly confused as morning approached. At 4 a.m., his wife could no longer wake him up, even with a loud shout, and she called the emergency medical service. On arrival in the hospital, the patient was first admitted to the medical service, where various tests, including an ECG, were performed but yielded no clear diagnosis. A neurologist was consulted. The patient could barely cooperate with the examination and seemed not to know what he was being asked to do, but the neurologist was able to get him to follow a moving flashlight with his eyes, and was thus able to detect a gaze-evoked nystagmus. He ordered an emergency MRI scan of the head, which revealed a large infarct of the right cerebellar hemisphere, accompanied by edema that was already exerting considerable mass effect. In-

▷

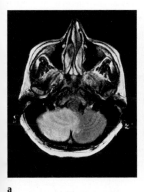 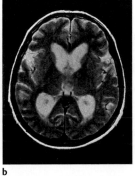

a   **b**

Fig. 11.**27 Cerebellar infarct**, as seen by MRI. **a** The axial T2-weighted image reveals a hyperintense (bright) infarct in the basal portion of the right cerebellar hemisphere, involving the inferior portion of the vermis. **b** Another axial image at the level of the lateral ventricles reveals marked dilatation of the inner CSF spaces. Increased pressure in the posterior fossa is impeding outflow of CSF, leading to hydrocephalus. At present, cerebellar infarcts can be demonstrated in an early phase with diffusion-weighted MRI (not shown here).

tensive treatment was given to combat brain edema, but the patient's state of consciousness failed to improve. He was therefore transferred to the neurosurgical service for operative decompression of the posterior fossa and insertion of a ventricular shunt. After surgery, his condition rapidly stabilized.

Cerebellar infarcts are often easy to misdiagnose initially because they often produce only mild limb ataxia along with the much more severe truncal ataxia. In such cases, the usual

cerebellar tests involving limb posture and intentional movement may yield no pathological findings. Vomiting may be ascribed to a gastrointestinal problem and the necessary imaging studies may not be performed until the increasing intracranial pressure finally causes the patient's state of consciousness to deteriorate. A CT scan obtained early in the course of the acute illness may be normal, but a diffusion-weighted MRI scan will reveal the cause of problem (Fig. 11.**27**).

The initial CT scan may not reveal a cerebellar stroke because it has been obtained very early in the course of infarction, or because there is too much artefact in the posterior fossa for the cerebellum to be seen clearly. As a result, even large cerebellar infarcts may escape diagnosis until the increasing cytotoxic edema of the damaged tissue causes *symptomatic brainstem compression*. This is manifest as *impairment of consciousness*, *vomiting*, and *cardiorespiratory disturbances*, up to and including *respiratory arrest*. Thus, whenever a cerebellar or brainstem stroke is suspected and the initial CT scan is normal, follow-up images should be obtained a few hours later, either by CT or, preferably, by diffusion-weighted MRI.

Anterior inferior cerebellar artery (AICA). Occlusions of this artery, like PICA occlusions, produce a wide variety of clinical manifestations, because its course and the extent of its territory vary widely across individuals. *Ipsilateral hemiataxia* and *nystagmus* may occur, and there may also be *deficits of cranial nerves VII and VIII*. Occlusion of the labyrinthine artery, a branch of the AICA, can cause *sudden deafness.*

Superior cerebellar artery (SCA). Occlusion of the superior cerebellar artery causes severe *ataxia* because of infarction of the superior cerebellar peduncle, as well as *astasia* and *abasia*. Tissue damage in the pontine tegmentum causes a *sensory deficit* in the ipsilateral half of the face and the contralateral half of the body, involving all qualities of sensation (syndrome of the oral pontine tegmentum, Fig. 4.**66**, p. 233).

Autopsy studies have shown that, in many persons, an elongated loop of the superior cerebellar artery comes into contact with the trigeminal nerve just distal to the exit of the nerve from the pons. It is of no clinical significance as an incidental finding, but its occurrence in many patients with *trigeminal neuralgia* suggests that it may be involved in the pathophysiology of this condition which is characterized by paroxysmal, extremely intense, lightninglike ("lancinating") pain on one side of the face. Trigeminal neuralgia usually responds well to medical therapy (e. g., with carbamazepine). In intractable cases, however, a neurosurgical operation can be performed in which the nerve and the vascular loop are separated by a pledget of synthetic material ("microvascular decompression," "the Jannetta procedure"). For more on the diagnosis and treatment of trigeminal neuralgia, see Chapter 4, p. 165.

Brainstem Vascular Syndromes

The many different vascular syndromes affecting the brainstem can only be understood on the basis of a thorough knowledge of its topographical anatomy. For this reason, they are discussed in the chapter on the brainstem (Chapter 4, p. 223 ff.), rather than here.

Impaired Venous Drainage from the Brain

Cerebral ischemia, as we have seen, is usually caused by an impairment of the arterial blood supply of the brain. It can also be caused by an impairment of the outflow of venous blood, though this situation is much less common. If a cerebral vein is blocked, the blood volume and venous pressure rise in the region of the brain that it normally drains. The arteriovenous pressure difference across the cerebral capillaries falls (the inflow of blood is "choked off"), leading to **diminished perfusion** and thus to diminished supply of oxygen and nutrients. Simultaneously, the transcapillary pressure gradient increases, leading to increased movement of water from the capillaries into the surrounding tissue (**vasogenic edema**). The neurons in the affected brain tissue lose the ability to function normally, and, if the problem persists, they die. *Venous infarction* is usually accompanied by the rupture of small vessels (probably veins) in the infarcted zone, producing *intraparenchymal hemorrhage* (so-called venous hemorrhage, which has a characteristic "salt-and-pepper" appearance in a CT scan).

Acute Venous Outflow Obstruction

Acute Thromboses of the Cerebral Veins and Venous Sinuses

Causes. The most common cause of acute obstruction of venous outflow from the brain is thrombosis of the dural venous sinuses and the parenchymal veins that drain into them (venous sinus thrombosis). Factors predisposing to this occurrence include coagulopathies such as protein S and C deficiency, factor V deficiency, and cardiolipin antibodies, as well as oral contraceptive use, cigarette smoking, steroid medication, dehydration, autoimmune diseases such as Behçet disease and Crohn disease, and the puerperium.

Manifestations. The clinical manifestations of venous sinus thrombosis are highly varied and depend on the site and extent of venous occlusion as well as on the degree to which collateral drainage is available. In one patient a relatively circumscribed occlusion may cause a major intraparenchymal hemorrhage, while in another an extensive occlusion may remain nearly asymptomatic. Prospective assessment is usually not possible in individual cases.

The general clinical manifestations of venous sinus thrombosis are *headache* and *epileptic seizures*. If the patient also develops *focal neurological deficits* that progress over the course of a few hours, rather than suddenly, then venous sinus thrombosis is the likely diagnosis. The diagnosis is further supported by evidence of *intracranial hypertension*, e. g., papilledema.

In cases of venous sinus thrombosis, marked clinical deterioration can occur in a very short time, perhaps over the course of an hour. Such occurrences are usually due to involvement of the internal cerebral veins or to extensive intraparenchymal venous hemorrhages.

Diagnostic evaluation. The diagnosis or exclusion of venous sinus thrombosis is often difficult even when modern imaging methods are used—CT, MRI, and digital subtraction angiography (DSA).

CT. Classic, acute cases can be diagnosed by CT, particularly when CT venography with contrast medium is performed. Problems are caused by congenital variants of the vascular anatomy, by less extensive occlusions, and by thromboses of the straight sinus and internal cerebral veins. Older venous sinus thromboses, too, are difficult to assess with CT.

MRI. MRI is currently the most important diagnostic technique for evaluation of the venous outflow of the brain. It reveals the veins in multiple planes, and it is performed with flow-sensitive sequences to demonstrate intravenous flow. Its resolution is high enough that the internal cerebral veins are well seen.

MRI also enables visualization of the brain parenchyma. The site and appearance of a parenchymal lesion may provide clues to the location of venous obstruction: occlusion of the internal cerebral veins, for example, produces characteristic thalamic lesions, while transverse sinus thrombosis produces characteristic lesions in the temporal lobe. The diagnostic power of MRI is reduced, however, by anatomical variants of the cerebral blood vessels (as in CT) and also by certain flow-related effects that are incompletely understood at present. MRI thus cannot detect every case of venous sinus thrombosis, and it occasionally yields false-positive findings as well. Furthermore, MRI scanning of uncooperative or unconscious patients is sometimes very difficult, and the resulting scans may be of marginal diagnostic value. In extreme cases, patients must be scanned under general anesthesia.

Case Presentation 8: *Superior Sagittal Sinus Thrombosis*

This 37-year-old secretary had a generalized epileptic seizure at work. After a postictal twilight phase lasting about 20 minutes, she regained full alertness and complained of a severe holocephalic headache. On admission to the hospital, she was awake, but abnormally slow. She continued to complain of severe headache. An MRI scan was obtained at once: the T2-weighted image revealed a left frontal parenchymal lesion (Fig. 11.**28a**), while MR venography (Fig. 11.**28b**, **c**) revealed thrombotic occlusion of the rostral portion of the superior sagittal sinus. The sinus thrombosis was treated with full heparinization followed by oral warfarin administration, and anticonvulsants were given to prevent further seizures. The headache improved rapidly with analgesics, and the patient was asymptomatic a few days later. Further diagnostic testing revealed no underlying hypercoagulable state. The only identifiable risk factor for venous sinus thrombosis was the use of oral contraceptives.

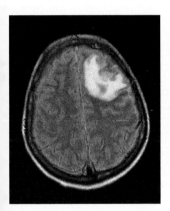

a

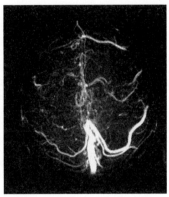

b

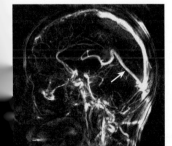

c

Fig. 11.**28 Venous sinus thrombosis. a** The T2-weighted FLAIR image reveals a hyperintense lesion in the left frontal lobe: this is an infarct due to venous obstruction. **b** MR venography reveals brisk flow in the posterior portion of the superior sagittal sinus (bright) and in the large tributary veins that join it. The rostral portion of the sinus, however, is devoid of signal, indicating lack of flow. There is also poor flow in the tributary veins that enter this portion of the sinus. **c** The same findings are evident in lateral projection: there is flow in the posterior portion of the superior sagittal sinus, as well as in the straight sinus (arrow) and the internal cerebral veins, but not in the rostral portion of the superior sagittal sinus.

Intra-arterial DSA. Intra-arterial angiography or DSA was once the only method of diagnosing venous sinus thrombosis with certainty. Unfortunately, the usefulness of this method is limited in precisely the same situations where the other methods fail to provide conclusive findings. DSA is no longer used to diagnose venous sinus thrombosis, except in rare cases, because it carries a much higher risk of complications than MRI.

Clinical course, treatment, and prognosis. The spontaneous course of venous sinus thrombosis is not clear. It was once thought that most cases were fatal, probably because most less-extensive thromboses went undetected and only the cases that turned out unfavorably were, in the end, correctly diagnosed. Occlusion of the straight sinus and/or internal cerebral veins is particularly ominous; this type of venous obstruction is still highly lethal, because it often leads to necrosis in the diencephalon to an extent that is incompatible with life. It can also cause cerebellar hemorrhage with mass effect. The straight sinus and the internal cerebral veins sometimes undergo thrombosis in isolation, but more often do so as a later stage in the progression of extensive thrombosis of the remaining venous sinuses.

The prognosis of venous sinus thrombosis has improved markedly since the introduction of **therapeutic anticoagulation with heparin**. Heparin is given even in the face of a parenchymal hemorrhage due to venous sinus thrombosis. In such cases, the correct interpretation of the hemorrhage as a sequela of thrombosis is essential, because it would otherwise absolutely contraindicate anticoagulation. Fibrinolytic techniques have not been shown to be of value in the treatment of venous sinus thrombosis. Surgical resection of venous hemorrhages is also not indicated.

Therapeutic anticoagulation is thought to halt the progression of venous sinus thrombosis, to promote the opening of collateral venous pathways, and to promote microcirculation. Intravenous heparin is given in the acute phase, then converted to oral anticoagulation for a further six months. Follow-up examinations are performed to detect recurrences early, particularly when known risk factors are present. Patients found to have suffered venous sinus thrombosis because of an underlying hypercoagulable disorder must be therapeutically anticoagulated for life.

Chronic Venous Outflow Obstruction

The manifestations of chronic venous outflow obstruction differ markedly from those of acute thrombosis.

The causes of chronic venous outflow obstruction are many, including medication side effects and bilateral stenosis of the venous outflow channels. In one published case, a patient with a congenitally hypoplastic transverse sinus on one side developed obstruction of the transverse sinus on the opposite side because of a slowly growing meningioma of the sinus wall.

Manifestations. The characteristic manifestations of chronic venous outflow obstruction are *headache* and *papilledema*, possibly accompanied by *impaired visual acuity*. Focal neurological deficits or epileptic seizures are usually not a component of the clinical picture.

Diagnostic evaluation. No parenchymal lesions are seen in the brain (in contrast to acute venous outflow obstruction). **MRI** sometimes reveals dilatation of the optic nerve sheaths as a result of intracranial hypertension and pressure-related changes of the sella turcica, but it generally does not show the cause of the impairment of venous outflow. In such cases, **intra-arterial digital subtraction angiography** is indispensable for the demonstration of circumscribed stenoses and for the assessment of venous flow dynamics. The diagnosis can be confirmed by lumbar puncture with **measurement of the cerebrospinal fluid pressure**.

Treatment. If etiological treatment is not possible, chronic elevation of the cerebrospinal fluid pressure can be treated by a **permanent CSF deviation procedure** (lumboperitoneal or ventriculoperitoneal shunt).

Differential diagnosis. Chronic intracranial hypertension is seen with increased frequency in young, overweight women in the absence of an obstruction to venous outflow. The cause of this condition is unknown. Its poorly descriptive traditional name is *pseudotumor cerebri*.

Intracranial Hemorrhage

Spontaneous, i.e., nontraumatic, bleeding in the brain parenchyma (**intracerebral hemorrhage**) or the meningeal compartments around it (**subarachnoid, subdural, and epidural hemorrhage**) accounts for 15-20% of clinical strokes, in the wider sense of the term. Although headache and impairment of consciousness occur in intracranial hemorrhage more commonly than in cerebral infarction, clinical criteria alone cannot reliably distinguish hemorrhagic from ischemic stroke. The diagnostic procedure of choice is CT.

An understanding of subarachnoid, subdural, and epidural hemorrhage requires knowledge of the anatomy of the meninges, as described on p. 402 ff.

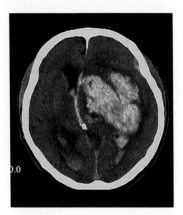

Fig. 11.**29 Large left basal ganglionic hemorrhage**
with midline shift and intraventricular hemorrhage

Intracerebral Hemorrhage (Nontraumatic)

Hypertensive Hemorrhage

Etiology. The most common cause of intracerebral hemorrhage is **arterial hypertension**. Pathologically elevated blood pressure damages the walls of smaller arteries, creating **microaneurysms** (Charcot aneurysms) that can rupture spontaneously. Sites of predilection for hypertensive intracerebral hemorrhage are the *basal ganglia* (Fig. 11.**29**), the *thalamus*, the *cerebellar nuclei*, and the *pons*. The deep cerebral white matter, on the other hand, is only rarely involved.

Manifestations. The manifestations of intracerebral hemorrhage depend on its location. Basal ganglionic hemorrhage with destruction of the internal capsule usually produces *severe contralateral hemiparesis*, while pontine hemorrhage produces *brainstem signs*.

The main danger in intracerebral hemorrhage is *intracranial hypertension* due to the mass effect of the hematoma. Unlike an infarct, which raises the intracranial pressure slowly as the associated cytotoxic edema worsens, an intracerebral hemorrhage raises it very rapidly. *Intraventricular rupture* of an intracerebral hemorrhage can cause hydrocephalus, either by obstructing the ventricular outflow with blood clot or by impairing CSF resorption from the arachnoid granulations; if present, hydrocephalus raises the intracranial pressure still further. There is hardly any free space in the posterior fossa, so intraparenchymal hemorrhages below the tentorium rapidly elevate the local intracranial pressure, possibly resulting in herniation of the posterior fossa con tents, either upward through the tentorial notch, or downward into the foramen magnum. Thus, an intraparenchymal hemorrhage in the brainstem or cerebellum carries a much worse prognosis than an equal-sized hemorrhage in a cerebral hemisphere.

Prognosis and treatment. The brain tissue in an area of hemorrhage (as opposed to an infarct) is generally not totally destroyed; living brain tissue can often be found amid the extravasated blood. This explains why the patient's neurological deficits usually resolve more rapidly, as the hematoma is resorbed, than they would if produced by an ischemic stroke.

The goal of treatment is, therefore, to preserve whatever brain tissue remains viable in the area of hemorrhage. **Persistent intracranial hypertension must be treated** to prevent secondary damage, not only of the brain tissue inside and around the hematoma but also of distant tissue. The intracranial pressure can be lowered by **pharmacotherapy** and/or by **neurosurgical removal of the hematoma**. Surgery should be performed only when indicated according to strict criteria, taking the patient's age into account, as well as the location and size of the hematoma. Large-scale studies have shown a therapeutic benefit only from the removal of large hematomas (>20 cm^3). The operative removal of smaller hematomas may actually be detrimental, as it may destroy more viable brain tissue than it saves; and the operative removal of hematomas deep within the brain always involves the destruction of some normal brain tissue along the neurosurgeon's path to the hematoma. For these reasons, the neurosurgical treatment of smaller intraparenchymal hematomas is limited to the treatment of hydrocephalus (if present) with external ventricular drainage, which can be performed with minimal injury to normal brain tissue. Patients with very large hematomas (>60 cm^3) will not benefit from removal of the hematoma because too much brain tissue has already been destroyed.

Nonhypertensive Intracerebral Hemorrhage

Intracerebral hemorrhage may be due to many causes besides arterial hypertension. The more important ones are *arteriovenous malformations*, *tumors*, *aneurysms*, *vascular diseases* including vasculitis and amyloid angiopathy, *cavernomas*, and *venous outflow obstruction* (as discussed above). An intracerebral hemorrhage is likely to have been caused by something other than arterial hypertension when it is not located at one of the sites of predilection for hypertensive hemorrhage, or when the patient does not suffer from marked arterial hypertension. In such cases (at least), a follow-up MRI scan should be performed once the hematoma is resorbed to detect the underlying cause of hemorrhage. Digital subtraction angiography is sometimes indicated as well.

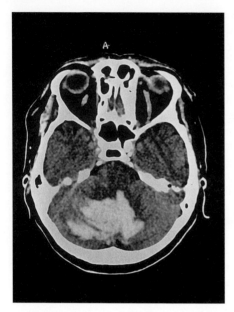

Fig. 11.**30 Cerebellar hemorrhage.** CT scan of a hypertensive patient who suddenly complained of an intense headache and then became less responsive. A large, hyperdense (bright) hemorrhage is seen in the region of the deep cerebellar nuclei. The brainstem is ventrally displaced and pushed against the clivus, and the prepontine cistern is markedly narrowed.

Cerebellar Hemorrhage

The cerebellar nuclei lie within the distribution of the superior cerebellar artery. One particular branch of this artery, which supplies the dentate nucleus, is particularly susceptible to rupture. In hypertensive individuals, hemorrhage from this vessel is more common than ischemia in its territory (Fig. 11.**30**).

Hemorrhage in this region often causes acute mass effect in the posterior fossa, with all of its attendant consequences (herniation of the brainstem and cerebellum upward through the tentorial notch and downward into the foramen magnum). The clinical manifestations are *severe occipital headache, nausea and vomiting,* and *vertigo,* generally accompanied by *unsteady gait, dysarthria,* and *head turning* and *gaze deviation to the side opposite the lesion.* Large hemorrhages rapidly produce somnolence, stupor, or coma. In the late phase, patients manifest extensor spasms, hemodynamic instability, and, finally, respiratory arrest, unless the posterior fossa can be operatively decompressed.

Smaller hemorrhages, particularly in the cerebellar hemispheres, produce focal manifestations including *limb ataxia, a tendency to fall to the side of the lesion,* and *deviation of gait to the side of the lesion.* These manifestations resolve incompletely when the deep cerebellar nuclei are damaged.

Further causes of cerebellar hemorrhage include the rupture of an arteri-ovenous malformation or aneurysm, and bleeding into a tumor (usually a metastasis).

Subarachnoid Hemorrhage

Aneurysms

The most common cause of spontaneous subarachnoid hemorrhage is the rup-ture of an aneurysm of one of the arteries of the base of the brain. There are different types of aneurysms.

Saccular ("berry") aneurysms are found at **points of bifurcation** of the in-tracranial arteries. They form on the basis of a prior lesion of the vessel wall, which is either a (usually congenital) structural defect, or an injury due to hy-pertension. The **common sites** of saccular aneurysms are the *anterior com-municating artery* (40%), the *bifurcation of the middle cerebral artery* in the sylvian fissure (20%), the *lateral wall of the internal carotid artery* (at the origin of the ophthalmic or posterior communicating artery, 30%), and the *basilar tip* (10%) (Fig. 11.**31**). Aneurysms at other sites, such as the origin of

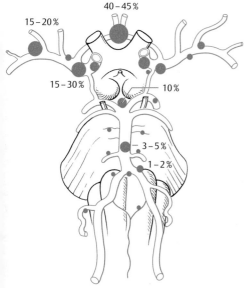

40–45%

15–20%

15–30%

10%

3–5%

1–2%

Fig. 11.**31 Common sites of intra-cranial aneurysms**

the PICA, the P2 segment of the posterior cerebral artery, or the pericallosal segment of the anterior cerebral artery, are rare. Aneurysms can produce neurological deficits by pressing on neighboring structures even before they rupture. For example, an aneurysm of the posterior communicating artery can compress the oculomotor nerve, causing a third nerve palsy (the patient complains of diplopia).

Fusiform aneurysms. An elongated ("spindle-shaped") enlargement of a vessel is called a fusiform aneurysm. Such aneurysms preferentially involve the *intracranial segment of the internal carotid artery*, *the main trunk of the middle cerebral artery*, and the *basilar artery*. They are usually caused by atherosclerosis and/or hypertension, and they are only rarely a source of hemorrhage. Large fusiform aneurysms of the basilar artery can compress the brainstem. Slow flow inside a fusiform aneurysm can promote intra-aneurysmal clot formation, particularly at the sides, with subsequent embolic stroke or cut-off of perforating vessels by the direct extension of thrombus. These aneurysms usually cannot be treated neurosurgically, because they are elongated enlargements of normal vessels, rather than pathological structures (like saccular aneurysms) making no contribution to the cerebral blood supply.

Mycotic aneurysms. Aneurysmal dilatations of intracranial blood vessels are sometimes the result of sepsis with bacterially induced damage to the vascular wall. Unlike saccular and fusiform aneurysms, these mycotic aneurysms are preferentially found on *small arteries* of the brain. The treatment consists of treatment of the underlying infection. Mycotic aneurysms sometimes regress spontaneously; they very rarely cause subarachnoid hemorrhage.

Case Presentation 9: *Multiple Unruptured Aneurysms*

This previously healthy 43-year-old mechanic was briefly unconscious after an automobile accident (front-end collision) and was taken to the hospital for observation. A CT scan of the head was performed to rule out intracranial injury. The noncontrast images revealed no hemorrhage or other abnormality, but the contrast-enhanced images revealed a possible aneurysm of the right middle cerebral artery as an incidental finding. This was followed up by cerebral angiography, which confirmed the presence of an aneurysm at the bifurcation of the right middle cerebral artery, as well as further aneurysms of the left internal carotid artery and the tip of the basilar artery (Fig. 11.**32a**). The MCA and ICA aneurysms were clipped in an open neurosurgical operation. The basilar tip aneurysm, however, was not amenable to surgical treatment with an acceptably low risk. Instead, it was treated with an interventional neuroradiological procedure: a microcatheter was inserted into it under angiographic control, and its lumen was filled with metal coils (Fig. 11.**32b**).

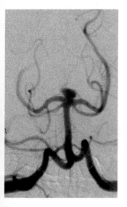
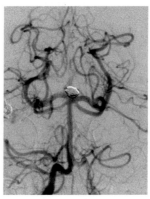

a   b

Fig. 11.**32 Basilar tip aneurysm.** Intra-arterial digital subtraction angiography before (**a**) and after (**b**) the aneurysm was filled with coils. The basilar tip aneurysm is well seen on the angiogram; it is narrower at its base (neck). Coiling excludes the aneurysm from the circulation. (Images courtesy of PD Dr. Skalej and Dr. Siekmann, Tübingen.)

Acute Nontraumatic Subarachnoid Hemorrhage

Nontraumatic subarachnoid hemorrhage (SAH) is usually caused by the **spontaneous rupture of a saccular aneurysm**, with escape of blood into the subarachnoid space.

Manifestations. The leading symptom of a subarachnoid hemorrhage is a **sudden, very intense headache** ("the worst headache of my life"). Meningeal irritation by subarachnoid blood causes **nuchal rigidity** (differential diagnosis: meningitis). **Consciousness may be impaired** immediately or within the first few hours. *Cranial nerve palsies* and *focal neurological signs* may be present, depending on the site and extent of the hemorrhage. The grading scheme proposed by Hunt and Hess in 1968 is still useful in clinical practice, as it gives a rough indication of the patient's prognosis (Table 11.**2**).

Diagnostic evaluation. CT sensitively detects acute subarachnoid hemorrhage (Fig. 11.**33**); yet, the longer the interval between the acute event and the CT scan, the more likely it is that the scan will be negative. If SAH is suspected despite a negative CT scan, a lumbar puncture must be performed. This will enable the direct demonstration of blood or siderophages in the cerebrospinal fluid.

Once SAH has been diagnosed, the source of bleeding must be identified. This can only be done reliably by *intra-arterial digital subtraction angiography*, which

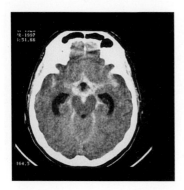

Fig. 11.**33 Acute subarachnoid hemorrhage.** The basal cisterns are filled with hyperdense (bright) blood. The temporal horns of the lateral ventricles are dilated because of an obstruction of CSF outflow (hydrocephalus). Because there is no blood in the ventricles, the internal CSF spaces are dark, while the external CSF spaces are bright.

should, however, be performed only if the patient is a candidate for a surgical procedure to clip the aneurysm or to close it with the methods of interventional neuroradiology (see below). DSA reliably demonstrates the presence of an aneurysm and illustrates its spatial relationship to the neighboring vessels. All four great vessels supplying the brain are studied with contrast medium, because about 20 % of patients with aneurysms have more than one aneurysm.

Treatment. Aneurysms can be treated with a neurosurgical operation in which the neck of the aneurysm is closed with a metal *clip.* The aneurysm is thereby permanently excluded from the circulation, so that it cannot bleed again. This form of treatment is definitive, but the disadvantage is that it requires operative opening of the skull (craniotomy) and neurosurgical manipulations around the base of the brain that may cause further complications. Surgery should be performed in the first 72 hours after subarachnoid hemorrhage, i.e., before the period of greatest risk for the development of vasospasm (see

Table 11.2 Grading of Subarachnoid Hemorrhage According to Hunt and Hess

Grade	Clinical features
1	Asymptomatic or mild headache and meningeal irritation
2	Moderate or severe headache (worst headache of life), meningismus, cranial nerve deficits (abducens palsy is common)
3	Drowsiness, confusion, mild focal neurological signs
4	Stupor, severe neurological deficits (e. g., hemiparesis), autonomic manifestations
5	Coma, decerebration

below). Early surgery has been shown to improve the prognosis of patients who present with SAH in Hunt and Hess grades 1, 2, or 3. It is the most important form of treatment for the prevention of rebleeding.

An alternative, less invasive form of treatment is the *filling of the aneurysm with metal coils* ("coiling," a procedure belonging to the field of interventional neuroradiology). The coils are delivered from the tip of a specialized angiographic catheter, which is inserted transfemorally and advanced to the level of the aneurysm. Coiling obviates the need for craniotomy, but it may not be an equally reliable method of permanently obliterating the aneurysm.

Clinical course, prognosis, and complications. Subarachnoid hemorrhage usually stops spontaneously, probably because it is tamponaded by the rising intracranial pressure. Only patients in whom the aneurysm has stopped bleeding survive to be transported to the hospital; the prehospitalization lethality of aneurysmal SAH is approximately 35 %.

After the acute event, the patient faces the risk of three potentially fatal complications:

- Hydrocephalus
- Vasospasm
- Rebleeding

Hydrocephalus (impaired CSF circulation and/or resorption), if it develops, appears very rapidly after the initial SAH. The resulting intracranial hypertension often impairs the patient's consciousness and may also cause focal neurological deficits. Hydrocephalus can be effectively treated by external ventricular drainage. Lumbar drainage is less commonly used.

Vasospasm occurs a few days later, presumably through the effect of vasoactive substances contained in the extravasated subarachnoid blood. The risk of vasospasm can be reduced by the removal of as much subarachnoid blood as

Case Presentation 10: *Acute Subarachnoid Hemorrhage due to Aneurysmal Rupture*

This previously healthy 46-year-old man suddenly experienced the worst headache of his life, combined with profound anxiety and a sense of impending doom. He also complained of double vision, particularly on looking to the right. The physician who admitted him to the hospital examined him neurologically and found a stiff neck and a right partial third cranial nerve palsy, but no other neurological deficits.

The presumptive diagnosis of acute subarachnoid hemorrhage was confirmed by CT scan and lumbar puncture. The patient was stable enough to be considered a candidate for surgery, and cerebral angiography was therefore performed at once, revealing an aneurysm of the internal carotid artery arising at the origin of the posterior communicating artery (Fig. 11.**34a**). This aneurysm proved to be amenable to treatment by interventional neuroradiological methods: immediately after the lesion was identified by angiography, a microcatheter was introduced into it under angiographic guidance, and its lumen was filled with platinum coils (Fig. 11.**34b**, **c**).

Because coiling does not immediately reduce the volume of the aneurysm, immediate improvement of the cranial nerve palsy was not expected. In the further course, however, the aneurysm may shrink, leading to symptomatic improvement. This took six weeks in the present case.

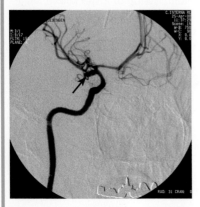

a

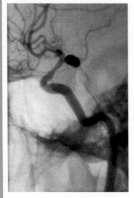

b

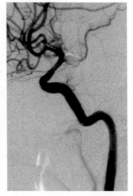

c

Fig. 11.**34 Acute nontraumatic subarachnoid hemorrhage due to rupture of an aneurysm of the internal carotid artery at the origin of the posterior communicating artery. a** Conventional angiography, lateral view. The internal carotid artery aneurysm is seen at the origin of the posterior communicating artery. **b** The aneurysm has been excluded from the circulation by coiling. The metal coils strongly absorb x-rays and therefore appear dark in the nonsubtracted images. **c** The coils are barely seen in the subtracted image, but the dome of the aneurysm is clearly no longer filled with blood. (Images courtesy of MD Dr. Skalej and Dr. Siekmann, Tübingen).

possible during surgery, and by therapeutically induced hypertension. These measures usually suffice to prevent the development of vasospastic infarcts, a much-feared complication. Vasospasm is a serious impediment to the effective diagnosis and treatment of aneurysmal subarachnoid hemorrhage.

Rebleeding, if it occurs, is more often lethal (50%) than the initial subarachnoid hemorrhage. The risk of rebleeding is 20% in the first 14 days after the initial SAH, and 50% in the first six months, if the aneurysm has not been obliterated. Unlike the initial SAH, rebleeds often produce large intraparenchymal hematomas, because the subarachnoid space around the aneurysm is partly sealed by adhesions resulting from the initial bleed. In such cases, the clinical manifestations and course of the aneurysmal rebleed are as described above for spontaneous intracerebral hemorrhage.

Subdural and Epidural Hematoma

Subdural Hematoma

In subdural hematoma, the collection of blood lies in the normally only virtual space between the dura mater and the arachnoid. The cause is usually trauma.

Acute Subdural Hematoma

Acute subdural hematoma (Fig. 11.**35**) is found in severe head trauma. It carries a poor prognosis, not because of the subdural blood itself but because it is very often associated with an underlying parenchymal injury. Its lethality may be as high as 50%. Its clinical manifestations are determined by the site and extent of the associated parenchymal injury.

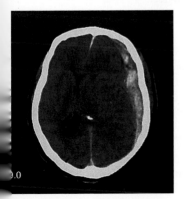

Fig. 11.**35 Acute subdural hematoma.** The space-occupying lesion is concave in shape and poorly demarcated from the underlying brain tissue. There is a pronounced mass effect with midline shift.

Treatment is directed both at the hematoma itself and at the associated parenchymal injury. If open neurosurgical removal of the hematoma is necessary, contused brain tissue must often be resected as well. At surgery, a duraplasty may be performed, and the bone plate may be left out, rather than put back in its original position, in order to provide room for the swollen brain and prevent potentially lethal intracranial hypertension—a similar procedure to decompressive craniectomy for massive ischemic stroke. The current trend in neurosurgery is to perform such decompressions more frequently, both for stroke and for head trauma.

Chronic Subdural Hematoma

The etiology of chronic subdural hematoma remains incompletely understood. There is often an antecedent history of one or more minor traumatic episodes. The fluid collection lies between the inner dural membrane and the arachnoid and is probably derived from an initial hemorrhage of the bridging veins. In the chronic phase, granulation tissue is found in the wall of the hematoma. This tissue is thought to be the source of repeated, secondary bleeding into the fluid collection, so that it slowly expands, rather than being resorbed.

The manifestations of chronic subdural hematoma are produced by pressure on the underlying brain tissue and depend on the site of the hematoma. A chronic subdural hematoma overlying the central region may be clinically indistinguishable from an infarct.

The treatment consists of **operative removal** or **percutaneous drainage**. There is a relatively high recurrence rate. The presence of a subdural hematoma contraindicates therapeutic anticoagulation, which may cause additional bleeding into the hematoma cavity, producing mass effect.

Epidural Hematoma

In epidural hematoma, the blood collection lies between the dura mater and the periosteum (Fig. 11.**36**). It is classically produced by traumatic laceration of a meningeal artery. Because the dura mater is tightly attached to the inner surface of the skull, a great deal of pressure is required to create a fluid collection at this site. The cause is almost always a skull fracture with a tear in the middle meningeal artery, the largest of the meningeal vessels. Such fractures often occur without producing any serious injury to the brain; thus, many patients with epidural hematoma remain awake immediately after the traumatic event and do not lose consciousness until some time later (after the so-called "lucid interval"). They may then die from the rapidly rising intracranial pressure un-

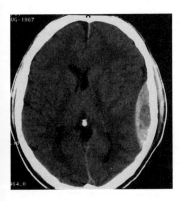

Fig. 11.**36 Acute epidural hematoma, left.** The hematoma is convex. The central hypodensity is due to blood that has not yet clotted. There is a pronounced mass effect with midline shift.

less the hematoma is rapidly diagnosed and operatively removed. Prompt treatment affords a good prognosis.

Vascular Syndromes of the Spinal Cord

Arterial Hypoperfusion

Spinal cord infarcts are much rarer than cerebral infarcts because of the extensive anastomotic network linking the arteries of the spinal cord. Large emboli cannot lodge in the small arteries of the cord, and the very small particles that can do so cause no clinically significant damage. Even aortic aneurysms or occlusions rarely cause damage to the spinal cord.

The symptoms of spinal cord infarction depend on the vascular territory involved.

Infarction in the territory of the anterior spinal artery. The clinical manifestations depend on the segmental level of the lesion. An infarct in the upper cervical spinal cord produces the following deficits: damage to the anterior horns and anterior roots causes *flaccid paresis of the arms*; damage to the decussating fibers of the lateral spinothalamic tract causes *analgesia and thermanesthesia* in the upper limbs; and damage to the corticospinal tracts causes *spastic paraparesis. Bladder and bowel dysfunction* are common. Because the posterior columns lie outside the territory of the anterior spinal artery, there may be no deficit of epicritic and proprioceptive sensation. The deficits typically appear suddenly and are accompanied by pain.

Infarction in the territory of the posterolateral spinal artery produces deficits resulting from damage to the posterior columns, posterior roots, and posterior horns. The corticospinal tracts may also be damaged. There is thus an *impairment of epicritic sense and proprioception below the level of the lesion*. At the level of the lesion, damage to the posterior roots causes an additional *segmental sensory deficit*. If the corticospinal tracts are involved as well, spastic paraparesis results.

Diagnostic evaluation. The diagnosis of spinal cord infarction is usually difficult. Even with *MRI*, infarcts often cannot be reliably distinguished from other types of myelopathy. An important clue to the presence of a spinal cord infarct, in addition to the typical history and physical findings, is the *radiological demonstration of ischemic changes in a vertebral body*, because the spinal cord and the vertebral body are supplied by the same radicular artery. The blood-CNS barrier is not demonstrably disrupted within the lesion until a few days after the acute event (that is, the lesion is not contrast-enhancing until this time). The final step of the diagnostic evaluation is a lumbar puncture to rule out an infectious process.

For technical reasons, diffusion-weighted MRI, which reliably demonstrates acute ischemia in the brain, is difficult to perform in the spinal cord.

Impaired Venous Drainage

The most common cause of elevated venous pressure in the spinal veins is a dural arteriovenous fistula.

Congestive Myelopathy

Etiology. The cause of congestive myelopathy (*Foix-Alajouanine disease*), a disorder that mainly affects elderly men, was first recognized in the 1980s: an **arteriovenous fistula**, usually located on a spinal nerve root. Arterial blood passes through the fistula directly into the intradural veins. The fistula remains clinically silent as long as the excess flow of blood into the veins (the *shunt volume*) does not exceed their drainage capacity. As soon as it does, however, the venous pressure rises, and the spinal cord, which is very sensitive to such increases, is damaged.

Manifestations. The initial manifestations are *unsteady gait* and *spastic paraparesis*, sometimes accompanied by *radicular pain*. If the disease progresses, *autonomic deficits* appear, including bladder, bowel, and sexual dysfunction. The *sensory deficit* at first mainly concerns the protopathic modalities; later, epicritic sensation and proprioception are also affected. Further progression

Case Presentation 11: **Spinal Dural Arteriovenous Fistula**

This 53-year-old woman noticed increasing weakness of both legs for several months. She had no pain, but complained of a "woolly" feeling in the legs, and also had increasing difficulty with urination and defecation. Peripheral neuropathy was diagnosed at first, but, when her leg weakness continued to progress, an MRI scan of the spinal cord was ordered (Fig. 11.**37**). This was performed in an outlying hospital and was initially interpreted as showing a tumor of the spinal cord.

The patient was transferred to the neurosurgical service. The patient's clinical history and MRI findings were considered to be more consistent with a spinal dural arteriovenous fistula than with an intramedullary tumor. This suspicion was confirmed by angiography, and the fistula was surgically excised. The patient's signs and symptoms resolved completely, except for residual bladder dysfunction.

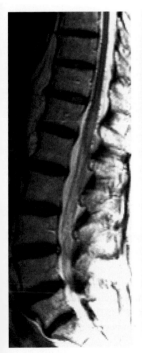
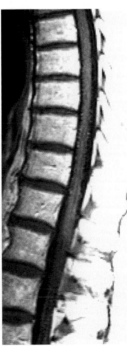

a   b

Fig. 11.**37 Spinal arteriovenous (AV) fistula. a** Sagittal T2-weighted image. Intramedullary edema is seen in the lower portion of the spinal cord, including the conus medullaris. Dilated epimedullary veins appear as dark, rounded structures. **b** In this T1-weighted image obtained after the administration of intravenous contrast, some vessels appear bright, others dark. There is no contrast enhancement within the spinal cord.

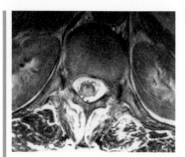

(Continued) Fig. 11.**37 Spinal arteriovenous (AV) fistula. c** This axial T2-weighted image of the spinal cord, obtained just above the level of the conus medullaris, reveals intramedullary edema sparing the ventral portion of the cord. This is an important criterion for the differential diagnosis of AV fistula versus arterial ischemia, in addition to the patient's clinical manifestations and the dilated epimedullary veins that were seen in the other MR images (above).

c

with necrosis of the anterior horns converts the spastic paraparesis into a *flaccid paraparesis.*

Diagnostic evaluation. *MRI* reveals dilated epimedullary veins and edema of the spinal cord. The fistula itself cannot be seen. It may also be very difficult to demonstrate by *angiography*, because the shunt volume may be very low, and the clinical manifestations of congestive myelopathy may be mainly due to impaired venous drainage.

Even today, arteriovenous fistulas causing congestive myelopathy are often not recognized before the appearance of irreversible neurological deficits. This is regrettable, because such fistulas are a potentially treatable cause of progressive paraparesis.

Treatment. The treatment consists of operative obliteration of the fistula after it has been localized by angiography.

Spinal Cord Hemorrhage and Hematoma

Hematomyelia—a hematoma within the spinal cord—is usually of traumatic origin, and is only rarely due to an aneurysm or vascular malformation. Because the blood usually tracks longitudinally (i.e., up and down) in the spinal gray matter, a clinical syndrome resembling that of syringomyelia results (cf. p. 74).

Spinal epidural hematoma usually occurs at thoracic levels, producing acute radicular pain at the level of the hematoma, as well as a subacute spinal cord transection syndrome that begins with paresthesiae, sensory deficits, and weakness in the feet and toes, and then rapidly ascends to the level of the hematoma. Symptomatic spinal epidural hematoma is an acute neurosurgical emergency: it must be evacuated immediately to prevent irreversible paraplegia.

Further Reading

Barth, A., J. Bogousslavsky, F. Regli: The Clinical and Topographic Spectrum of Cerebellar Infarcts: A Clinical-Magnetic Resonance Imaging Correlation Study. Annals of Neurology 33 (1993) 451-456

Bartholow, R.: Experimental investigations into the functions of the human brain. Amer. J. med. Sci 67 (1874) 305-313

Bassetti, C., J. Bogousslavsky, A. Barth, F. Regli: Isolated infarcts of the pons. Neurology 46 (1996) 165-175

Beevor, C. E., V. A. Horsley: An experimental investigation into the arrangement of th exitable fibres of the bonnet monkey. Phil. Trans. 181 B (1890) 49-68

Bookheimer, S.: Functional MRI of Language. New Approaches to Understanding the Cortical Organization of Semantic Processing. Annual Rev. of Neuroscience 25 (2002) 151-188

Brandt T., Kaplan, J. Dichgans, H. C. Diener, C. Kennard: Neurological Disorders, Course and Treatment. 2nd ed., Academic Press 2003

Brazis, P. W., I. C. Masdeu, I. Biller: Localization in Clinical Neurology. Little Brown & Co., Boston, New York, Toronto, London 1996

Broca, P.: Rémarques sur le siège de la faculté du langage articulé. Bull. Soc. anat. Paris 36 (1861) 330-357

Broca, P.: Recherches sur la localisation de la faculté du langage articulé. Exposé des titres et travaux scientifiques 1868

Broca, P.: Anatomie comparée circonvolutions cérébrales. Le grand lobe limbique et la scissure limbique dans la série des mammifères. Rev. anthropol. Ser. 2, 1 (1878) 384-498

Brodal, A.: Neurological Anatomy. Oxford University Press, Oxford 1981.

Brodmann, K.: Vergleichende Lokalisationslehre der Großhirnrinde in ihren Prinzipien dargestellt auf Grund des Zellaufbaus. Barth, Leipzig 1909; Neudruck 1925

Bucy, P. C.: Cortical extirpation in the treatment of involuntary movements. Res. Publ. Ass. nerv. ment. Dis. 21 (1942) 551

Bucy, P. C.: The Precentral Motor Cortex. University of Illinois Press, Urban/Ill. 1944

Burnstock, G., M. Costa: Adrenergic Neurons. Chapman & Hall, London 1975

Cajal, S. R.: Histologie du système nerveux de l'homme et des vértébrés. Maloine, Paris 1909-1911

Cajal, S. R.: Texture of the Nervous System of Man and the Vertebrates. Vol. I. [Annotated and edited translation of the original Spanish text with the additions of the French version]. P. Pasik, T. Pasik (eds.). Springer, Berlin 1999

Campbell, A. W.: Histological Studies on the Localisation of Cerebral Function. Cambridge University Press, Cambridge 1905

Carpenter, M. B.: Core Text of Neuroanatomy. Williams & Wilkins, Baltimore 1978

Chan-Palay, V., C. Köhler (eds.): The Hippocampus - New Vistas. Neurology and Neurobiology. Vol. 52, Alan R. Liss, Inc. New York 1989

Creutzfeld, O. D.: Cortex Cerebri. Springer, Berlin, Heidelberg, New York, Tokyo 1983

Cushing, H.: The field defects produced by temporal lobe lesions. Brain 44 (1922) 341-396

Cushing, H.: Intracranial Tumors: Notes upon a Series of Two Thousand Verified Cases. Thomas, Springfield/Ill, 1932

Duane, E., E. Haines: Fundamental Neuroscience. Churchill Livingstone 1997

Dejerine, J., G. Roussy: Le syndrome thalamique. Rev. neurol. 14 (1906) 521-532

Denny-Brown, D.: The nature of apraxia. J. nerv. ment. Dis. 126 (1958) 9-32

Dusser de Barenne, I. G.: Experimental researches on sensory localisations in the cerebral cortex. Quart. J. exp. Physiol. 9 (1916) 355-390

Duvernoy, H. M.: Human Brainstem Vessels. Springer, Berlin 1978

Eccles, J. C.: The physiology of synapses. Springer, Berlin, Göttingen, Heidelberg, New York 1964

Eccles, J. C., M. Ito, J. Szentágothai: The Cerebellum as a Neuronal Machine. Springer, Berlin 1967

v. Economo, C.: Zellaufbau der Großhirnrinde des Menschen. Springer, Berlin 1927

v. Economo, C., G. N. Koskinas: Die Cytoarchitektonik der Hirnrinde des erwachsenen Menschen. Springer, Wien 1925

Edinger, L.: Bau der nervösen Zentralorgane des Menschen und der Tiere. Bd. I und II, 7. Aufl., Vogel, Leipzig 1904

Feneis, H., W. Dauber: Pocket Atlas of Human Anatomy, Based on the International Nomenclature. 4th ed., revised and enlarged. 2000 Thieme, Stuttgart 2000

Fetter, M., J. Dichgans: Oculomotor Abnormalities in Cerebellar Degeneration. In: Cerebellar Degenerations: clinical Neurobiology. A. Plaitakis (ed.), Kluwer Academic Publishers, Boston 1992

Flechsig, F.: Anatomie des menschlichen Gehirns und Rückenmarks auf myelogenetischer Grundlage. Bd. I., Thieme, Leipzig 1920

Flourens, P.: Recherches expérimentales sur les propriétés et les fonctions du système nerveux dans les animaux vertébrés. Crevot, Paris 1824

Foerster, O.: Motorische Felder und Bahnen. In Bumke, O., O. Foerster: Handbuch der Neurologie, Bd. VI, Springer, Berlin 1936

Freeman, W., I. W. Watts: Psychosurgery. Thomas, Springfield/Ill. 1942

Freeman, W., J. W. Watts: Psychosurgery in the Treatment of Mental Disorders and Intractable Pain. Thomas, Springfield/Ill. 1950

Freund, T. F., G. Buzsáki (eds.): Interneurons of the Hippocampus. Hippocampus 6 (1996) 347-473

Friede, R. L.: Developmental Neuropathology. Springer, Berlin 1975

Frotscher, M., P. Kugler, U. Misgeld, K. Zilles: Neurotransmission in the Hippocampus. Advances in Anatomy, Embryology and Cell Biology, Vol. 111, Springer, Berlin, Heidelberg 1988

Gazzaniga, M. S., I. E. Bogen, R. W. Sperry: Observation on visual perception after disconnection of the cerebral hemispheres in man. Brain 88 (1965) 221-236

Gazzaniga, M. S., R. W. Sperry: language after section of the cerebral commissures. Brain 90 (1967) 131-148

Gerstmann, J.: Syndrome of finger agnosia, disorientation for right or left, agraphia and acalculia: local diagnostica value. Arch. Neurol. Psychiat. (Chic.) 44 (1940) 389-408

Geschwind, N.: Disconnection syndrome in animals and man, Part. I., Part II. brain 88 (1965) 237-294, 585-644

Geschwind, N.: W. Levitsky: Human brain, left-right asymmetries in temporal speech region. Science 16 (1968) 168-187

Geschwind, N.: Language and the brain. Sci. Amer. 226 (1972) 76-83

Gilman, S., J. R. Bloedel, R. Lechtenberg: Disorders of the Cerebellum. Davis, Philadelphia 1981

Grünbaum, A. S. F., C. S. A. Sherrington: Observations on the physiology of the cerebral cortex of some of the higher apes. Proc. roy. Soc. Ser. B. 69 (1901) 206-209

Gudden, B.: Experimentaluntersuchungen über das periphere und centrale Nervensystem. Arch. Psychiat. Nervenkr. 1870, 693-723

Guillain, G., P. Mollaret : Deux cas de myoclonies synchrones et rythmées vélopharyngolaryngo-oculo-diaphragmatiques. Rev. neurol. 2 (1931) 245-566

Hassler, R.: Fiber connections within the extrapyramidal system. Confin. neurol. 36 (1974) 237-255

Hassler, R., T. Riechert: Klinische und anatomische Befunde bei stereotaktischen Schmerzoperationen im Thalamus. Arch. Psychiat. Nervenkr. 200 (1959) 93-122

Heiss, W.D., G. Pawlik, K. Herholz, K. Wienhard (eds.): Clinical Efficacy of Positron Emission Tomography (Proceedings of a Workshop held 23-25 Oct. 1986 in

Cologne, FRG; sponsored by the Commission of the European Communities as Advised by the Committee on Medical and Public Health Research). Developments in Nuclear Medicine, Vol. 12. Springer, Berlin 1987

Hirsch, M. C., T. Kramer (Hrsg.): Neuroanatomy 3 D, Stereoscopy. Atlas of the Human Brain. Springer, Berlin, Heidelberg 1999

Hubel, D. H., T. N. Wiesel: Ferrier lecture: Functional architecture of macaque monkey visual cortex. Proc. roy. Soc. Serv. B 198 (1977) 1-59

Hubel, D. H., T. N. Wiesel, P. M. Stryker: Anatomical demonstration of orientation columns in macaque monkey. J. comp. Neurol. 177 (1978) 361-397

Jacobsen, C. F.: Functions of frontal association areas in primates. Arch. Neurol. Psychiat. (Chic.) 33 (1935) 558-569

Jannetta, P. J.: Arterial compression of the trigeminal nerve at the pons in patients with trigeminal neuralgia. J. Neurosurg. 26 (1967) 150-162

Jannetta, P. J., M. H. Benett: The Pathophysiology of Trigeminal Neuralgia. In: The Cranial Nerves, ed. by M. Samii and P. J. Jannetta, Springer 1981, 312-315

Jannetta, P. J.: Vascular Decompression in the Trigeminal Neuralgia. In: The Cranial nerves, ed. By M. Samii and P. J. Jannetta, Springer 1981, 331-340

Jones, E. G., A. Peters: Cerebral Cortex. Vol. 1-6, Plenum, New York 1984-1987

Jung, R., R. Hassler: The extrapyramidal motor system. In: Handbook of Physiology, Section 1, Bd. 2, hrsg. von J. Field, H. W. Magoun, V. E. Hall, American Physiological Society, Washington 1960

Kandel, E. R., J. H. Schwartz, T. M. Jessell: Principles of Neural Science. 3rd Edition, Appleton & Lange 1991

Kahle, W., M. Frotscher: Color Atlas and Textbook of Human Anatomy. 5th ed. Vol. 3: Nervous System and Sensory Organs. Thieme, Stuttgart 2003

Klüver, H.: "The temporal lobe syndrome" produced by bilateral ablations. In: Neuro-

logical Basis of Behaviour (pp. 175-182), Ciba Found. Symp. Churchill, London 1958

Klüver, H., P. Bucy: Preliminary analysis of functions of the temporal lobes in monkeys. Arch. Neurol. Psychiat. (Chic.) 42 (1939) 979-1000

Kolb, B., I. Whishaw (Hrsg.): Fundamentals of Human Neuropsychology. 4. Aufl., W. H. Friedman & Company, New York 1996

Kretschmann H. J., W. Weinrich: Cranial Neuroimaging and Clinical Neuroanatomy, Magnetic Resonance Imaging and Computed Tomography. 3rd ed., revised and expanded. Thieme, Stuttgart 2004

Lang, J.: Topographical Anatomy of the Cranial Nerves. In: The Cranial Nerves, ed. by M. Samii and P. J. Jannetta, Pringer, 1981, 6-15

Luria, A.: Higher Cortical Function in Man. Basic Books, New York 1966

Masur, H.: Scales & Scores in Neurology. Thieme, Stuttgart 2004

Milner, B.: Brain mechanisms suggested by studies of temporal lobes. In Millikan, C. H., F. L. Darley: Brain Mechanism Underlying Speech and Language. Grune & Stratton, New York 1967

Milner, B., W. Penfield: The effect of hippocampal lesion on recent memory. Trans. Amer. neurol. Asso. 80 (1955) 42-48

Mishkin, M.: Memory in monkeys severely impaired by combined but not by separate removal of amygdala and hippocampus. Nature 273 (1978) 297-298

Mumenthaler, M.: Neurologic Differential Diagnosis. 2nd ed. Thieme, Stuttgart 1992

Nissl, F.: Experimentalergebnisse zur Frage der Hirnrindenschichtung. Mschr. Psychiat. Neurol. 23 (1908) 186-188

Ojemann, G. A., P. Fedio, J. M. van Buren: Anomia from pulvinar and subcortical parietal stimulation. Brain 91 (1968) 99-116

Orrison, W. W. jun.: Atlas of Brain Functions. Thieme, Stuttgart 1995

Papez, J. W.: A proposed mechanism of emotion. Arch. Neurol. Psychiat. (Chic.) 38 (1937) 725-43

Penfield, W., B. Milner: Memory deficit produced by bilateral lesions in the hippocampal zone. Arch. Neurol. Psychiat. (Chic.) 79 (1958) 475-497

Penfield, W., T. Rasmussen: The Cerebral Cortex of Man. Macmillan, New York 1950

Penfield, W., L. Roberts: Speech and Brain Mechanisms. Princeton University Press, Princetown/N.J. 1959

Peters, A., S. L. Palay, H. F. Webster: The Fine Structure of the Nervous System. Oxford University Press, New York 1991

Ross, A. T., W. E. De Myer: Isolated syndrome of the medial longitudinal fasciculus in man. Arch. Neurol. (Chic.) 15, 1966

Samii, M., P. J. Jannetta, ed.: The Cranial Nerves. Springer, Berlin, Heidelberg, New York 1981

Sherrington, C. S.: The Integrative Action of the Nervous System. Scribner, New York 1906; Cambridge University Press, London 1947

Smith, A., C. Burklund: Dominant hemispherectomy. Science 153 (1966) 1280-1282

Sperry, R. W.: Cerebral organization and behavior. Science 133 (1961) 1749-1757

Sperry, R. W.: The great cerebral commissure. Sci. Amer. 210 (1964) 42-52

Stephan, H.: Allocortex, In: Handbuch der mikroskopischen Anatomie, Bd. IV/9, ed. by W. Bargmann, Springer, Berlin 1975

Tessier-Lavigne, M., C. S. Goodman: The molecular biology of axon guidance. Science 274 (1996) 1123-1133

Tatu, L., T. Moulin, J. Bogousslavsky, H. Duvernoy: Arterial territories of the human brain. Neurology 50 (1998), 1699-1708

Thompson, P. D., B. L. Day: The Anatomy and Physiology of Cerebellar Disease. Advances in Neurology, Raven Press 1993

Vogt, O., C. Vogt: Allgemeine Ergebnisse unserer Hirnforschung. J. Psych. 25, Erg. H. 1, 1925

Wall, M., S. H. Wray: The "One and a Half" syndrome. A unilateral disorder of the pontine tegmentum. Neurology (Chic.) 33 (1983) 971-980

Warwick, R.: Representation of the extraocular muscles with oculomotorius nuclei of the monkey. J. comp. Neurol. 98 (1953) 449-503

Warwick, R.: Oculomotor organization. In: Bender, M. B.: The Oculomotor System, Harper & Row, New York 1964

Wässle, H., B. B. Boycott: Functional architecture of the mammalian retina. Physiol. Rev. 71 (1991) 447-480

Wernicke, C.: Der aphasische Symptomenkomplex, eine psychologische Studie auf anatomischer Basis. Cohn & Weigert, Breslau 1874.

Zigmond, M. J., F. E. Bloom, S. C. Landis, J. L. Roberts, L. R. Squire: Fundamental Neuroscience. Academic Press, San Diego, London, Boston 1999

Index

Fossa
  interpeduncular 120
  rhomboid 117
Fovea 131, 132
Foville syndrome 231
Friedreich ataxia 76-78
Functional magnetic reso-
  nance imaging (fMRI)
  371, 378, 383
Funicular myelosis 72, 74-75
Funiculus, posterior 44, 45,
  49

G

G-protein-coupled recep-
  tors 8, 12
Gagging 222
Galactorrhea 286
Gamma-aminobutyric acid
  (GABA) 11
  receptors 12
Ganglion
  celiac 290, 294, 298-299
  cervical
    inferior 298-299
    middle 293, 298-299
    superior 100, 293, 298-
      299
  cervicothoracic (stellate)
    293
  ciliary 156, 158, 161, 290,
    296, 298
  dorsal root (spinal) 18, 27
    syndrome of 71-72
  geniculate 168, 169, 171,
    172-173
  glossopharyngeal
    inferior 196, 202
    superior 196, 203
  hypogastric 299
  lumbar, lower 299
  mesenteric
    inferior 290, 294, 297,
      299
    superior 290, 294, 298
  otic 290, 296, 298
  pterygopalatine 161, 168,
    173, 290, 296, 298
  sacral, upper 299
  spiral 179, 180, 181

submandibular 173, 290,
  296
thoracic, upper 298-299
trigeminal (gasserian)
  123, 127, 138, 160, 161,
  216
vagal
  inferior 197
  superior 197
vestibular 180, 187
see also Basal ganglia
Gastrointestinal motility
  222
Gaze
  horizontal 146-149
    disturbances 148-149
  vertical 149-150
    disturbances 270
Gaze center
  lesions 150-151
  pontine 146, 151
  vertical 149
Genitalia
  dysfunction 307
  innervation 296, 299, 306
Genu
  corpus callosum 334
  facial nerve
    external 167
    internal 167
  internal capsule 58
Gerstmann syndrome 396
Gland(s)
  adrenal, innervation 299
  Bowman's 128
  lacrimal 173, 175, 298
  nasal 175
  parotid 175, 298
  pineal (epiphysis) 261,
    272-273, 407
  pituitary
    anterior lobe (adenohy-
      pophysis) 262, 280,
      281, 284
    posterior lobe (neuro-
      hypophysis) 261,
      274-275, 278, 280,
      284
    tumor 287-288
  sublingual 173, 175, 298
  submandibular 173, 175,
    298

Glial cells 13
Glioarchitecture 362
Globus pallidus 62, 262,
  266-268, 273-274, 330-
  337
  connections 337, 338-339
Glutamate 11
  receptors 11-12
Glycine 11
  receptors 12
Golgi tendon organs 20, 21,
  34
Golgi-Mazzoni corpuscle
  20, 21, 44
Gonadotropin-releasing
  hormone (GnRH) 284
Gordon reflex 64
Gradenigo syndrome 166
Granulations, arachnoid
  403, 408, 410
Granule cells 243, 244, 317,
  359-361
Gray matter 358
  spinal cord 70
  syndrome 74, 75
Gray type II synapses 8
Growth hormone (GH) 284
Growth-hormone-releasing
  hormone (GHRH) 284
Guillain Barré syndrome
  410
Gustatory pathway 174
Gynecomastia 286
Gyrus
  ambient 128, 129
  cingulate 130, 268, 313,
    315
    isthmus 356
  dentate 315-317, 356
  fusiform 357
  lingual 357
  occipitotemporal
    lateral 357
    medial 357
  of insula
    long 358
    short 358
  orbital 357
  parahippocampal 128,
    316, 357
  postcentral 18, 44, 46-48,
    50, 354-357, 372